D1374079

Medically Challenging Patients Undergoing Cardiothoracic Surgery

Edited by

Neal H. Cohen, MD, MPH, MS

Professor, Department of Anesthesia and Perioperative Care
and Department of Medicine
Vice Dean, School of Medicine
University of California San Francisco

with 23 contributors

Wolters Kluwer | Lippincott Williams & Wilkins
Health

Medically Challenging Patients Undergoing Cardiothoracic Surgery

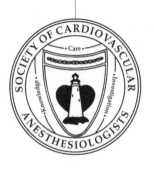

A Society of
Cardiovascular Anesthesiologists
Monograph

Accurate indications, adverse reactions, and dosage schedules for drugs are provided in this book, but it is possible that they may change. The reader is urged to review the package information data of the manufacturers of the medications mentioned.

Printed in the United States of America
ISBN-10: 1608312992
ISBN-13: 9781608312993

Preface

Improvements in anesthesia care and technology have facilitated major advances in cardiothoracic surgery. The surgical options have expanded and, in many cases the complexity of the procedures increased. At the same time, the patient population presenting for these procedures has also become more complex; many patients have significant co-morbidities that must be considered during the perioperative period. In order to care for this increasingly complex and diverse group of patients, the anesthesiologist must understand the relationship between the underlying pathophysiology and its impact on clinical care. For some of the most complex patients, the anesthetic management and perioperative care must be modified to optimize the likelihood of a positive outcome. This monograph provides a review of selected topics related to the care of the medically challenging patient who presents for cardiothoracic surgery. It includes a discussion of management strategies to optimize neurologic outcome and clinical considerations for patients with coexisting medical conditions, such as carotid disease, hypertension, hyperglycemia, dialysis-dependent renal disease and pulmonary hypertension. It also includes a review of the clinical considerations when caring for the patient with heparin-induced thrombocytopenia, the pregnant patient requiring cardiac surgery with cardiopulmonary bypass and the obese patient. The monograph also provides a discussion of some of the considerations that must be taken into account when caring for selected patient populations requiring thoracic surgery, such as the patient who requires lung isolation, but has a difficult airway, the patient with an anterior mediastinal mass or the patient with an invasive tumor of the vena cava. Finally a discussion of the issues related to the care of the patient who refuses transfusion addresses some of the ethical and legal implications of the patient's choice and the clinical options available to optimize care.

Contributors

Martin Abel, MD
Professor of Anesthesiology
Department of Anesthesiology
College of Medicine
Mayo Clinic
Rochester, MN

Katherine Arendt, MD
Instructor in Anesthesiology
Department of Anesthesiology
College of Medicine
Mayo Clinic
Rochester, MN

Solomon Aronson, MD, FACC,
    FCCP, FAHA., FASE
Professor of Anesthesiology
Executive Vice Chair
Department of Anesthesiology
Duke University Health System
Durham, NC

Jeremy L. Bricker, MD, MS
Associate Professor of Clinical
    Anesthesiology
Richard L Roudebush VA
    Medical Center
Department of Anesthesia
Indiana University School
    of Medicine
Indianapolis, IN

John Butterworth, MD
Robert K. Stoelting Professor
    Chairman, Department of
    Anesthesia
    Indiana University School
    of Medicine
    Indianapolis, IN

Javier H. Campos, MD
Professor of Anesthesia
Vice Chair of Clinical Affairs

Director of Cardiothoracic Anesthesia
Medical Director Operating Rooms
Department of Anesthesia
University of Iowa Hospitals
    and Clinics
Iowa City, IA

Neal H. Cohen, MD, MPH, MS
Professor
Department of Anesthesia
    and Perioperative Care and
    Department of Medicine
Vice Dean, School of Medicine
University of California San Francisco
San Francisco, CA

Thomas J. Ebert, MD, PhD
Professor
Department of Anesthesiology
The Medical College of Wisconsin
Milwaukee, WI

John E. Ellis, MD
Adjunct Professor
Department of Anesthesiology
    and Critical Care
University of Pennsylvania
Philadelphia, PA

Brenda G. Fahy, MD, FCCM
Professor
Department of Anesthesiology
College of Medicine
University of Kentucky
Lexington, KY

Pedram Fatehi, MD
Clinical Fellow
Division of Critical Care Medicine
Departments of Medicine and
    Anesthesia and Perioperative Care
University of California
San Francisco, CA

Kevin W. Hatton, MD
Assistant Professor
Department of Anesthesiology
College of Medicine
University of Kentucky
Lexington, KY

Steven E. Hill, MD
Professor
Department of Anesthesiology
Duke University Medical Center
Durham, NC

Charles W. Hogue, MD
Associate Professor of
Anesthesiology and Critical
Care Medicine
Department of Anesthesiology
and Critical Care Medicine
The Johns Hopkins Medical
Institutions
and The Johns Hopkins Hospital
Baltimore, MD

Julie L. Huffmyer, MD
Assistant Professor
Department of Anesthesiology
University of Virginia
Charlottesville, VA

Kathleen D. Liu, MD
Assistant Professor
Critical Care Medicine
Department Anesthesia and
Perioperative Care
and Department of Medicine
Division of Nephrology
University of California
San Francisco, CA

Jutta Novalija, MD, PhD
Assistant Professor
Department of Anesthesiology
The Medical College of Wisconsin
Milwaukee, WI

E. Andrew Ochroch, MD, MSCE
Associate Professor
Department of Anesthesiology
and Critical Care
University of Pennsylvania
Philadelphia, PA

Audrey Oware, MD
Fellow
Department of Anesthesiology
and Critical Care
University of Pennsylvania
Philadelphia, PA

George F. Rich, MD, PhD
Harrison Medical Teaching Professor
and Chair
Department of Anesthesiology
University of Virginia
Charlottesville, VA

David C. Sane, MD
Associate Professor, Section
on Cardiology
Department of Internal Medicine
Wake Forest University School
of Medicine
Winston-Salem, NC

Thomas F. Slaughter, MD
Professor and Section Head,
Cardiothoracic Anesthesiology
Wake Forest University School
of Medicine
Winston-Salem, NC

Peter Slinger, MD, FRCPC
Professor
Department of Anesthesia
University of Toronto
Toronto, Canada

Joshua D. Stearns, MD
Assistant Professor
Department of Anesthesiology
and Critical Care Medicine
The Johns Hopkins Medical
Institutions
and The Johns Hopkins Hospital
Baltimore, MD

Jerry V. Young, PharMD, MD
Professor of Clinical Anesthesia
Director of Thoracic Anesthesia
Indiana University School
of Medicine
Director of Anesthesia
University Hospital
Clarian Partners
Indianapolis, IN

Contents

Preface

Contributors

1   1
Protecting the Brain During Cardiac Surgery
Joshua D. Stearns and Charles W. Hogue

2   29
Management of Blood Pressure in the Patient Requiring Cardiothoracic Surgery: What's the Correct End Point?
Solomon Aronson

3   69
Carotid Stenosis and Coronary Disease: Understanding the Disease Processes and Defining How to Approach Them
E. Andrew Ochroch, Audrey Oware, and John E. Ellis

4   109
Glucose Control for the Diabetic Patient Requiring Cardiothoracic Surgery: Does It Matter?
Kevin W. Hatton and Brenda G. Fahy

5   129

Perioperative Management of the Patient with Dialysis-Dependent Renal Failure Requiring Cardiac Surgery
Pedram Fatehi, Kathleen D. Liu, and Neal H. Cohen

6   163

Heparin-Induced Thrombocytopenia in Patients Requiring Cardiovascular Surgery
Thomas F. Slaughter and David C. Sane

7   185

Managing the Patient with Pulmonary Hypertension Who Requires Cardiac Surgery
Julie L. Huffmyer and George F. Rich

8   215

The Pregnant Patient and Cardiopulmonary Bypass
Katherine Arendt and Martin Abel

9   245

Anesthetic Management of the Extremely Obese Patient Undergoing Cardiovascular Surgery
Jutta Novalija and Thomas J. Ebert

10   267

Lung Isolation in a Patient with a Difficult Airway
Peter Slinger

11   285

Managing the Patient with an Anterior
Mediastinal Mass

Javier H. Campos

12   303

The Patient with a Tumor Invading the
Vena Cava

Jerry L. Bricker, Jerry V. Young, and John Butterworth

13   327

Care of the Cardiothoracic Surgical Patient
Refusing Transfusion

Steven E. Hill

Joshua D. Stearns, MD
Charles W. Hogue, MD

1 | Protecting the Brain During Cardiac Surgery

INTRODUCTION

Neurological complications after cardiac surgery remain a major source of patient morbidity that is associated with high mortality, prolonged hospitalization, and impaired postoperative quality of life (1–4). These complications have a range of manifestations, including clinically detected stroke affecting 1% to 3% of patients and alterations in mental status, including delirium, that affect 8.4% to 32% of patients (5). Postoperative brain injury may have other manifestations, depending on the size and location of ischemic injury (e.g., motor cortex vs. brain areas involved with cognition). The reported incidence of postoperative neurologic deficits is also influenced by the extent of diagnostic testing. More intense monitoring may identify deficits that are not detected by routine clinical evaluation. For example, clinical series that obtain brain magnetic resonance imaging (MRI) have revealed new brain ischemic injury in as many as 45% of patients after cardiac surgery (3, 6). Detailed psychometric testing may also reveal subtle deterioration in cognitive function manifest as alterations in attention, concentration, memory, or visual motor performance. The frequency of postoperative cognitive dysfunction varies depending on the patient populations tested, cognitive testing battery employed, timing of the testing, and definition of cognitive decline. Most contemporary investigations report a frequency of cognitive dysfunction of 10% to 30% when patients are evaluated 1 month after cardiac surgery (5). Although these findings are noted within the first few months after

Medically Challenging Patients Undergoing Cardiothoracic Surgery, edited by Neal H. Cohen, MD, MPH, MS, Lippincott Williams & Wilkins, Baltimore © 2009.

cardiac surgery, the impact of postoperative cognitive dysfunction on long-term cognitive function remains incompletely defined. Seminal investigations by Newman et al. (2) showed that patients with cognitive dysfunction at hospital discharge had a greater risk for cognitive deterioration 5 years after cardiac surgery than did patients without postoperative cognitive dysfunction. In contrast, Selnes et al. (7) found no differences in the rate of cognitive deterioration at 1-, 3-, or 6-year intervals between patients who underwent coronary artery bypass graft (CABG) surgery with cardiopulmonary bypass (CPB) and those who had angiographically documented coronary artery disease and were undergoing medical management. Furthermore, van Dijk et al. (8) found that the cognitive performance of patients 5 years after CABG surgery was no different than that of an aged-matched control group. Thus, emerging data suggest that, in an aging surgical population, progression of underlying cerebral vascular disease is a better determinant of long-term cognitive deterioration than is cardiac surgery. Regardless, when considering approaches to brain protection during cardiac surgery, the goal is to reduce the frequency of all forms of ischemic brain injury and cognitive dysfunction (including clinically manifested and more subtle manifestations) at any time in the postoperative period.

MECHANISMS OF PERIOPERATIVE BRAIN INJURY

The aim of brain protection during cardiac surgery is to prevent primary injury and/or limit its extent by attenuating secondary injury that results from the activation of multiple neuronal injury pathways (i.e., ischemic cascade) (9). The primary causes of perioperative brain injury are cerebral embolism and cerebral hypoperfusion; primary cerebral hemorrhage is unusual during surgery (3, 5). Brain ischemic injury is likely exacerbated by inflammatory processes that result from cardiac surgery and ischemia/reperfusion injury (3). Furthermore, growing evidence suggests that susceptibility to brain injury may be modified by genotype (10–16). Regardless, approximately one-half of strokes that occur after cardiac surgery are reported to be caused by cerebral macroemboli that likely arise from an atherosclerotic ascending aorta (3,17–20). Microemboli, which might result in subtle manifestations of brain injury, may be composed of atherosclerotic debris, particulate matter, fat globules arising from shed mediastinal blood, or air (3).

Brain O_2 supply/demand mismatch may occur in 27% to 43% of patients during CPB, as documented by jugular venous bulb or near-infrared spectroscopy (NIRS)-detected O_2 desaturation (21, 22). Cerebral hypoperfusion during CPB might be a more likely clinical problem in modern cardiac surgery practices because of the rising prevalence of eld-

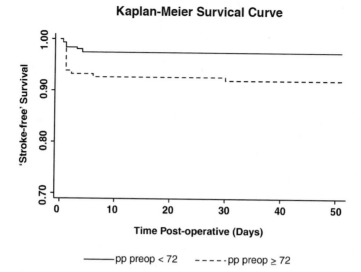

Kaplan-Meier Survical Curve

FIGURE 1–1. Comparison of stroke-free survival between patients with pulse pressure (pp) <72 mmHg and those with pp ≥72 mmHg after cardiac surgery. Reprinted with permission from (24).

erly patients with cerebral vascular disease (3, 23–26). Studies by Benjo et al. (24) (Figure 1–1) and Fontes et al. (25) (Figure 1–2) have demonstrated an independent relationship between elevated pulse pressure, an indicator of vascular stiffness and compensatory microvascular changes, and risk for perioperative stroke. In a review of 98 patients who experienced a stroke after cardiac surgery, Gottesman et al. (23) reported that 68% of strokes detected with sensitive MRI brain-imaging methods were hypoperfusion-related watershed strokes. Moreover, in a study of 82 patients without prior stroke or transient ischemic attack who were scheduled for elective CABG surgery, Moraca et al. (26) found that 75% had impaired regional cerebral perfusion before surgery based on brain single photon emission computed tomography imaging (Figure 1–3). Perioperative stroke occurred in 5% of patients, but only in those with abnormal preoperative cerebral perfusion. Importantly, it is not likely that cerebral embolism and hypoperfusion occur in isolation; they more likely contribute to brain injury synergistically often associated with pre-existing cerebrovascular abnormalities (27, 28). Thus, a comprehensive brain protection strategy must address both etiologies of injury.

Although CPB is considered a risk factor for neurologic injury, the mechanisms of brain injury are most likely similar for "off-pump" surgery and surgery with CPB, although the frequency of microemboli

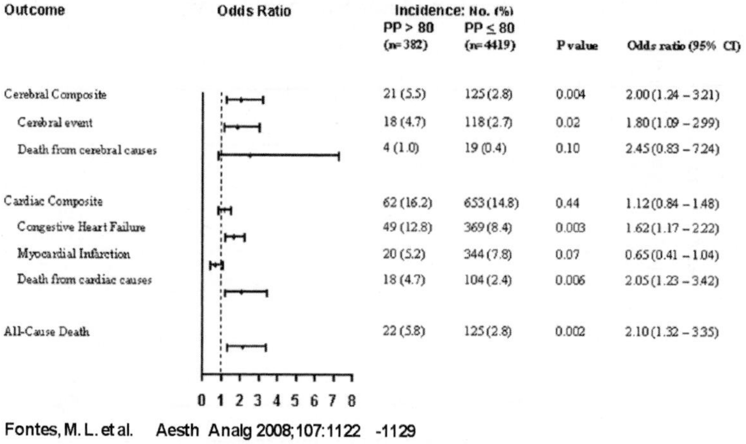

Outcome	Odds Ratio	Incidence: No. (%) PP > 80 (n=382)	PP ≤ 80 (n=4419)	P value	Odds ratio (95% CI)
Cerebral Composite		21 (5.5)	125 (2.8)	0.004	2.00 (1.24 – 3.21)
Cerebral event		18 (4.7)	118 (2.7)	0.02	1.80 (1.09 – 2.99)
Death from cerebral causes		4 (1.0)	19 (0.4)	0.10	2.45 (0.83 – 7.24)
Cardiac Composite		62 (16.2)	653 (14.8)	0.44	1.12 (0.84 – 1.48)
Congestive Heart Failure		49 (12.8)	369 (8.4)	0.003	1.62 (1.17 – 2.22)
Myocardial Infarction		20 (5.2)	344 (7.8)	0.07	0.65 (0.41 – 1.04)
Death from cardiac causes		18 (4.7)	104 (2.4)	0.006	2.05 (1.23 – 3.42)
All-Cause Death		22 (5.8)	125 (2.8)	0.002	2.10 (1.32 – 3.35)

0 1 2 3 4 5 6 7 8

Fontes, M. L. et al.   Aesth Analg 2008;107:1122 -1129

FIGURE 1–2.   Fatal and nonfatal outcomes after cardiac surgery for patients with a pulse pressure (PP <80 mmHg or ≥80 mmHg. Reprinted with permission from (25).

detected with transcranial Doppler monitoring is lower when CPB is avoided (29, 30). Marked hemodynamic changes associated with cardiac manipulation during off-pump CABG may expose some patients to reduced cerebral perfusion [i.e., low mean arterial pressure (MAP) with high central venous pressure] for varying periods of time. Nonetheless, data from detailed studies designed to evaluate the etiology of neurological complications associated with the surgical technique are limited. Prospectively randomized trials have failed to show that off-pump CABG surgery substantially reduces the frequency of neurological complications compared to surgery with CPB (31, 32). Whether it is beneficial to avoid CPB in older and higher-risk patients, however, has not been extensively studied (33).

BRAIN PROTECTION

Although the time of the events surrounding CPB might be the time of greatest risk for those patients for whom CPB is used, brain injury can occur any time perioperatively and if surgery is off-pump. The onset of the abnormality can occur at any time in the perioperative period, including postoperatively after tracheal intubation. Our data and those of others suggest that >20% of strokes occur after the first postoperative day (5, 34, 35). Despite the variable time of onset or recognition of the injury, brain-protective strategies used during the surgical procedure are effective (3, 5). A number of recommended brain-protective strategies

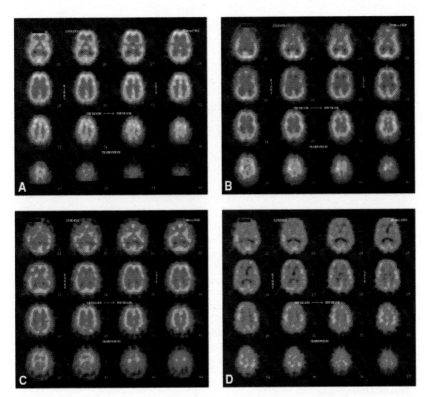

FIGURE 1–3. Regional cerebral perfusion measured with single photon emission computed tomographic brain imaging in 82 patients before coronary artery bypass graft (CABG) surgery. Images are from patients with (A) normal perfusion ($n = 25\%$ of patients) (A), mild perfusion defects ($n = 25\%$ of patients) (B), moderate perfusion defects ($n = 24\%$ of patients) (C), and severe regional cerebral perfusion defects ($n = 24\%$ of patients) (D). Reprinted with permission from (28).

implemented during cardiac surgery are listed in Table 1–1. These recommendations are based on an objective evidence-based assessment of the data as previously described (3, 5). The studies evaluated included those in which patients undergoing cardiac surgery were assessed for the primary outcomes of clinical stroke and/or neurocognitive dysfunction.

Atherosclerosis of the Aorta

Multiple investigations have convincingly linked atherosclerosis of the ascending aorta and risk for stroke and cognitive dysfunction after cardiac surgery (1, 3, 17, 19). Avoiding trauma to atheroma during aortic manipulations (e.g., cannulation, cross-clamping) may reduce the risk

TABLE 1-1.   **Strategies for lowering the risk of brain injury during cardiac surgery**

Class I Recommendations

A membrane oxygenator and an arterial line filter (≤40 μM) should be used for cardiopulmonary bypass (CPB) (Level A)

Epiaortic ultrasound should be used for detection of atherosclerosis of the ascending aorta (Level B)

Hyperthermia should be avoided during and after CPB (Level B)

Class IIa Recommendations

A single aortic cross-clamp technique should be used for patients at risk for atheroembolism (Level B)

Arterial line temperature during CPB rewarming should be limited to 37°C (Level B)

Class IIb Recommendations

Nonpulsatile (vs. pulsatile) perfusion (Level B)

α-stat (vs. pH-stat) acid–base management (Level A)

Near-infrared spectroscopy monitoring should be considered, especially in high-risk patients (Level B)

Arterial blood pressure should be maintained at >70 mmHg during CPB in high-risk patients (Level B)

Serum glucose should be kept to <140 mg/dL with an infusion of insulin (Level C)

Transfusion of packed red blood cells should be considered in high-risk patients when hemoglobin is ≤7 g/dL or higher, depending on other patient-specific considerations (Level C)

Processing cardiotomy suction aspirate with a cell-saver device as a means for preventing neurocognitive dysfunction (Level A)

Class Indeterminate

Systemic hypothermia during CPB (Level A)

Pharmacologic neuroprotection (Level B)

The data are ranked based on the methods used by the American Heart Association as Level A (the data come from multiple randomized clinical trials or meta-analyses), Level B (the data are from a single randomized trial or nonrandomized studies), and Level C (case studies, expert opinion, or standard of care). Based on this hierarchy of evidence, recommendations are made as follows: *Class I*: always acceptable, proven safe, and definitely useful; *Class IIa*: acceptable, safe, and useful. Reasonably prudent physicians can choose. Considered the intervention of choice by a majority of physicians. *Class IIb*: acceptable, safe, and useful. Considered optional or alternative treatment by most experts; *Class III*: no evidence of benefit. *Class Indeterminate:* Intervention can be used, but evidence is insufficient to support efficacy.

Table adapted from (3).

of cerebral embolization (17–21). The primary factors that influence management decisions for the clinician include 1) detection of atherosclerotic lesions in the ascending aorta, and 2) management strategies to avoid them. Traditionally, direct palpation of the aorta was the primary method for detecting an atheromatous aorta. Although palpation remains a mainstay of surgical assessment, epiaortic ultrasound has been demonstrated consistently to be the most sensitive method for detecting atherosclerosis of the ascending aorta (3, 17, 36–39). Many surgeons now utilize this technique to optimize their assessment of the aorta.

A number of surgical management options can also be employed to minimize the risks associated with manipulation of atherosclerotic lesions of the ascending aorta. They include 1) utilizing off-pump surgery rather than CPB; 2) cannulation of the axillary artery or femoral artery for CPB; 3) placement of a single aortic cross-clamp, whereby proximal bypass graft anastomosis is performed during aortic cross-clamping to avoid partial occlusion clamps; 4) initiation of fibrillatory arrest during the surgical procedure to avoid the need for cross-clamping; 5) avoiding proximal aortic anastomosis by use of all in situ arterial bypass grafts; and 6) performing circulatory arrest for the procedure including the option to replace the ascending aorta with a graft, if the atherosclerotic disease is extensive (3). A prospectively randomized study of 169 high-risk patients found a lower incidence of cognitive dysfunction in patients after CABG surgery when a single cross-clamp technique was used than when a partial occlusion clamp was used for proximal bypass graft anastomosis (40).

Aortic atheroma can be dislodged during other aspects of the surgical procedure in addition to the direct injury that can occur at the time of cannulation or cross-clamping. One form of atheroma embolization is referred to as the "sandblasting" effect from the arterial CPB return flow in which there is a showering of embolic material caused by the high flow (41, 42). In addition, neurologic injury can occur based on other factors related to, but not directly caused by, emboli. For many patients, undergoing cardiac surgery under CPB atherosclerosis of the ascending aorta is a marker of more widespread vascular disease and cerebrovascular disease. These patients may be more prone to brain injury from cerebral emboli from other sources or cerebral hypoperfusion because of a variety of reasons, rather than from embolization associated with direct cannulation. For example, data from the Aortic Plaque and Risk of Ischemic Stroke (APRIS) study in nonsurgical patients with stroke suggest an association between aortic atherosclerosis and hypercoagulability (43). Aortic plaque injury during surgery in patients with hypercoagulability might also be synergistic with and account for some postoperative neurologic deficits.

CPB Flow Management

The impact of the characteristics of the CPB circuit and flow on postoperative neurologic dysfunction has been of concern since the technique was first used in humans. The potential merits and risks of pulsatile versus nonpulsatile CPB in particular have been sources of considerable debate, not only with respect to the potential neurologic sequelae, but also with respect to perfusion to other organs. Experimentally, pulsatile CPB has been found to attenuate the neurohumoral response to CPB and lower systemic and organ vascular resistance, thus increasing visceral, renal, and liver blood flow compared with that achieved by nonpulsatile flow (44, 45). Furthermore, pulsatile perfusion improves the distribution of blood flow to the microcirculation in the brain, enhancing blood O_2 delivery to experimental ischemic brain regions (46). Moreover, compared with nonpulsatile perfusion, pulsatile flow promotes capillary patency, lowers venous "sludging," attenuates inflammatory responses to CPB, lessens endothelial injury, reduces edema formation, increases endothelial nitric oxide release, attenuates endothelin-1 release, increases cerebral blood flow (CBF) to pressure-dependent brain regions, lessens neuronal loss in the ischemic penumbra of a cerebral infarction, and reduces hippocampal cell and caudate nucleus cell loss after cerebral ischemia (44, 47–52). At the same time, nonpulsatile flow is more common, in large part because it is easier to initiate, but it does have some potential limitations. Although theoretically more "physiologic," pulsatile flow does not, in fact, effectively transmit physiologic pulse pressures because of inherent resistance from the CPB circuitry and arterial cannulae. Furthermore, it is associated with higher CPB "line" pressure and an increased potential to cause hemolysis because of red blood cell (RBC) trauma (44, 45).

Despite the theoretical advantages of pulsatile flow, there is a dearth of data from adequately powered, prospectively randomized studies in humans that documents its advantages, particularly related to neurologic outcomes (3). In a study of 316 patients, there were no differences in frequency of postoperative cognitive dysfunction between patients randomized to receive pulsatile or nonpulsatile CPB (53, 54). In that study, the use of pulsatile flow was associated with a significantly lower rate of death and myocardial infarction than was the use of nonpulsatile perfusion. However, the study did not adequately address whether pulsatile CPB was advantageous in patients at high risk for brain injury, as there were few such patients enrolled. Pulsatile flow has been shown to attenuate global cerebral O_2 demand/supply imbalance during rewarming (55). Changing from nonpulsatile to pulsatile CPB was effective in correcting regional cerebral O_2 imbalance detected with NIRS in 17% of patients with cerebral O_2 desaturation during CABG surgery (56). The choice of pulsatile or nonpulsatile CPB, thus, has not been clearly delineated. Although nonpulsatile flow is most commonly used and may have limited disadvantages for most patients, pulsatile CPB may have some value in selective clinical situations.

pH Management During Hypothermia

Another long debated topic in the management of patients undergoing CPB relates to acid–base balance. Acid–base management during hypothermic CPB utilizes either α-stat or pH-stat strategy. The difference in the two approaches is related to the increase in CO_2 solubility that naturally occurs with declining blood temperatures (3). These fundamental physicochemical changes result in a decrease in $PaCO_2$ and an increase in pH with a fall in temperature, but no change in total CO_2 content. When utilizing α-stat pH management, there is no correction for the decreased $PaCO_2$ that occurs with body cooling (3). The target during CPB is a pH of ~7.4 and a $PaCO_2$ of ~35–40 mmHg measured at 37°C (as is reported routinely by the blood gas machine). With pH-stat management, $PaCO_2$ is kept at 40 mmHg *regardless* of blood temperature. When pH-stat is the strategy used during CPB, the $PaCO_2$ is maintained at the normal level by adding CO_2 to the CPB circuit to compensate for the rising CO_2 solubility and decreasing $PaCO_2$. Because arterial blood gases are measured at 37°C, the $PaCO_2$ at the patient's body temperature must be calculated or corrected at the time of measurement.

The debate as to which technique is most appropriate for patients undergoing cooling under CPB depends on interpretation of a number of factors. The α-stat pH management approach mimics acid–base changes that occur in poikilothermic animals such as reptiles in which the absolute CO_2 content stays constant over a range of temperatures, and the slope of the change in pH versus temperature is similar to that of the pH of water (pN) (3, 57). The term "α-stat," in fact, is based on the α-imidazole moiety of protein-bound histidine, the main buffer for the temperature changes in pH that maintains protein pKa in parallel with pN over a wide range of temperatures. These acid–base changes are believed to maintain cellular pH near the optimum level for enzyme function. Hibernating mammals, however, increase intracellular CO_2 and H^+ content by hypoventilation, thus using a pH-stat strategy to reduce cellular metabolism of some tissues (3, 57).

Several factors should be considered with regard to CBF and brain tissue oxygenation when selecting the approach to pH management during hypothermic CPB. First, CO_2 is a cerebral vasodilator, such that CBF directly relates to total CO_2 content. Consequently, CBF is higher with pH-stat than with α-stat management (58–62). However, CBF remains coupled to cerebral metabolic rate for O_2 ($CMRO_2$) with α-stat pH management, but not with pH-stat management (60). Thus, the use of α-stat pH management may cause CBF to decrease during CPB to compensate for reduced cerebral metabolic demand. Because CBF–MAP autoregulation is maintained using α-stat pH management, cerebral tissue O_2 supply is believed to be appropriate for tissue O_2 demand. In contrast, with pH-stat management, CBF is pressure-dependent and not autoregulated; hence, CBF may exceed tissue O_2 demands (60). The higher CBF obtained with pH-stat management, as compared to that with α-stat pH management, may increase the risk of injury associated with cerebral microembolism, may potentially cause cerebral arterial "steal" if associated with intracerebral vascular disease, and may potentially contribute to cerebral edema in light of the potential for "leaky" capillaries as a result of the inflammatory responses to CPB (63). At the same time, the higher CO_2 brain tissue content obtained with pH-stat has some theoretical advantages, including 1) rightward shift of the oxyhemoglobin dissociation curve promoting O_2 unloading to tissues, 2) reduced $CMRO_2$, 3) modulation of the N-methyl-D-aspartate (NMDA) receptor to limit the neurotoxic effects of excitatory amino acids, and 4) improved tolerance to cerebral ischemia (3, 64–66).

Despite these theoretical advantages of one approach to blood gas management versus another, results from prospectively randomized trials are conflicting on whether α-stat or pH-stat management during hypothermic CPB reduces neurological complications in adults after cardiac surgery (3, 67–69). Limitations to these studies include 1) the small number of patients enrolled, 2) the use of bubble oxygenators in at least one of the studies, 3) the reporting of only short-term neurologic endpoints, and 4) the use of post hoc statistical analyses when the primary endpoints did not differ between randomized groups (3). Murkin et al. (53) found, on secondary analysis of their randomized trial, that patients undergoing CPB for more than 90 minutes had a lower frequency of postoperative neurocognitive dysfunction when α-stat pH management was used than when pH-stat management was used. Similarly, Patel and Drummond (69) found a greater benefit to neurological outcomes with α-stat than with pH-stat management, but only on secondary analysis that included modifying the definition of cognitive dysfunction. One study in pediatric patients demonstrated lower morbidity and earlier return of first electroencephalogram (EEG) activity after deep hypothermic CPB when pH-stat management was used than when α-stat pH management was used (70). However, these same investigators reported that neurological examination and neurodevelopment were not markedly different 1 year after cardiac surgery in infants randomized to pH-stat or α-stat management (71). Thus, the role of α-stat versus pH-stat management during hypothermic CPB has not been clearly defined, particularly in adults.

Pericardial Suction Aspirate

Another potential cause for neurologic injury in patients undergoing CPB is related to the shed blood from the surgical field. Shed mediasti-

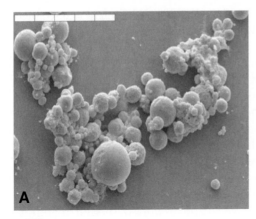

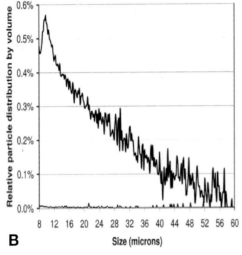

FIGURE 1–4. A: Scanning electron microscopy images of particles in the supernatant of shed mediastinal blood obtained during coronary artery bypass graft (CABG) surgery. The scale bar is 100 μm and divided into 20-μm intervals. B: The size distribution of the particles determined with Coulter counter analysis from the supernatant of arterial (bottom curve) and shed mediastinal blood (top curve) from 24 patients undergoing CABG surgery with cardiopulmonary bypass (CPB). The level of particles in the 10- to 60-μm range was higher in mediastinal blood than in arterial catheter blood. Most particles were approximately 10 μm, consistent with the size of microemboli. Reprinted with permission from (82).

nal blood contains high levels of lipid globules (Figure 1–4) that are a likely source of lipid-laden cerebral emboli found in the brains of patients at autopsy after cardiac surgery (72–77). These lipid globules are not removed from the systemic circulation with the usual CPB arterial line filters, leading many to advocate that cardiotomy suction aspirate be processed with a cell saver prior to return to the CPB circuit. Although processing pericardial suction blood was found to reduce blood lipid content significantly compared with controls (filtering only), other studies could not reproduce these findings (75–77).

The impact of shed blood on neurologic outcome remains undefined. Data are contradictory on whether processing of shed mediastinal blood with a cell saver improves neurological outcomes after cardiac surgery. Rubens et al. (78) prospectively randomized patients undergoing CABG surgery with or without aortic valve replacement to have shed mediastinal blood processed through a cell saver prior to its return to the CPB circuit ($n = 132$) or to have cardiotomy suction aspirate returned unprocessed to the CPB circuit ($n = 134$). The frequency of neurocognitive dysfunction at hospital discharge (cell-saver group, 45.3% vs. standard care, 39.0%) and 3 months after surgery (16.7% vs. 15.9%) was not different between the two groups. In contrast, Djaiani et al. (79) reported that processing cardiotomy suction with a continuous cell saver during cardiac surgery resulted in a lower frequency of cognitive dysfunction 6 weeks after cardiac surgery compared with patients who had pericardial aspirate returned unprocessed to the CPB reservoir (6% with continuous cell saver vs. 15% if returned unprocessed to CPB reservoir, $P < .05$). These investigators have recently reported, though, that these benefits to cognitive function in the cell-saver group were not sustained 1 year after surgery (80).

Processing large quantities of blood using a cell saver is not without consequences. It might predispose patients to bleeding and blood transfusion because the discarded supernatant contains blood-clotting proteins and platelets. Both Rubens et al. (78) and Djaiani et al. (79) found higher rates of non-RBC transfusion in patients who received cell-saver treatment than in controls whose shed mediastinal blood was returned unprocessed to the CPB circuit. This finding is a concern because transfusion of platelets is associated with risk for stroke in patients undergoing cardiac surgery (81).

Blood Pressure Management

CBF autoregulation is maintained during CPB when α-stat pH management is used, but it is directly related to MAP with pH-stat blood gas management (3, 82). Thus, standard practice using the α-stat approach is designed to maintain MAP at some level >50 mmHg, which is generally acknowledged as the lower limit of CBF–MAP autoregulation, at least for patients with normal blood pressure. This practice fails to take into account that, in many patients (such as those with hypertension or prior stroke), the lower CBF autoregulatory threshold might be higher (i.e., shifted to the right) (83, 84). Furthermore, this practice is based on data derived mostly from patients with few risk factors for perioperative brain injury (85). Another approach for managing elderly patients and those with cerebral vascular disease is to target MAP during CPB to levels >70–80 mmHg. This approach is supported by data from Gold et al. (86) in patients undergoing CABG surgery, which showed that the combined endpoint of myocardial infarction and/or stroke was less common in patients randomized to have high MAP (80–100 mmHg) compared with those maintained with low MAP (50–60 mmHg; $P = .026$). Other retrospective data support the strategy of maintaining higher MAP during CPB to reduce the risk of brain injury in *high-risk* patients (87).

A potential problem associated with routinely targeting higher MAP during CPB is that, in some patients, these MAP values might be higher than the upper CBF autoregulatory threshold, as volatile anesthetics in clinical concentrations shorten the autoregulatory plateau (69). Increasing CBF during CPB above that necessary to ensure cerebral metabolic demands might paradoxically pose a risk for brain injury by increasing cerebral embolic load (3, 58). In patients with systemic inflammatory response to CPB and leaky capillaries, higher CBF might further promote cerebral edema formation. Additionally, rewarming from hypothermic CPB might potentially disrupt normal CBF reactivity and impair autoregulation (88).

Clinical monitoring of CBF autoregulation is increasingly employed in neurosurgical ICUs for patients with traumatic brain injury and as a means to monitor for cerebral arterial vasospasm after subarachnoid hemorrhage (89–92). Targeting cerebral perfusion pressure to an optimal range based on continuous measurement of CBF reactivity was found to lead to improved outcomes after head injury and is now recommended in treatment guidelines for traumatic brain injury (92, 93). These methods are based on continuous monitoring of a moving linear regression correlation coefficient between cerebral perfusion pressure and CBF (such as transcranial Doppler–measured CBF velocity of the middle cerebral arteries) (94, 95). More recently, NIRS has been shown to be a suitable surrogate for more direct CBF measurement for autoregulation monitoring (96, 97). When CBF is autoregulated, the correlation coefficient between MAP and transcranial Doppler CBF velocity or NIRS signals, termed *mean velocity index* (Mx) and *cerebral oximetry index* (COx), respectively, are near 0. In contrast, when MAP is outside the CBF autoregulatory limits, Mx and COx become markedly positive (indicating correlation between MAP and CBF; Figure 1–5). These methods hold promise to provide a monitoring means for individualizing MAP during cardiac surgery.

Mediastinal CO$_2$ Insufflation

A number of techniques have been used to reduce the risk of cerebral microemboli associated with CPB. Carbon dioxide is more soluble in blood than is air; thus, insufflation of CO$_2$ into the pericardium during surgery has been used to increase the rate of absorption of intravascular emboli and reduce cerebral air microembolism (14). Limited data are available to show a benefit of this approach for improving neurological

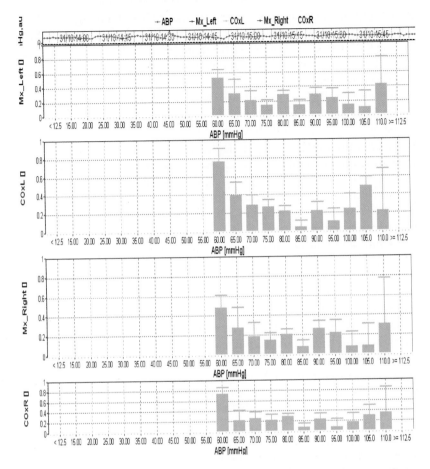

FIGURE 1–5. Dynamic monitoring of cerebral blood flow (CBF) autoregulation in the left and right cerebral hemispheres of an 86-year-old male undergoing coronary artery bypass graft (CABG) surgery. The term Mx represents the correlation coefficient between transcranial Doppler-derived CBF velocity and mean arterial pressure (MAP), and COx represents the correlation coefficient between near-infrared spectroscopy signals and MAP. A marked increase in Mx and COx, which indicates that CBF is pressure passive or dysregulated, is observed at a MAP of 65–70 mmHg. An optimal MAP in this patient might be >70 mmHg to ensure stable CBF commensurate with metabolic demand. These Mx and COx data are provided in real time, allowing for detailed patient monitoring.

outcomes after cardiac surgery. Martens et al. (98) randomly assigned 80 patients undergoing valve surgery to receive mediastinal CO_2 insufflation or no insufflation. Five days after surgery, P300 auditory-evoked potentials indicated less brain damage in the group that received CO_2

insufflation than in the group that did not, but there were no differences in rates of cognitive dysfunction or clinical neurological events between groups. Hence, few risks appear to be associated with this practice.

Hemoglobin/Hematocrit Targets

Perioperative anemia has been identified as an independent risk factor for operative morbidity and mortality (99–103). In particular, low hematocrit during CPB has been linked to adverse events, including perioperative stroke and mortality (100–103). Habib et al. (102) found that a hematocrit <22% during CPB was independently associated with stroke after cardiac surgery. Karkouti et al. (103) found that the odds of stroke increased 10% for each 1% decrease in hematocrit during CPB.

It is not known whether the relationship between anemia and adverse perioperative outcomes is merely a statistical association or whether anemia itself is the cause of adverse outcomes. With respect to the brain, decreased blood O_2 carrying capacity caused by anemia leads to a compensatory increase in CBF and increased tissue O_2 extraction. In canine models of CPB, brain tissue oxygenation is adequate at hematocrits down to 12% at 12°C and 18% at 38°C (104). However, these compensatory responses might be ineffective for ischemic neurons when the hematocrit is <30% (105). Data are limited on the optimal hematocrit levels during CPB with respect to neurological outcomes (106, 107). Mathew et al. (108) reported on a trial of 107 patients undergoing CABG surgery who were randomized to target hematocrits of either 27% or 15% to 18% during CPB. Because of higher adverse events in the low hematocrit group, the study was stopped by the safety committee. Subanalysis of the data showed an interaction between age and the lower hematocrit levels and risk for postoperative neurocognitive dysfunction.

Guidelines for blood transfusion from the Society of Thoracic Surgeons and the Society of Cardiovascular Anesthesiologists suggest that it is "reasonable" to transfuse RBCs during CPB when hemoglobin is <6 g/dL or when hemoglobin is <7 g/dL postoperatively (109). The targets are modified to 7 and 8 g/dL, respectively, when there is risk for end-organ ischemia. These guidelines state, however, that the patient's clinical situation is the most important component of the transfusion decision process.

Temperature Management

Experimentally, hypothermia provides clinically significant protection against ischemic brain injury by reducing cerebral O_2 demands and attenuating excitotoxicity, as well as by other mechanisms (3). Deliberate hypothermia initiated after cardiac arrest has also been shown to improve neurological outcomes and survival (110, 111). In contrast, after stroke, fever is associated with poor functional outcome, increased hospital length of stay, and mortality (112). The data regarding temperature regulation during CPB are not as definitive. Even though hypothermia is a basic tenet of organ protection during CPB, little evidence supports its efficacy for providing protection against brain injury (3, 113). The failure of hypothermia to improve neurological outcomes after cardiac surgery might be explained in part by inadvertent cerebral hyperthermia during rewarming (114). Cerebral hyperthermia can occur easily with excessive blood temperatures from the CPB arterial return, as the aortic cannulae are most often placed at the origin of the cerebral vessels. Usual clinical temperature-monitoring sites (e.g., nasopharynx, esophagus) underestimate brain temperature, a phenomenon which might result in failure to detect brain hyperthermia (114). In a series of studies, Nathan et al. (115) and Boodhwani et al. (116) reported that rewarming to a nasopharyngeal temperature of 34°C rather than to 37°C after hypothermic CPB (32°C) led to a lower frequency of neurocognitive dysfunction 1 week and 3 months after CABG surgery.

Glucose Management

Hyperglycemia should be avoided during CPB. Even mild hyperglycemia (i.e., >140 mg/dL) is associated with worsening of experimental brain injury and with poor outcome after stroke via activation of multiple neuronal injury pathways (3). Data from clinical trials in surgical intensive care units (ICUs) showed that mortality decreased by 34% (8% vs 4.6%, $P = .04$) when patients were given intensive insulin infusion to maintain plasma glucose between 80 and 110 mg/dL instead of being given insulin therapy only when glucose exceeded 215 mg/dL (117). However, these improved outcomes were observed only in patients who were in the ICU for more than 5 days. A recent meta-analysis of 29 randomized controlled studies involving 8432 patients found that tight glucose control was not associated with significantly reduced hospital mortality but was associated with increased risk of hypoglycemia (118). However, risk for septicemia (relative risk [RR], 0.76; 95% confidence interval [CI], 0.59-0.97) was lower with intensive insulin infusions.

Whether the findings from studies of glucose control in the ICU patient population can be extrapolated to acute glycemic control during cardiac surgery is not known. A prospectively randomized trial in nondiabetic patients undergoing CABG surgery found that intraoperative insulin given when glucose was >100 mg/dL did not lower the frequency of neurological complications 6 weeks or 6 months after surgery compared with standard care (insulin was begun when glucose was

>200 mg/dL) (119). Furthermore, the findings of a randomized study of 400 patients undergoing cardiac surgery showed that, compared with controls who were given insulin when glucose was >200 mg/dL, patients who received intensive insulin infusion to maintain glucose between 80 and 100 mg/dL had a higher composite outcome of death, cardiac morbidity, stroke, or renal failure ($P = .02$) (120).

At the same time, hyperglycemia (>200 mg/dL) during the first 24 hours after stroke is an independent predictor of larger stroke and poor outcome (121). Guidelines for management of acute ischemic stroke from the American Heart Association (122) suggest that it is reasonable to initiate insulin therapy when glucose is >140–185 mg/dL, even if the exact target glucose levels are not precisely known. In a clinical trial of patients whose glucose levels were between 108 and 308 mg/dL after acute stroke, there were no differences in 90-day mortality or functional outcome between patients prospectively randomized to receive glucose–potassium–insulin infusion for 24 hours and those who received no treatment (123). Clearly, additional study of the risks and benefits of glycemic control for patients with brain injury is needed to guide clinical practice. In addition, although glucose control may have some benefits, hypoglycemia must be avoided.

PHARMACOLOGIC BRAIN PROTECTION

There has been expansive growth in the understanding of the basic mechanisms of secondary neuronal death following ischemic injury (10). These data provide a sound basis for the development of pharmacologic strategies for brain protection during cardiac surgery (3). The various compounds tested have included NMDA receptor antagonists, calcium channel blockers, agents that block oxidant stress, gamma-aminobutyric acid (GABA) receptor agonists, and others. The results of these studies have been mostly negative; thus, there are no currently accepted pharmacologic agents with proven benefit for reducing brain injury from cardiac surgery (3). It is likely that, for such a strategy to be beneficial, agents that block multiple pathways, including apoptosis, will be needed.

NEUROMONITORING

NIRS-detected O_2 desaturation during cardiac surgery is associated with risk for stroke and neurocognitive dysfunction (124, 125). Two U.S. Food and Drug Administration (FDA)-approved devices are available in the United States for monitoring oxygen saturation in the brain. The INVOS device (Somanetics Corp, Troy, MI) provides a continuous-wave spectrometer from two-channel, light-emitting diodes that measure relative changes in regional O_2 saturation of the frontal lobe. The FORE-SIGHT™ Cerebral Oximeter (CAS Medical Systems, Branford, CT) utilizes fiberoptic light from four channels to monitor phase shifts at 754 nm, 785 nm, and 816 nm in reference to 780 nm to measure brain tissue oxygenation (126). In a prospectively randomized study of 200 patients undergoing CABG surgery, various strategies for managing NIRS-detected regional brain O_2 desaturation were compared with standard care (56). The interventions for treating low regional brain O_2 desaturation in order of efficacy were 1) ensuring adequate CPB flow, 2) raising the MAP, 3) ensuring normocarbia (reducing gas inflow during CPB or "sweep"), 4) deepening anesthesia, 5) raising the F_1O_2, and 6) initiating pulsatile CPB flow. Patients in the intervention group had a lower rate of major organ injury (death, myocardial infarction, stroke) and shorter ICU length of stay than did those in the control group. However, this study was not powered to evaluate isolated neurological complications.

SUMMARY

Brain injury from cardiac surgery is an important source of patient morbidity and mortality. The relationship between risk for brain injury and advanced age portends a rising frequency of these complications because of an increasing proportion of elderly patients undergoing cardiac surgery. A comprehensive strategy of brain protection must address its two main precipitants: cerebral embolism and cerebral hypoperfusion. Evaluation of the available evidence suggests that brain protective measures during cardiac surgery include the use of membrane oxygenator, arterial line filter, epiaortic ultrasound, and avoidance of hyperthermia during rewarming. Other common management principles during CPB (Table 1–1) can be considered, but the data are insufficient to definitively conclude that these measures will reduce the frequency of neurological complications. Newer methods of patient monitoring hold promise for providing an improved method of individualizing blood pressure management to ensure that it remains within CBF autoregulatory limits during surgery.

References

1. Roach GW, Kanchuger M, Mora-Mangano C, et al.: Adverse cerebral outcomes after coronary bypass surgery. N Engl J Med 1996; 335:1857–63
2. Newman MF, Grocott HP, Mathew JP, et al.: Longitudinal assessment of neurocognitive function after coronary-artery bypass surgery. N Engl J Med 2001; 344:395–402

3. Hogue CW, Jr., Palin CA, Arrowsmith JE.: Cardiopulmonary bypass management and neurologic outcomes: an evidence-based appraisal of current practices. Anesth Analg 2006; 103:21–37
4. McKhann GM, Grega MA, Borowicz LE, Jr., et al.: Stroke and encephalopathy after cardiac surgery: an update. Stroke 2006; 37:562–71
5. Grogan K, Stearns J, Hogue C.: Brain protection in cardiac surgery. Anesthesiol Clin North America 2008; 26:521–38
6. Leary MC, Caplan L.: Technology insight: brain MRI and cardiac surgery-detection of postoperative brain ischemia. Nat Clin Pract Cardiovasc Med 2007; 4:379–88
7. Selnes O, Grega M, Bailey M, et al.: Cognition 6 years after surgical or medical therapy for coronary artery disease. Ann Neurol 2008; 63:581–90
8. van Dijk D, Moons K, Nathoe H, et al.: Cognitive outcomes five years after not undergoing coronary artery bypass graft surgery. Ann Thorac Surg 2008; 85:60–4
9. Mergenthaler P, Dirnagl U, Meisel A.: Pathophysiology of stroke: lessons from animal models. Metab Brain Dis 2004; 19:151–67
10. Abildstrom H, Christiansen M, Siersma VD, Rasmussen LS.: Apolipoprotein E genotype and cognitive dysfunction after non-cardiac surgery. Anesthesiology 2004; 101:855–61
11. Tardiff BE, Newman MF, Saunders AM, et al.: Preliminary report of a genetic basis for cognitive decline after cardiac operations. Ann Thorac Surg 1997; 64:715–20
12. Robson MJ, Alston RP, Andrews PJ, et al.: Apolipoprotein E and neurocognitive outcome from coronary artery surgery. J Neurol Neurosurg Psychiatry 2002; 72:675–6
13. Askar FZ, Cetin HY, Kumral E, et al.: Apolipoprotein E epsilon4 allele and neurobehavioral status after on-pump coronary artery bypass grafting. J Card Surg 2005; 20:501–5
14. Heyer EJ, Wilson DA, Sahlein DH, et al.: APOE-epsilon4 predisposes to cognitive dysfunction following uncomplicated carotid endarterectomy. Neurology 2005; 65:1759–63
15. Grocott HP, White WD, Morris RW, et al.: Genetic polymorphisms and the risk of stroke after cardiac surgery. Stroke 2005; 36:1854–8
16. Mathew JP, Podgoreanu MV, Grocott HP, et al.: Genetic variants in P-selectin and C-reactive protein influence susceptibility to cognitive decline after cardiac surgery. J Am Coll Cardiol 2007; 49:1934–42
17. Wareing TH, Dávila-Román VG, Barzilia B, et al.: Management of the severely atherosclerotic ascending aorta during cardiac operations. J Thorac Cardiovasc Surg 1992; 103:453–62

18. Blauth CI, Cosgrove DM, Webb BW, et al.: Atheroembolism from the ascending aorta: an emerging problem in cardiac surgery. J Thorac Cardiovasc Surg 1992; 103:1104–12
19. Lilosky DS, Marrin CA, Caplan LR, et al.: Determination of etiologic mechanism of strokes secondary to coronary artery bypass graft surgery. Stroke 2003; 34:2830–4
20. Djaiani G, Fedorko L, Borger M, et al.: Mild to moderate atheromatous disease of the thoracic aorta and new ischemic brain lesions after conventional coronary artery bypass graft surgery. Stroke 2004; 35:e356–8
21. Croughwell ND, Newman MF, Blumenthal JA, et al.: Jugular bulb saturation and cognitive dysfunction after cardiopulmonary bypass. Ann Thorac Surg 1994; 58:1702–8
22. Edmonds HJ: Protective effect of neuromonitoring during cardiac surgery. Ann N Y Acad Sci 2005; 1053:12–9
23. Gottesman R, Sherman P, Grega M, et al.: Watershed strokes after cardiac surgery: diagnosis, etiology, and outcome. Stroke 2006; 37:2306–11
24. Benjo A, Thompson RE, Fine D, et al.: Pulse pressure is an age-independent predictor of stroke development after cardiac surgery. Hypertension 2007; 50:630–5
25. Fontes M, Aronson S, Mathew J, et al.: Pulse pressure and risk of adverse outcome in coronary bypass surgery. Anesth Analg 2008; 7:1122–9
26. Moraca R, Lin E, Holmes J, et al.: Impaired baseline regional cerebral perfusion in patients referred for coronary artery bypass. J Thorac Cardiovasc Surg 2006; 131:540–6
27. Caplan L, Hennerici M.: Impaired clearance of emboli (washout) is an important link between hypoperfusion, embolism, and ischemic stroke. Arch Neurol 1998; 55:1475–82
28. Ogasawara K, Suga Y, Sasaki M, et al.: Intraoperative microemboli and low middle cerebral artery blood flow velocity are additive in predicting development of cerebral ischemic events after carotid endarterectomy. Stroke 2008; 39:3088–91
29. Kotoh K, Fukahara K, Doi T, et al.: Predictors of early postoperative cerebral infarction after isolated off-pump coronary artery bypass grafting. Ann Thorac Surg 2007; 83:1679–83
30. Ascione R, Ghosh A, Reeves B, et al.: Retinal and cerebral microembolization during coronary artery bypass surgery: a randomized, controlled trial. Circulation 2005; 112:3833–8
31. Van Dijk D, Jansen EW, Hijman R, et al.: Cognitive outcome after off-pump and on-pump coronary artery bypass graft surgery. JAMA 2002; 287:1405–12

32. Cheng DC, Bainbridge, D, Martin JE, et al.: Does off-pump coronary artery bypass reduce mortality, morbidity, and resource utilization when compared with conventional coronary artery bypass? A meta-analysis of randomized trials. Anesthesiology 2005; 102:188–203

33. Biancari F, Mosorin M, Rasinaho E, et al.: Postoperative stroke after off-pump versus on-pump coronary artery bypass surgery. J Thorac Cardiovasc Surg 2007; 133:169–73

34. Hogue C, Jr., Murphy S, Schechtman K, Dávila-Román V.: Risk factors for early or delayed stroke after cardiac surgery. Circulation 1999; 100:642–7

35. McKhann G, Grega M, Borowicz L, et al.: Encephalopathy and stroke after coronary artery bypass grafting: incidence, consequences, and prediction. Arch Neurol 2002; 59:1422–8

36. Davila-Roman VG, Murphy SF, Nickerson NJ, et al.: Atherosclerosis of the ascending aorta is an independent predictor of long-term neurologic events and mortality. J Am Coll Cardiol 1999; 33:1308–16

37. Katz ES, Tunick PA, Rusinek H, et al.: Protruding aortic atheromas predict stroke in elderly patients undergoing cardiopulmonary bypass: experience with intraoperative transesophageal echocardiography. J Am Coll Cardiol 1992; 20:70–7

38. Katz ES, Tunick PA, Rusinek H, et al.: Protruding aortic atheromas predict stroke in elderly patients undergoing cardiopulmonary bypass: experience with intraoperative transesophageal echocardiography. J Am Coll Cardiol 1992; 20:70–7

39. Ribakove GH, Katz ES, Galloway AC, et al.: Surgical implications of transesophageal echocardiography to grade the atheromatous aortic arch. Ann Thorac Surg 1992; 53:758–61

40. Hammon JW, Stump DA, Butterworth JR, et al.: Single cross-clamp improves 6-month cognitive outcome in high-risk coronary bypass patients: the effect of reduced aortic manipulation. J Thorac Cardiovasc Surg 2006; 131:114–21

41. Swaminathan M, Grocott HP, Mackensen GB, et al.: The "sandblasting" effect of aortic cannulation on arch atheroma during cardiopulmonary bypass. Anesth Analg 2007; 104:1350–1

42. Ura M, Sakata R, Nakayama Y, Goto T.: Ultrasonographic demonstration of manipulation-related aortic injuries after cardiac surgery. J Am Coll Cardiol 2000; 35:1303–10

43. Di Tullio M, Homma S, Jin Z, Sacco R.: Aortic atherosclerosis, hypercoagulability, and stroke the APRIS (Aortic Plaque and Risk of Ischemic Stroke) study. J Am Coll Cardiol 2008; 52: 855–61

44. Taylor K.: The hemodynamics of cardiopulmonary bypass. Semin Thorac Cardiovasc Surg 1990; 2:300–12

45. Undar A, Lodge A, Daggett C, et al.: The type of aortic cannula and membrane oxygenator affect the pulsatile waveform morphology produced by a neonate-infant cardiopulmonary bypass system in vivo. Artif Organs 1998; 22:681–6

46. Matsumoto T, Wolferth C, Perlman M.: Effects of pulsatile and non-pulsatile perfusion upon cerebral and conjunctival micro-circulation in dogs. Ann Surg 1971; 37:61–4

47. Watanabe T, Orita H, Kobayashi M, et al.: Brain tissue pH, oxygen tension, and carbon dioxide tension in profoundly hypothermic cardiopulmonary bypass: comparative study of circulatory arrest, nonpulsatile low-flow perfusion, and pulsatile low-flow perfusion. J Thorac Cardiovasc Surg 1989; 97:396–401

48. Sadahiro M, Haneda K, Mohri H.: Experimental study of cerebral autoregulation during cardiopulmonary bypass with or without pulsatile perfusion. J Thorac Cardiovasc Surg 1994; 108:446–54

49. Anstadt M, Stonnington M, Tedder M, et al.: Pulsatile reperfusion after cardiac arrest improves neurologic outcome. Ann Surg 1991; 214:478–88

50. Champsaur G, Vedrinne C, Martinot S, et al.: Flow-induced release of endothelium-derived relaxing factor during pulsatile bypass: experimental study in the fetal lamb. J Thorac Cardiovasc Surg 1997; 114:738–45

51. Orime Y, Shiono M, Hata H, et al.: Cytokine and endothelial damage in pulsatile and nonpulsatile cardiopulmonary bypass. Artif Organs 1999; 23:508–12

52. Trammer B, Gross C, Kindt G, Adey G.: Pulsatile versus nonpulsatile blood flow in the treatment of acute cerebral ischemia. Neurosurgery 1986; 19:724–31

53. Murkin JM, Martzke JS, Buchan AM, et al.: A randomized study of the influence of perfusion technique and pH management strategy in 316 patients undergoing coronary artery bypass surgery. I. Mortality and cardiovascular morbidity. J Thorac Cardiovasc Surg 1995; 110:340–8

54. Murkin JM, Martzke JS, Buchan AM, et al.: A randomized study of the influence of perfusion technique and pH management strategy in 316 patients undergoing coronary artery bypass surgery. II. Neurologic and cognitive outcome. J Thorac Cardiovasc Surg 1995; 110:349–62

55. Mutch W, Lefevre G, Thiessen D, et al.: Computer controlled cardiopulmonary bypass increases jugular venous oxygen saturation during rewarming. Ann Thorac Surg 1998; 65:59–65

56. Murkin J, Adams S, Novick R, et al.: Monitoring brain oxygen saturation during coronary bypass surgery: a randomized, prospective study. Anesth Analg 2006; 104:51–8
57. Rahn H, Reeves R, Howell B.: Hydrogen ion regulation, temperature, and evolution. Am Rev Resp Disease 1975; 112:165–72
58. Henriksen L, Hjelms E, Lindeburgh T.: Brain hyperperfusion during cardiac operations. J Thorac Cardiovasc Surg 1983; 86:202–8
59. Prough D, Stump D, Roy R, et al.: Response of cerebral blood flow to changes in carbon dioxide tension during hypothermic cardiopulmonary bypass. Anesthesiology 1986; 64:576–81
60. Murkin J, Farrar J, Tweed A, et al.: Cerebral autoregulation and flow/metabolism coupling during cardiopulmonary bypass: the influence of $PaCO_2$. Anesth Analg 1987; 66:825–32
61. Lundar T, Lindegaard KF, Froysacker T, et al.: Dissociation between cerebral autoregulation and carbon dioxide reactivity during non-pulsatile cardiopulmonary bypass. Ann Thorac Surg 1985; 40:582–7
62. Henriksen L.: Brain luxury perfusion during cardiopulmonary bypass in humans: a study of the cerebral blood flow response to changes in CO_2, O_2, and blood pressure. J Cereb Blood Flow Metab 1986; 6:366–78
63. Laffey J, Boylan J, Cheng D.: The systemic inflammatory response to cardiac surgery. Anesthesiology 2002; 97:215–52
64. Dexter F, Hindman B.: Effect of haemoglobin concentration on brain oxygenation in focal stroke: a mathematical modeling study. Br J Anaesth 1997; 79:346–51
65. Duebener L, Hagino I, Sakamoto T, et al.: Effects of pH management during deep hypothermic bypass on cerebral microcirculation: alpha-stat versus pH-stat. Circulation 2002; 106(Suppl I):I103–8
66. Tombaugh G, Sapolsky R.: Evolving concepts about the role of acidosis in ischemic neuropathology. J Neurochem 1993; 61: 793–803
67. Bashein G, Townes B, Nessly M, et al.: A randomized study of carbon dioxide management during hypothermic cardiopulmonary bypass. Anesthesiology 1990; 72:7–15
68. Stephan H, Weyland A, Kazmaier S, et al.: Acid-base management during hypothermic cardiopulmonary bypass does not affect cerebral metabolism but does affect blood flow and neurological outcome. Br J Anaesth 1992; 69:51–7
69. Patel P, Drummond J.: Cerebral physiology and the effects of anesthetics and techniques, 6th Edition. Philadelphia, PA, Elsevier Churchill Livingstone, 2005
70. du Plessis A, Jonas R, Wypij D, et al.: Perioperative effects of alpha-stat versus pH-stat strategies for deep hypothermic cardiopul-

monary bypass in infants. J Thorac Cardiovasc Surg 1997; 114: 991–1001

71. Bellinger D, Wypij D, du Plessis A, et al.: Developmental and neurologic effects of alpha-stat versus pH-stat strategies for deep hypothermic cardiopulmonary bypass in infants. J Thorac Cardiovasc Surg 2001; 121:374–83

72. Moody DM, Brown WR, Challa VR, et al.: Brain microemboli associated with cardiopulmonary bypass: a histologic and magnetic resonance imaging study. Ann Thorac Surg 1995; 59:1304–7

73. Eyjolfsson A, Sciclunaa S, Johnsson P, et al.: Characterization of lipid particles in shed mediastinal blood. Ann Thorac Surg 2008; 85:978–81

74. Brooker RF, Brown WR, Moody DM, et al.: Cardiotomy suction: a major source of brain lipid emboli during cardiopulmonary bypass. Ann Thorac Surg 1998; 65:1651–5

75. Kincaid EH, Jones TJ, Stump DA, et al.: Processing scavenged blood with a cell saver reduces cerebral lipid microembolization. Ann Thorac Surg 2000; 70:1296–300

76. Jewell AE, Akowuah EF, Suvarna SK, et al.: A prospective randomised comparison of cardiotomy suction and cell saver for recycling shed blood during cardiac surgery. Eur J Cardiothorac Surg 2003; 23:633–6

77. Kaza AK, Cope JT, Fiser SM, et al.: Elimination of fat microemboli during cardiopulmonary bypass. Ann Thorac Surg 2003; 75:555–9

78. Rubens FD, Boodhwani M, Mesana T, et al.: The cardiotomy trial. A randomized, double-blind study to assess the effect of processing of shed blood during cardiopulmonary bypass on transfusion and neurocognitive function. Circulation 2007; 116(11 Suppl):I-89–7

79. Djaiani G, Fedorko L, Borger MA, et al.: Continuous-flow cell saver reduces cognitive decline in elderly patients after coronary bypass surgery. Circulation 2007; 116:1888–95

80. Djaiani G, Van Rensburg A, Fedorko L, et al.: Early benefit of preserved neurocognitive function is not sustained at 1-year after cardiac surgery. Orlando, FL, 2008 Annual Meeting of the American Society of Anesthesiologists

81. Spiess BD, Royston D, Levy JH, et al.: Platelet transfusions during coronary artery bypass graft surgery are associated with serious adverse outcomes. Transfusion 2004; 44:1143–8

82. Murkin JM, Farrar JK, Tweed A, et al.: Cerebral autoregulation and flow/metabolism coupling during cardiopulmonary bypass: the influence of $PaCO_2$. Anesth Analg 1987; 66:825–32

83. Davis S, Ackerman R, Correia J, et al.: Cerebral blood flow and cerebrovascular CO_2 reactivity in stroke-age normal controls. Neurology 1983; 33:391–9

84. Yamamoto M, Meyer J, Sakai F, Yamaguchi F.: Aging and cerebral vasodilator responses to hypercarbia. Responses in normal aging and in persons with risk factors for stroke. Arch Neurol 1980; 37:489–96

85. Schell R, Kern F, Greeley W, et al.: Cerebral blood flow and metabolism during cardiopulmonary bypass. Anesth Analg 1993; 76:849–65

86. Gold JP, Charlson ME, Williams-Russo P, et al.: Improvement of outcomes after coronary artery bypass: a randomized trial comparing intraoperative high versus low mean arterial pressure. J Thorac Cardiovasc Surg 1995; 110:1302–11

87. Hartman GS, Yao FS, Bruefach M, et al.: Severity of aortic atheromatous disease diagnosed by transesophageal echocardiography predicts stroke and other outcomes associated with coronary artery surgery: a prospective study. Anesth Analg 1996; 83:701–8

88. Lavinio A, Timofeev I, Nortje J, et al.: Cerebrovascular reactivity during hypothermia and rewarming. Br J Anaesth 2007; 99:237–44

89. Steiner L, Coles J, Johnston A, et al.: Assessment of cerebrovascular autoregulation in head-injured patients: a validation study. Stroke 2003; 34:2404–9

90. Soehle M, Czosnyka M, Pickard J, Kirkpatrick P.: Continuous assessment of cerebral autoregulation in subarachnoid hemorrhage. Anesth Analg 2004; 98:1133–9

91. Ragauskas A, Daubaris G, Petkus V, et al.: Clinical study of continuous non-invasive cerebrovascular autoregulation monitoring in neurosurgical ICU. Acta Neurochir 2005; 95:367–70

92. Bratton S, Chestnut R, Ghajar J, et al.: Guidelines for the management of severe traumatic brain injury. IX. Cerebral perfusion thresholds. J Neurotrauma 2007; 24:S59–64

93. Steiner LA, Czosnyka M, Piechnik S, et al.: Continuous monitoring of cerebrovascular pressure reactivity allows determination of optimal cerebral perfusion pressure in patients with traumatic brain injury. Crit Care Med 2002; 30:733–8

94. Lang EW, Mehdorn HM, Dorsch NW, et al.: Continuous monitoring of cerebrovascular autoregulation: a validation study. J Neurol Neurosurg Psychiatry 2002; 72:583–6

95. Minhas PS, Smielewski P, Kirkpatrick PJ, et al.: Pressure autoregulation and positron emission tomography-derived cerebral blood flow acetazolamide reactivity in patients with carotid artery stenosis. Neurosurgery 2004; 55:63–8

96. Brady K, Lee J, Kibler K, et al.: Continuous time-domain analysis of cerebrovascular autoregulation using near-infrared spectroscopy. Stroke 2007; 38:2818–25

97. Steiner L, Pfister D, Strebel S, et al.: Near-infrared spectroscopy can monitor dynamic cerebral autoregulation in adults. Neurocrit Care 2009; 10(1):122–8. Epub 2008 Sep 20

98. Martens S, Neumann K, Sodemann C, et al.: Carbon dioxide field flooding reduces neurologic impairment after open heart surgery. Ann Thorac Surg 2008; 85:543–7

99. Kulier A, Levin J, Moser R, et al.: Impact of preoperative anemia on outcome in patients undergoing coronary artery bypass graft surgery. Circulation 2007; 116:471–9

100. DeFoe GR, Ross CS, Olmstead EM, et al.: Lowest hematocrit on bypass and adverse outcomes associated with coronary artery bypass grafting. Ann Thorac Surg 2001; 71:769–76.

101. Fang WC, Helm RE, Krieger AH, et al.: Impact of minimum hematocrit during cardiopulmonary bypass on mortality in patients undergoing coronary artery surgery. Circulation 1997; 96:II194–9

102. Habib RH, Zacharias A, Schwann TA, et al.: Adverse effects of low hematocrit during cardiopulmonary bypass in the adult: should current practice be changed? J Thorac Cardiovasc Surg 2003; 125:1438–50

103. Karkouti K, Djaiani G, Borger MA, et al.: Low hematocrit during cardiopulmonary bypass is associated with increased risk of perioperative stroke in cardiac surgery. Ann Thorac Surg 2005; 80:1381–7

104. Cook DJ, Huston J III, Trenerry MR, et al.: Postcardiac surgical cognitive impairment in the aged using diffusion-weighted magnetic resonance imaging. Ann Thorac Surg 2007; 83:1389–95

105. Dexter F, Hindman B.: Effect of haemoglobin concentration on brain oxygenation in focal stroke: a mathematical modelling study. Br J Anaesth 1997; 79:346–51

106. Johnson RG, Thurer RL, Kruskall MS, et al.: Comparison of two transfusion strategies after elective operations for myocardial revascularization. J Thorac Cardiovasc Surg 1992; 104:307–14

107. Bracey AW, Radovancevic R, Riggs SA, et al.: Lowering the hemoglobin threshold for transfusion in coronary artery bypass procedures: effect on patient outcome. Transfusion 1999; 39:1070–7

108. Mathew JP, Mackensen GB, Phillips-Bute B, et al.: Extreme hemodilution is associated with increased cognitive dysfunction in the elderly after cardiac surgery. Anesthesiology 2007; 107:577–84

109. Ferraris VA, Ferraris SP, Saha SP, et al.: Perioperative blood transfusion and blood conservation in cardiac surgery: the Society of Thor-

acic Surgeons and The Society of Cardiovascular Anesthesiologists clinical practice guideline. J Thorac Cardiovasc Surg 2007; 83:S27–86

110. Minamisawa H, Smith ML, Siejö BK.: The effect of mild hyperthermia and hypothermia on brain damage following 5, 10, and 15 minutes of forebrain ischemia. Ann Neurol 1990; 28:26–33

111. Bernard SA, Gray TW, Buist MD, et al.: Treatment of comatose survivors of out-of-hospital cardiac arrest with induced hypothermia. N Engl J Med 2002; 346:557–63

112. Greer DM, Funk SE, Reaven NL, et al.: Impact of fever on outcome in patients with stroke and neurologic injury. Stroke 2008; 39:3029–35

113. Rees K, Beranek-Stanley M, Burke M, Ebrahim S.: Hypothermia to reduce neurological damage following coronary artery bypass surgery (Cochrane Review). Chichester, UK, John Wiley & Sons, 2004

114. Grocott HP, Mackensen GB, Grigore AM, et al.: Postoperative hyperthermia is associated with cognitive dysfunction after coronary artery bypass graft surgery. Stroke 2002; 33:537–41

115. Nathan HJ, Wells GA, Munson JL, Ebrahim S.: Neuroprotective effect of mild hypothermia in patients undergoing coronary artery surgery with cardiopulmonary bypass: a randomized trial. Circulation 2001; 104:I85–91

116. Boodhwani M, Wozny D, Rubens FD, et al.: Effects of sustained mild hypothermia on neurocognitive function after coronary artery bypass surgery: a randomized, double-blind study. J Thorac Cardiovasc Surg 2007; 134(6):1443–50; discussion 1451–2. Epub 2007 Oct 29

117. van den Berghe G, Wilmer A, Hermans G, et al.: Intensive insulin therapy in the medical ICU. N Engl J Med 2006; 354:449–61

118. Wiener R, Wiener D, Larson R.: Benefits and risks of tight glucose control in critically ill adults: a meta-analysis. JAMA 2008; 300:933–44

119. Butterworth J, Wagenknecht LE, Legault C, et al.: Attempted control of hyperglycemia during cardiopulmonary bypass fails to improve neurologic or neurobehavioral outcomes in patients without diabetes mellitus undergoing coronary artery bypass grafting. J Thorac Cardiovasc Surg 2005; 130:1319–25

120. Gandhi FY, Nuttall GA, Abel MD, et al.: Intensive intraoperative insulin therapy versus conventional glucose management during cardiac surgery. Ann Intern Med 2007; 146:233–43

121. Baird TA, Parsons MW, Phanh T, et al.: Persistent poststroke hyperglycemia is independently associated with infarct expansion and worse clinical outcome. Stroke 2003; 34:2208–14

122. Adams HP, Jr., del Zoppo G, Alberts MJ, et al.: Guidelines for the early management of adults with ischemic stroke: a guideline from

the American Heart Association/American Stroke Association Stroke Council, Clinical Cardiology Council, Cardiovascular Radiology and Intervention Council, and the Atherosclerotic Peripheral Vascular Disease and Quality of Care Outcomes in Research Interdisciplinary Working Group. Stroke 2007; 38:1655–711

123. Gray CS, Hildreth AJ, Sandercock PA, et al.: Glucose-potassium-insulin infusions in the management of post-stroke hyperglycaemia: the UK Glucose Insulin in Stroke Trial (GIST-UK). Lancet Neurol 2007; 6:397–406

124. Yao FS, Tseng CC, Ho CY, et al.: Cerebral oxygen desaturation is associated with early postoperative neuropsychological dysfunction in patients undergoing cardiac surgery. J Cardiothorac Vasc Anesth 2004; 18:552–8

125. Goldman S, Sutter F, Ferdinand F, Trace C.: Optimizing intraoperative cerebral oxygen delivery using noninvasive cerebral oximetry decreases the incidence of stroke for cardiac surgical patients. Heart Surg Forum 2004; 7:E376–81

126. Kurth CD, Thayer WS.: A multiwavelength frequency-domain near-infrared cerebral oximeter. Phys Med Biol 1999; 44:727–40

Solomon Aronson

Management of Blood Pressure in the Patient Requiring Cardio-thoracic Surgery: What's the Correct End Point?

2

"A man is as old as his arteries." — Sir William Osler, 1898

INTRODUCTION

Hypertension remains one of the most important preventable risk factors for heart disease and stroke, accounting for 14% of cardiovascular deaths worldwide (1), yet nearly one third of the population in the United States (70 million) has some form of the disease (2–5). In general, among the hypertensive population, approximately 25% are not treated, 50% are inadequately treated, and 25% are undiagnosed (3, 6). Data from National Health and Nutrition Examination Survey/National Center for Health Statistics (NHANES/NCHS) 2005–2006 showed that, of persons $\geq$20 years of age who are hypertensive, 78.7% were aware of their condition, 69.1% were under current treatment, 45.4% had blood pressure (BP) under control, and 54.6% did not have it controlled (7). According to several estimates, 90% of people in the United States will be diagnosed with hypertensive disease by their sixth to seventh decade of life (3, 8), which coincidentally is the fastest growing segment of the general population (9) (Figure 2–1). Furthermore, it is projected that more than 1.5 billion people worldwide will suffer from the condition by 2025 (10). Cardiovascular disease, a cause and consequence of hypertension, accounts for ~30% of all deaths worldwide and is expected to remain the most serious public health challenge in the decades to come (11). It is estimated that there are as many deaths and hospital readmissions attrib-

Medically Challenging Patients Undergoing Cardiothoracic Surgery, edited by Neal H. Cohen, MD, MPH, MS, Lippincott Williams & Wilkins, Baltimore © 2009.

utable to acute BP crises (8.8% and 37.2%, respectively) as to acute coronary syndromes (ACS; 5%–7% and 21%, respectively) and congestive heart failure (CHF; 8.5% and 25.7%, respectively) (12–17). Intensive BP control saves approximately $2000 per quality-adjusted life-year (18). Despite these alarming statistics about the prevalence of hypertension and its consequences, treatment is effective. It comes at significant finan-

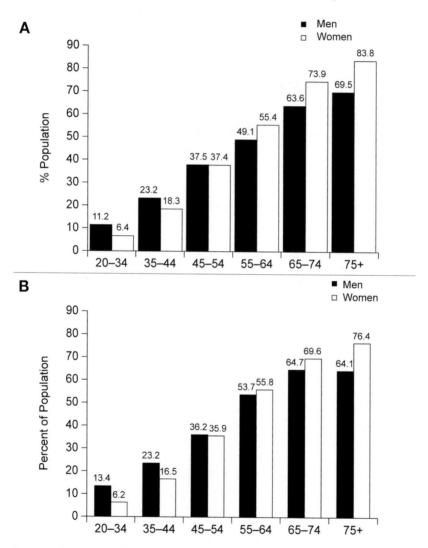

FIGURE 2–1. Prevalence of high blood pressure (BP) in adults aged ≥20 years by age and sex (NHANES: 2005 to 2006) (7). Hypertension is defined as systolic BP ≥140 mm Hg or diastolic BP ≥90 mm Hg, taking antihypertensive medication, or being told twice by a physician or other professional that one has hypertension.

cial cost. The costs associated with the clinical manifestations of untreated hypertension are even greater. The annual cost of hypertension management is estimated to be nearly $70 billion per year in the Unites States alone (18).

Taking into account the fact that up to 64 million people per year in the United States have surgery requiring anesthesia (19), the increasing incidence of hypertension, and that hypertension is an established risk factor for adverse outcome following surgery, it should come as no surprise that poorly controlled hypertension remains one of the most common medical indications for deferring elective surgery (20–22). This chapter provides an overview of the risks associated with pathophysiology of hypertension and strategies for managing the hypertensive patient requiring cardiac surgery.

UNDERSTANDING THE RISK

Old Questions with New Answers for Acute BP Control

The Seventh Report of the Joint National Committee on Prevention, Detection, Evaluation, and Treatment of High Blood Pressure classifies BP as normal, prehypertension, and stages 1 and 2 hypertension (3) (Table 2–1). Prehypertension (formally known as "high normal" BP) also is associated with increased cardiovascular morbidity and mortality, as well as subclinical atherosclerosis and target-organ damage (23, 24).

Hypertension represents a major risk factor for coronary artery disease (CAD), dyslipidemia (25–27), CHF (26–28), renal dysfunction (29–31), cerebral dysfunction, dementia (25, 29, 32–35), and diabetes (35). A number of studies have established that cardiovascular morbidity and mortality risk increases continuously with increasing BP at levels well below thresholds for "standard" definitions of hypertension (25). The higher the BP, the higher the risk, such that between the ages of 40 and 69 years, for each 20-mm Hg increase in systolic BP (SBP) or 10-mm Hg increase in diastolic BP (DBP), the chance of developing cardiovascular disease doubles across the BP range of 115/75 to 185/115 (25).

TABLE 2–1. Classification of hypertension subtypes

Systolic BP (mm Hg)	Diastolic BP (mm Hg)	Category
<120	and <80	Normal
120–139	or 80–89	Prehypertension
140–159	or 90–99	Stage 1 hypertension
>160	or >100	Stage 2 hypertension

From (3).

TABLE 2–2.   Characteristics of systolic and diastolic blood pressure levels

Characteristics	Blood pressure (mm Hg)
Optimal	<120 SBP/80 DBP
ISH	>140 SBP/<90 DBP
IDH	<140 SBP/>90 DBP
Combined hypertension	>140 SBP/>90 DBP
Mean PP	Mean SBP − mean DBP
MAP	1/3 SBP + 2/3 DBP

From (31, 36).

Over the years, much has been learned about the characterization of hypertensive states, associated morbidity and mortality, and efficacy and safety of antihypertensive therapy. During this period of time, we have gained a better understanding of the relative importance of mean, systolic, diastolic, and pulse pressure (PP) and the impact of each on management. These hypertension subtypes (or phenotypes) have been appreciated to reflect specific manifestations of underlying cardiovascular disease status (Table 2–2). There is irrefutable evidence that these BP phenotypes are independently associated with adverse cardiovascular outcomes (3, 27, 31, 35).

Curiously, we accept disease-specific treatment strategies for subtypes of heart failure (e.g., left vs. right, systolic vs. diastolic) or cancer (e.g., type, stage, and grade); however, we typically don't tailor BP management or routinely distinguish one form of hypertensive disease from another for risk stratification or as a part of the plan for perioperative care. Yet the specific hypertensive characterization (phenotype) is a signature of underlying vascular pathophysiology that should govern our management strategy for BP control (Figure 2–2).

Isolated systolic hypertension (ISH) increases in prevalence with age (37) whereas the prevalence of isolated diastolic hypertension (IDH) decreases. Combined ISH and IDH also decrease with age. Adverse ischemic cardiac and cerebral vascular diseases also increase with age-adjusted increases in SBP.

Systolic hypertension is more prevalent than diastolic hypertension, particularly in individuals older than 60 years, and is associated with greater risks of both fatal and nonfatal outcomes, including cerebral and cardiac dysfunction (25, 32, 37, 38).

Multiple studies have documented that the specific BP phenotype also conveys an independent risk for adverse perioperative outcomes (29–31, 39, 40) (Figures 2–3 and 2–4). For many years, preoperative DBP has served

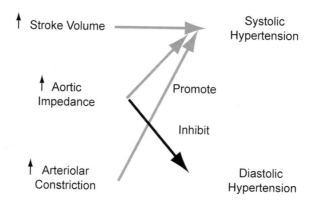

FIGURE 2–2. Pathogenesis of systolic and diastolic hypertension.

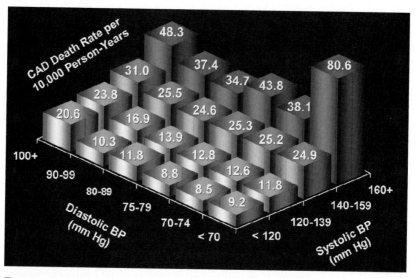

FIGURE 2–3. Age-adjusted coronary heart disease death rates per 10,000 person-years from the Multiple Risk Factor Intervention Trial (37).

as the underpinning for defining perioperative risk and the success or failure of antihypertensive therapy and clinical trial design (41, 42).

Mean arterial pressure (MAP) also has been extensively evaluated as an intraoperative indicator of perioperative risk associated with noncardiac (43, 44) as well as cardiac surgery involving cardiopulmonary bypass (CPB) (45). High risk patients who experience a drop in MAP of >20 mm Hg for more than 1 hour or the same decrease in addition to an increase in MAP >20 mm Hg for more than 15 minutes from baseline (BP lability)

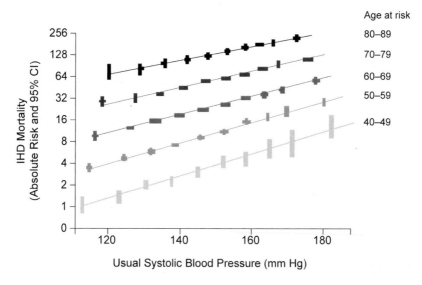

FIGURE 2–4. Prospective study collaboration of 1 million patients (25).

while undergoing elective noncardiac surgery had the greatest risk of complications (44). Additionally, a drop in MAP from baseline during CPB in patients undergoing cardiac surgery is associated with an increased risk of cognitive dysfunction and bilateral watershed strokes (46–48).

Recently, data on the relationship between preoperative ISH and perioperative outcome have been reported in cardiac and noncardiac surgery (29, 39). In these studies, ISH was associated with a 40% increase in perioperative cardiovascular morbidity following coronary artery bypass graft procedures (Table 2–3). Interestingly, this risk remained, regardless of preoperative antihypertension medication, anesthetic techniques, or other perioperative cardiovascular risk factors (29).

Among patients undergoing cardiac surgery, the mean PP was greater in those patients who suffered renal dysfunction (Table 2–4) or a stroke (81 vs. 65 mm Hg), and each additional increase of 10 mm Hg contributed additional risk (odds ratio [OR], 1.35; 95% confidence interval [CI], 1.13–1.62; $P = .001$) (40). An additional independent observation was that death from cardiac and cerebral causes was directly associated to preoperative PP in this patient population (Figure 2–5, 2–6).

Despite efforts to understand the contribution of BP phenotype in an individual patient on clinical decision making, we still do not have a definitive perioperative BP management strategy to optimize outcome. Recognizing that for many organ systems there is autoregulation of blood flow over a range of BPs, it is likely that an autoregulatory range is distinctly different for patients with different hypertension phenotypes. Surgery and

Table 2–3. Rate of adverse outcomes following CABG[29]

	No ISH (n = 1457)	ISH (n = 612)	OR (95% CI)
Renal failure/insufficiency - (injury)	6.7%	8.8%	1.3 (0.9–1.9)
Stroke	6.3%	10.1%	1.7 (1.2–2.3)
LV dysfunction	29.1%	34.3%	1.3 (1.0–1.6)
Renal injury, stroke, LV dysfunction, death	33.2%	40.9%	1.4 (1.1–1.7)

From (29).
CABG = coronary artery bypass graft.
PP has also been shown to be an independent predictor of postoperative renal dysfunction, adverse cardiac events, and stroke following cardiac surgery (30,31,40).

Table 2–4. Kidney injury after cardiac surgery is proportionate to PP

Preoperative Risk Factors	Score	Intraoperative Risk Factors	Score
Age >75 years	7	>2 Inotropes	10
PP (mm Hg)		Intra-aortic balloon pump	15
40	0		
41–60	4		
61–80	8		
81–100	12		
>100	16		
History		Cardiopulmonary bypass ≥122 min	6
CHF	9		
MI	6		
Renal disease	13		

From (30).

anesthesia will have additional affects on blood flow and autoregulation. The unique circumstances for each patient might lead to organ hypoperfusion in some despite what might be deemed to be a "clinically acceptable" BP in others.

THE CHANGING PARADIGM IN ACUTE HYPERTENSION MANAGEMENT

Although preexisting hypertension is a significant risk factor for perioperative outcome, it is important to recognize that hypertension is not a uniform process. In addition to chronic BP elevation, with or without treatment, some patients experience acute changes in BP that 1) must be

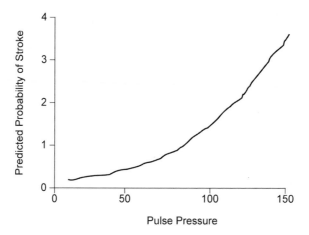

FIGURE 2–5. Stroke after cardiac surgery is proportionate to pulse pressure (40). **AQ:15**

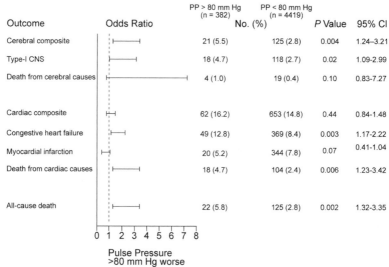

Incidence

Outcome	Odds Ratio	PP > 80 mm Hg (n = 382) No. (%)	PP < 80 mm Hg (n = 4419)	P Value	95% CI
Cerebral composite		21 (5.5)	125 (2.8)	0.004	1.24–3.21
Type-I CNS		18 (4.7)	118 (2.7)	0.02	1.09-2.99
Death from cerebral causes		4 (1.0)	19 (0.4)	0.10	0.83-7.27
Cardiac composite		62 (16.2)	653 (14.8)	0.44	0.84-1.48
Congestive heart failure		49 (12.8)	369 (8.4)	0.003	1.17-2.22
Myocardial infarction		20 (5.2)	344 (7.8)	0.07	0.41-1.04
Death from cardiac causes		18 (4.7)	104 (2.4)	0.006	1.23-3.42
All-cause death		22 (5.8)	125 (2.8)	0.002	1.32-3.35

Pulse Pressure
>80 mm Hg worse

FIGURE 2–6. Kaplan–Meier analysis. Cerebral and cardiac survival according to preoperative pulse pressure <80 mm Hg versus >80 mm Hg (n = 4801). CNS = central nervous system (31).

managed and 2) cause significant morbidity and mortality. For example, the acute hypertension syndrome, typically seen during surgery or post-surgery as well as in other conditions that result from these acute elevations in BP such as acute stroke, ACS, or acute decompensated heart

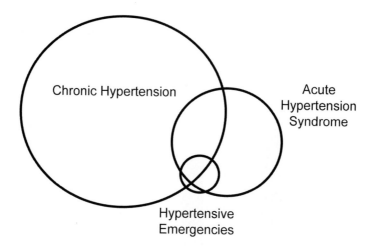

FIGURE 2–7. Prevalence of hypertension (HTN) type.

failure, may differ in mechanism and responsiveness to treatment modalities from the approaches used to treat patients with chronic preexisting hypertension. In addition, acute hypertension syndrome is not necessarily the same as other hypertensive emergencies, with the latter representing 1%–2% of the overall manifestation of hypertensive disease (i.e., 700,000 of 70 million cases) and often unassociated with anesthesia or surgery (Figure 2–7) (48).

Although there is overlap between the risk associated with hypertension that occurs in the setting of surgery and anesthesia from preexisting hypertension and/or some hypertensive emergencies, hypertension seen in surgery and postsurgery is typically independent of the underlying hypertensive conditions (Figure 2–8) and may differ mechanistically as well. In contrast, active management of BP during surgery is critical to outcome and essentially independent of the management strategies used to treat the underlying hypertension.

Whereas many patients who develop hypertension associated with surgery and anesthesia have underlying BP abnormalities, the acute changes seen in the perioperative period have ramifications for the overall care, both in the operating room and thereafter. Acute conditions that affect vascular tone during the perioperative period (whether neural, endothelial, or mechanical) can cause acute changes in regional and/or systemic hemodynamics as a result of dilatory or constrictive stimuli; these changes can trigger acute procoagulation or inflammatory reactions that affect outcomes after surgery (50, 51). The changes in stretch and/or stress, endothelial function, and central nervous system stimulation often exist in combination with one another. As a result, adverse

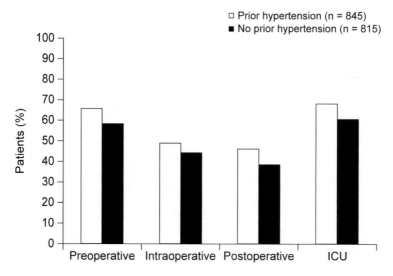

FIGURE 2–8. Patients requiring antihypertensive treatment. ICU = intensive care unit (49).

vascular outcomes associated with acute fluctuations in BP superimposed on preexisting hypertension may be accelerated in the setting of surgery, manifesting over days versus decades (31, 40, 52).

PATHOPHYSIOLOGY OF HYPERTENSION

State of the Knowledge

BP consists of a steady component (MAP) and a pulsatile component (PP). The fluid-pressure dynamic of BP is determined by different parameters depending on its component subtype; for example, the determinants of MAP are left ventricular (LV) ejection and peripheral vascular resistance, whereas the determinants of SBP are stroke volume, LV ejection, distensibility, and wave reflection. The determinants of PP are LV ejection, viscoelasticity, and wave reflection. The actual observed pulse contour that is displayed on a monitor is a summation of forward and returning pressure waves (Figure 2–9).

Adaptive changes in the vessel wall are dependent on BP load. The lumen-to-wall ratio is decreased in diastolic hypertension with inward (eutrophic) remodeling in small vessels. Vascular remodeling (characterized by outward hypertrophy), in contrast, occurs with PP hypertension, a disease of large conduit vessels (e.g., aorta) (Figure 2–10).

Acute changes in systemic hemodynamics during cardiothoracic surgery are common; the causes for these changes include alterations in systemic vascular resistance induced by anesthesia, surgical stimulation, aortic occlusive clamping and unclamping, fluid shifts, hemorrhage, and secondary drug effects, among others. These changes commonly occur in the setting of insufficient or acute changes in intravascular volume. They likely effect patients differently, depending on their underlying vascular physiology and compliance.

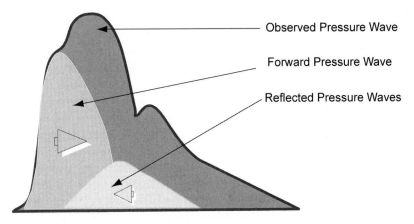

FIGURE 2–9.   Observed arterial pulse wave contour is the aggregate of forward and reflected waves

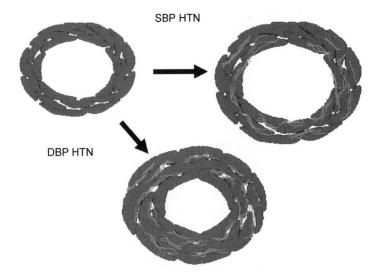

FIGURE 2–10.   Vascular remodeling occurs in an outward manner in systolic hypertension (SBP HTN) and inward manner in diastolic hypertension (DBP HTN).

Arterial compliance relates directly to the change in volume (stroke volume) and inversely to the ensuing change in pressure. PP, the difference between SBP and DBP, is an index of conduit vessel stiffness and the rate of pressure wave propagation within the arterial tree (53). When stiffening of the aorta occurs, propagated and reflected waves within the arterial tree travel much more rapidly, resulting in an early return of the propagated wave to the central aorta during late systole as opposed to early diastole (54). This augmented systolic component effectively increases afterload and compromises DBP augmentation, resulting in a decrease in organ perfusion, including coronary, cerebral, and renal perfusion pressure (55–58).

There is a close relationship between aging, long-standing arterial hypertension, vascular disease, and PP—all acting in concert to limit organ flow and reserve. The preexisting vasculopathy in conjunction with aortic-wall injury caused by surgical manipulation (aortic clamping/declamping and cannulation/decannulation), as well as the inflammatory response associated with CPB, provide a compelling pathophysiologic basis for the increased postoperative vascular complications seen in some patients after cardiac or major vascular surgery. The stiff vessels have altered vascular smooth muscle cell phenotypes with resultant arterial remodeling of the blood vessels in vital organs. In these cases, it is likely that the autoregulatory BP range is distinctly different across individuals with different vascular properties and is variously affected by different surgical procedures and anesthesia. As a result, any alteration in the autoregulatory range might lead to organ hypoperfusion in some individuals, despite maintenance of what is thought to be a "clinically acceptable" BP. Moreover, any increase in systolic load, along with a lower diastolic perfusion pressure and relative intravascular volume depletion, may create the pathophysiologic foundation for perioperative vascular injury and postoperative organ dysfunction.

Shear forces associated with hypertension, particularly when the upstroke on the arterial pressure waveform is present, may account for significant vascular damage, particularly in patients undergoing cardiac or major vascular surgery (Figure 2–11). In normal arteries, low shear has been shown to be atherogenic, whereas high shear in normal arteries appears to be atheroprotective. In contrast, in the patient populations who require cardiovascular interventions and in whom the arteries are not normal, shear has been demonstrated to promote vascular injury, plaque rupture, thrombosis, and neurohumoral activation. Wide PP is also known to augments oscillatory shear (59–64), and may therefore contribute to further injury (Figure 2–12).

In addition, increased BP directly contributes to vessel stretch (Figure 2–13), which can promote endothelial dysfunction, an inflammatory cas-

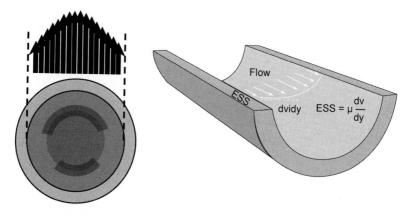

FIGURE 2–11. Pathogenic role of mechanical forces. Oscillatory shear or endothelial shear stress (ESS) is proportional to the product of blood viscosity (μ) and spatial gradient of blood velocity at the wall (dv/dy) (59).

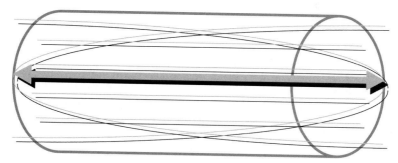

FIGURE 2–12. Oscillatory shear stress.

cade, and a procoagulation process. A local increase in pressure stretch can also contribute to plaque rupture.

Acute hemodynamic fluctuations also contribute to endothelial dysfunction because of loss of normal reparative mechanisms (65). In normal vessels, acute injury is overcome quickly by repair mechanisms in the media and endothelium; in abnormal vessels, however, acute injury cannot be fully repaired and adds to vascular pathology.

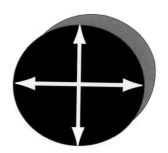

FIGURE 2–13. Elevated stretch.

Endothelial cells release various relaxing and constricting factors to maintain normal vascular tone (Figure 2–14). The impact that acute, hemodynamic fluctuations may have on endothelial function and potential destabilization of vulnerable plaque

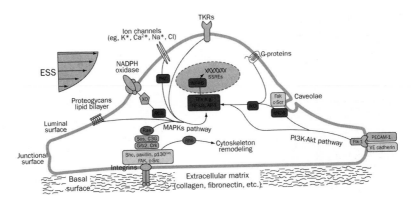

FIGURE 2–14. Endothelial mechanoreceptors sense changes in shear stress. AP-1 = activator protein-1; eNOS = endothelial nitric oxide synthase; ESS = endothelial shear stress; FAK = focal adhesion kinase; MAPKs = mitogen-activated protein kinases; NADPH = nicotinamide adenine dinucleotide phosphate; NO = nitric oxide; NOS = nitric oxide synthase; PECAM-1 = platelet endothelial cell adhesion molecule-1; PKC = protein kinase C; ROS = reactive oxygen species; SSREs = shear stress responsive elements; TFs = transcription factors; TKRs = tyrosine kinase receptors; XO = xanthine oxidase (59).

has been studied. An essential and common consequence of endothelial dysfunction is reduced endothelial nitric oxide synthase and the loss of a protective effect from nitric oxide with increased reactive oxygen species caused by decreased scavenging (66).

It has been postulated that changes in strain and shear stress on the endothelial wall in the setting of endothelial plaque may contribute to inflammation and the destabilization of vulnerable plaque (59–61, 67, 68). This procoagulation effect may be further enhanced by low and oscillatory shear stress forces that are exacerbated in noncompliant arteries (Figure 2–15). Importantly, the pulsatile stress that conduit vessels are exposed to may cause the elastic elements in the vessel wall to break down, thereby producing further vessel dilation and stiffening. As the vessel dilates, the stress on the wall worsens. Remodeling changes lead to vessel-wall medial necrosis, stiffening, increased vascular resistance, and reduced organ perfusion. Whereas the effects of laminar shear stress in normal vessels are atheroprotective, the effects of oscillatory and low shear stress promote atherosclerosis and plaque rupture (59, 61, 68).

BP MEASUREMENTS

The Closer You Look, the More You See

To appropriately manage hypertension and minimize the likelihood of adverse events requires accurate measurement of BP and an understand-

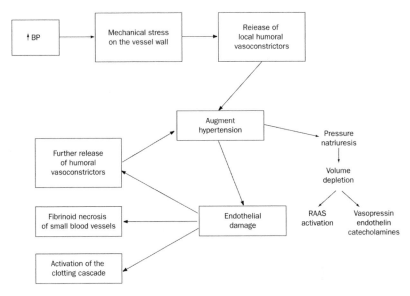

FIGURE 2–15. Pathophysiology of acute hypertensive syndromes. BP = blood pressure; RAAS = renin–angiotensin–aldosterone system.

ing of what is actually being measured. Although there are traditionally accepted methods for determining BP, recent evidence challenges these methods for BP evaluation, particularly for some of the components of the determination that affect management. For example, MAP is an integrated, static signal determined by multiplying cardiac output by systemic vascular resistance, whereas PP is a dynamic signal principally determined by the interaction of cardiac contractility and aortic impedance, which is reflective of large conduit artery compliance. The methods used to measure or calculate these parameters influence the accuracy.

Noninvasive BP measurements are typically obtained by placing the BP cuff over the brachial artery and providing direct and/or derived measurements of SBP, DPB, and MAP. SBP is dependent on stroke volume, rate of systolic ejection, arterial distensibility, and wave reflections. DBP is dependent on intravascular volume, aortic compliance, and pulse wave velocity. Moreover, it is an important determinant of augmentation index and pulse wave velocity. PP is dependent on ventricular ejection, viscoelastic properties of large arteries, and wave reflection. The determinants of MAP include ventricular ejection and SVR. The peripheral pressure indices, although associated with changes in cardiovascular outcome, are not necessarily the same marker of cardiovascular structure as are the central aortic pressure indices. Central aortic pressure parameters, in addition to being determined by cardiac output and SVR, are also

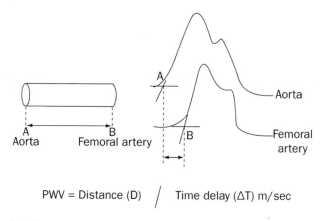

PWV = Distance (D) / Time delay (ΔT) m/sec

FIGURE 2–16. Determination of pulse wave velocity (PWV).

Simultaneous Recordings of the 2 Waves

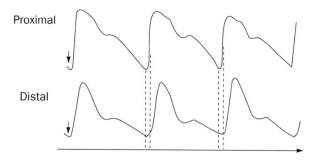

FIGURE 2–17. Calculating the pulse wave velocity from simultaneous recordings of proximal and distal wave forms.

dependent on arterial wall stiffness and pressure wave reflections (50). These latter parameters (particularly stiffness) can be isolated by measuring vascular reactivity (69–71), systolic augmentation (72–74), pulse wave velocity (72, 75) (Figures 2–16, 2–17, and 2–18), and other mechanical and bioassay parameters of clinical endothelial function (76, 77), which may be more sensitive markers for predicting adverse outcomes than is peripheral or brachial BP monitoring (Figure 2–19) (51).

The differentiation between central and peripheral BP has significant impact on both clinical management and outcomes after cardiac surgery. Unfortunately, in many clinical situations the difference between the measurement of BP centrally and peripherally has been virtually

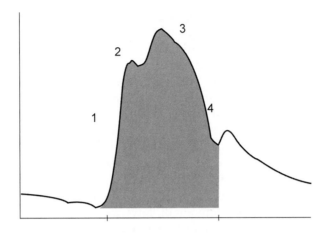

1 = systolic upstroke; 2 = systolic peak;
3 = systolic decline; 4 = dicrotic notch.
(Williams 2006)

FIGURE 2–18. Pulse wave contour. 1 = systolic upstroke; 2 = systolic peak; 3 = systolic decline; 4 = dicrotic notch.

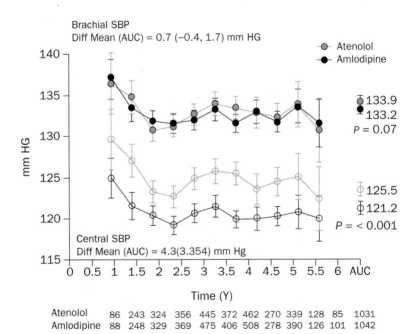

	86	243	324	356	445	372	462	270	339	128	85	1031
Atenolol												
Amlodipine	88	248	329	369	475	406	508	278	390	126	101	1042

FIGURE 2–19. Brachial and central systolic blood pressure (SBP) with atenolol versus amlodipine. AUC = area under the curve (78).

ignored. This finding is especially troubling given the growing numbers of elderly and diabetic patients who come for surgery for whom these discrepancies may have significance.

One study that helped clarify this issue is the Conduit Artery Function Evaluation (CAFE) study. The study evaluated more than 2000 patients as part of a subanalysis of the Anglo-Scandinavian Cardiac Outcomes Trial (ASCOT) (78). The CAFE study showed clearly that a pharmacological regimen (angiotensin-converting enzyme inhibition plus a calcium antagonist) that preferentially decreased central vascular pressures (and presumably central vascular stiffness) resulted in lower long-term cardiovascular event rates compared with a regimen (beta-blockers and diuretics) that did not decrease central pressures. It was demonstrated that different BP-lowering regimens, although causing equivalent peripheral reduction in BP, nonetheless showed different central BP-lowering effects (78). As a result, for many patients with severe vascular disease and hypertension, measurement of central arterial pressure may provide a more important assessment of hemodynamics than will peripherally measured BP (Figure 2–19).

SCIENCE TO STRATEGY

Do Current Behaviors and Options Meet Clinical Needs?

Often, physicians prefer to monitor BP rather than choose to control it. This therapeutic inertia is a behavior that may be a result of our lack of understanding or appreciation of optimal target BP levels, which help to avoid poor outcomes or a lack of acknowledgment of the consequences of alterations in BP. In addition, many clinicians are as concerned about "overtreating" and causing acute changes in BP, in either direction, do may delay interventions to "confirm" that the changes are real. This response is particularly true in the operating room, where rapid changes may be transient and, in some cases, require no intervention.

Furthermore, there are remarkably few data that help define the target BP for patients with acute hypertension (3, 79) in the setting of stroke, heart failure, dialysis, or surgery. In most cases, clinicians are inclined to avoid "hypotension," rather than to achieve specific therapeutic BP targets. This approach is based on a number of factors, not the least of which is the inability to define for an individual patient the BP range in which autoregulation is maintained. In addition, many of the pharmacologic options do not allow careful titration and risk rapid reductions in BP with significant potential consequences. For example, a review of patients treated for acute hypertensive emergencies at a university hospital revealed that 57% of patients meeting study criteria were excessively treated during the acute treatment period (80). The excessive reduction in MAP led to adverse outcomes (myocardial infarction or ischemic stroke) in 4% of the patients after initiation of overtreatment.

The significant inadequacy in the management of patients with acute hypertension has recently been highlighted (18, 48). As many as 25% of patients present to emergency departments with acute hypertension (90% with preexisting hypertension, 25% as a result of medication noncompliance, 27% with a history of prior hospitalization for acute hypertension) with symptoms such as chest pain, shortness of breath, and symptoms of stroke, with almost one quarter having a stroke at the time of presentation. The median time to achieve a SBP <160 mm Hg was 4 hours, with a high rate of overshoot (4% developing hypotension, necessitating intervention; 6.2% in subarachnoid hemorrhage patients) (81). In addition, 60% of patients had a bounce-back SBP >180 mm Hg after initial control (48). In another survey of current treatment patterns for acute hypertension (82), physicians reported an average of 4.9 patients per month being admitted to the intensive care unit with a hypertensive emergency. When reporting what drove their treatment decisions, 27% reported their institution's practice guidelines for hypertensive emergency in acute hemorrhagic stroke patients, and 10% reported the same for nonstroke patients. Their comments indicate that the algorithms for treatment of acute hypertension are either out of date or not supported by the literature. The researchers concluded that a national guideline for the pharmacotherapy of acute hypertension was needed (82).

Evidence now suggests that control of the BP rather than the specific antihypertension treatment leads to improved outcomes and mitigates risk (83, 84). A number of acute unstable BP syndromes such as ischemic and hemorrhagic stroke, subarachnoid hemorrhage, malignant hypertension associated with dialysis, dissecting aortic disease, perioperative hypertension, and others have specific and sometimes narrow BP therapeutic windows that may require a rapid-acting and easily titratable therapeutic agent with a rapid offset to optimally maintain the BP within this narrow bandwidth. Unfortunately there is no standard cocktail for every patient. Each patient and each clinical situation must be ideally managed to maintain the BP within this zone of tolerance (bandwidth) when acute BP management is needed. For many patients, this range is difficult to define, for many of the reasons mentioned above. Nonetheless, for each patient it is critical to attempt to determine "How high is too high?" and "How low can you go?" and define the "sweet spot" of tolerance to optimal BP conditions (or intolerance to suboptimal conditions, particularly in the cardiac surgical patient population in whom vascular disease and hypertension are common problems (83, 84).

The definition of hypertension and hypotension is also not standardized. In a literature review (85), a cohort of >15,000 patients was assessed for a definition of intraoperative hypotension. It was concluded that there is no widely accepted definition, and, as importantly, outcome associations are also variable. The data support the impression of most clinicians that a number of measures are important. Absolute BP values, percent change from baseline BP, duration of abnormal pressure, and BP index itself (SBP, MAP) all have been reported to be associated with undesirable outcomes (85), indicating that definitions for BP standards are still impossible to define. The same issues must be considered when evaluating hypertension.

HYPERTENSION AND CARDIOVASCULAR SURGERY

A Unique Environment with Unique Considerations

The need to actively manage high BP during cardiovascular surgery is a frequent occurrence (in as many as 88% of all cases) (49). Perhaps this need reflects the fact that alterations in BP during surgery are common and result from a number of interventions or underlying clinical problems, including ischemia, manipulations of the vasculature, including clamping and unclamping of the great vessels, alterations in BP during CPB, and changes in blood flow related to nonpulsatile CPB, acute hemorrhage, and fluid shifts. The same concerns exist in the postoperative period, when requirements for weaning from mechanical ventilation and analgesia are additional stresses that may compromise BP control. In addition, it is well recognized that perioperative hypertension increases myocardial oxygen consumption and LV end-diastolic pressure and contributes to subendocardial hypoperfusion and myocardial ischemia (86–88). It also increases the risk of stroke, neurocognitive dysfunction, and renal dysfunction and contributes to surgical bleeding from anastomotic sites (44, 89, 90). Finally, poorly controlled BP during surgery can trigger hyperinflammatory and procoagulation conditions (89) including platelet activation (91), which may compromise microvascular blood flow.

The assessment, characterization, and management of hypertension in the setting of cardiovascular surgery is confounded by acute mechanical and physiologic perturbation involving aortic occlusive clamps, excessive release of catecholamine, reperfusion injury, humoral and cellular inflammatory response, and platelet activation, which can compromise microvascular blood flow (89, 92–94). The severity of atherosclerosis—an important predictor of risk of stroke, myocardial infarction, and postoperative renal dysfunction—has been shown to be related to

BP as well (95–97). Acute circulatory dysfunction is a rapid change in BP, distinct from low-flow to no-flow conditions (i.e., shock), that can damage blood vessels and result in a procoagulation condition, inflammation, and leaking of fluid or blood into tissues. The heart, therefore, may not be able to maintain adequate circulation of blood, and irreversible organ damage may occur within the central nervous system, heart, vasculature, and kidneys.

Few data have reported or defined the morbidity associated with BP abnormality during CPB. In a recent study of 1395 patients who underwent CPB, using multivariate analysis applied to recorded intraoperative BP, Ganushchak and colleagues (98) reported an increased risk of postoperative neurologic complications as a result of large fluctuations in BP parameters. In a study by Fleischer (99), patients with normal preoperative renal function developed acute renal failure associated with longer CPB times and perfusion pressures <60 mm Hg.

ARTERIAL STIFFNESS AND SURGERY

The Plot Thickens

Patients with long-standing hypertension have stiff vessels that complicate management strategies. In the elderly population with PP hypertension, special attention should be paid to managing hemodynamics, because the constant pulsatile stress that conduit vessels are exposed to in this subset of patients may cause the elastic elements of the vessel wall to break down. These abnormal anatomic, chronic vascular changes with superimposed mechanical or local humoral acutely induced changes on arterial pathophysiology may cause increased vulnerability of these patients when they experience the surgical and anesthetic physiologic perturbations. The hemodynamic abnormality that occurs during surgery may further contribute to endothelial dysfunction, as well as to an increase in pulsatile load on these stiff vessels. These nondistensible vessels lose the buffering capacity that is inherent in the normal compliant aorta and minimizes the harmful acute pressure changes associated with ventricular ejection throughout the cardiac cycle. Conditions that contribute or predispose individuals to conduit artery stiffness include advanced age (100), hypertension (101), glucose intolerance (102), menopause (103), and CAD (104)—all common to patients who require cardiac surgery with CPB. In addition, pulsatile stress in central arteries may contribute to plaque rupture by a mechanical fatiguing effect. Perhaps nowhere are the assessment, characterization, and management of hypertension, therefore, more important than in the setting of cardiac or major vascular surgery, when acute

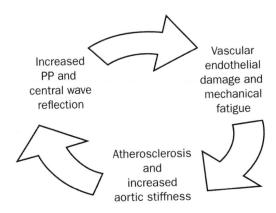

FIGURE 2–20.
Relationship between
pulse pressure (PP) and
atherosclerosis (105).

and stressful physiologic perturbations occur including excessive release of catecholamine, reperfusion injury, humoral and cellular inflammatory response, and platelet activation, with resultant reductions in microvascular blood flow (Figure 2–20).

CLINICAL MANAGEMENT STRATEGIES

Defining goals for BP control depends on a number of specific patient factors such as the presence of preexisting hypertensive disease, the specific acute-care situation that is being managed, and the vulnerable end organ(s). Specific BP goals need to be defined for each patient in each instance, recognizing the situation (type of surgery, CHF, stroke, etc.), the type of hypertension (i.e., phenotype: DBP, SBP, MAP, PP), and the condition (treatment effectiveness).

There is compelling evidence that patients with severe DBP elevations are more prone to perioperative ischemia, arrhythmia, and cardiovascular lability but less clear evidence that deferring anesthesia and surgery for these patients reduces perioperative risk. In the early 1970s, a series of studies by Prys-Roberts and colleagues on the interaction between hypertension and anesthesia were published. In the first of these studies (41), 29 patients undergoing elective surgery were evaluated. Although 7 patients were considered to have normal BP at the time of the study, all would qualify as hypertensive today. The remaining patients were treated or untreated hypertensive. The authors reported that the untreated hypertensive patients had a greater decrease in BP at induction and were more prone to intraoperative ischemia, arrhythmia, and hemodynamic lability. In the late 1970s and early 1980s, Goldman and colleagues (106) examined the risk of admission BP and perioperative risk and created the Goldman Risk Index. In a landmark study conducted from 1975 through 1976 (107), 617 patients were divided into 5 groups: 1) normotensive patients; 2) patients treated with diuretics; 3) controlled/treated hypertensive patients; 4) uncontrolled/treated hypertensive patients; and 5) untreated hypertensive patients. No difference was found between hypertensive patients and the remaining groups. However, the study lacked the power to confirm or refute an association; only 5 patients had a DBP >111 mm Hg.

In the early 1990s, Charlson and colleagues (44) examined the risk of intraoperative BP fluctuation and wide variation in BP over time. They reported that, among high-risk hypertensive patients undergoing elective surgery, those with a decrease in MAP >20 mm Hg for more than 1 hour and those with a decrease in MAP >20 mm Hg for less than 1 hour and an increase in MAP >20 mm Hg for more than 15 minutes had the greatest risk of adverse outcomes. Others, including Gold and colleagues (45), reported on BP management during specific times of the operation, including management of MAP during CPB and its association with renal and cerebral function outcomes.

Absolute DBP has traditionally served as the standard for BP management and has been a cornerstone for the evaluation of perioperative cardiovascular clinical risk. Both the sixth report of the Joint National Committee on Prevention, Detection, Evaluation, and Treatment of High Blood Pressure (JNC VI) (36) and the American College of Cardiology/çAmerican Heart Association guidelines (22) recommend a delay of surgery when preoperative DBP exceeds 110 mm Hg.

As additional data have become available, much has been learned about hypertensive physiology (the most appropriate BP parameter to follow) and associated morbidity, mortality, and therapy. PP has been identified as a better predictor of stroke than SBP or DBP in both normotensive and hypertensive individuals (108). Franklin and colleagues (108) reported that increases in PP at a fixed SBP are associated with a much greater risk of ischemic outcomes than increases in SBP at a fixed PP. Aggressive attempts to treat systolic hypertension or "normalize BP" may result in profound and clinically significant diastolic hypotension and coronary hypoperfusion. The potential for hypoperfusion is especially true in patients with significant atherosclerotic disease and stiffened arteries manifested as a wide PP (e.g., ≥80 mm Hg). Somes and colleagues (109) found that in treating ISH, lowering DBP as few as 5 mm Hg significantly increases the risk of coronary heart disease and stroke. Glynn and colleagues (110) reported that the death rate is highest in hypertensive individuals with an SBP ≥160 mm Hg and a DBP <70 mm Hg—a PP value >90 mm Hg. Lee and colleagues (111) demonstrated that markers of vascular thrombosis (plasma viscosity, fibrinogen levels, von Willebrand factor, flow-mediated dilatation, D-dimer, and platelet activation) were significantly elevated in patients with a PP >50 mm Hg compared with those without a high PP. It is possible that the combination of endothelial injury (e.g., surgical manipulation, inflammatory response associated with CPB) and a wide PP provide a trigger for the increased postoperative vascular complications observed in patients with increased PP.

Recently, the focus on BP management and risk assessment has supported the "sweet spot" concept mentioned previously. Gottesman and colleagues (46) reported that a drop in MAP of ≥27 mm Hg from baseline was associated with cerebral dysfunction. Aronson and colleagues (29), in a 2002 multicenter study of patients undergoing cardiac surgery, demonstrated that the presence of ISH was associated with a 30% increase in adverse cardiovascular events compared with normotensive patients. ISH, particularly in individuals older than 50 years, is much more prevalent than diastolic hypertension and is associated with a greater risk of both fatal and nonfatal stroke and coronary heart disease (112). In another study by Aronson and colleagues (30), PP was found to be associated with increased risk of renal dysfunction outcomes in patients undergoing cardiac surgery. These observations also were reported for cerebral dysfunction outcomes, including stroke and cardiac adverse events, in a similar group of patients (40). Fontes and colleagues (31) showed that PP was independently associated with an increased risk of developing a postoperative cerebral event, such that for every 10-mm Hg increment in PP (above a threshold of 40 mm Hg), the odds of experiencing a cerebral event increased by 12% (adjusted OR, 1.12; 95% CI, 1.002–1.28; $P = .026$). The incidence of a cerebral event and/or death from neurologic complications nearly doubled for patients with PP >80 mm Hg versus ≤80 mm Hg (5.5% vs. 2.8%; $P = .004$) (31).

Many studies have attempted to define treatment strategies to manage hypertension generally as well as in selected surgical patient populations. The Evaluation of Clevidipine in the Perioperative Treatment of Hypertension Assessing Safety Events (ECLIPSE) trial was performed to compare the safety and efficacy of clevidipine (CLV) with nitroglycerin (NTG), sodium nitroprusside (SNP), and nicardipine (NIC) in the treatment of perioperative acute hypertension. In the ECLIPSE trial, the largest randomized perioperative hypertension management trial (>1500 patients undergoing cardiac surgery), an overall treatment-independent evaluation of BP control to 30-day mortality was also conducted (Figure 2–21). BP control was assessed by area under the curve (AUC) analysis (Tables 10–5, 10–6, and 10–7). AUC was defined as the summation of the integrated SBP-time curve excursions (AUC_{SBP-D}), capturing the magnitude (mm Hg) times duration (minutes) of BP outside the predefined ranges (65–135 mm Hg intraoperatively [from chest incision through

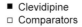

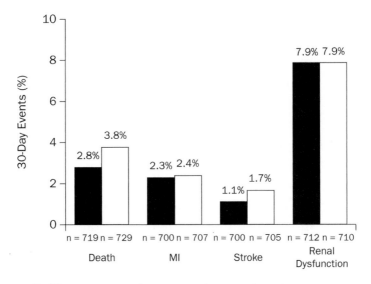

FIGURE 2–21. Summary of primary end point, Clinical Events Committee–adjudicated 30-day events (safety population) from the Evaluation of Clevidipine in the Perioperative Treatment of Hypertension Assessing Safety Events (ECLIPSE) trial. MI = myocardial infarction (113).

chest closure] and 75–145 mm Hg pre- and postoperatively). AUC was calculated based on BP recorded from the initiation of study drug infusion through either the permanent removal of the arterial line or 24 hours after drug initiation, whichever occurred first. AUC was normalized per hour and expressed as mm Hg × min/h. The total area of the SBP-time curve outside (either above or below) the predefined SBP ranges (AUC_{SBP-D}) was calculated, as well as by treatment group as the SBP range was narrowed by incrementally increasing the lower SBP limit by 10, 20, and 30 mm Hg (Figures 2–22, 2–23, and 2–24).

Results from the ECLIPSE trial demonstrated the safety of CLV (Figure 2–21). As importantly, the study demonstrated that SNP was associated with longer time periods outside of the predefined SBP range (Figure 2–22). The SNP group also exhibited a tendency toward increased mortality. This result may have a number of explanations, but could involve BP excursions outside the autoregulatory range. As a result, SNP, which has been the mainstay of treatment for hypertension, should be administered with caution.

TABLE 2–5. ECLIPSE: Predictors of 30-day mortality

	P value	OR	95% CI
Surgery duration (h)	<.0001	1.517	1.240–1.856
Age (y)	.0003	1.070	1.031–1.110
Pre-op creatinine ≥1.2 mg/dL	.0031	2.670	1.392–5.122
AUC (area outside the range)	.0069	1.003	1.001–1.004
Additional surgical procedures	.0089	2.409	1.246–4.655
Pre-op Hgb (g/dL)	.0135	0.824	0.707–0.961
Pre-op SBP >160 or DBP >105	.0228	2.386	1.147–4.963
History of COPD	.0228	2.326	1.125–4.812
History of recent MI (<6 mo prior)	.0312	2.197	1.073–4.497

From (52).
COPD = chronic obstructive pulmonary disease.

TABLE 2–6. ECLIPSE: Multiple logistic regression analysis results—predictors of 30-day mortality

Amount of average BP excursions over 60 minutes	OR	95% CI
1 mm Hg/min	1.20	1.06–1.27
2 mm Hg/min	1.43	1.13–1.61
3 mm Hg/min	1.71	1.20–2.05
4 mm Hg/min	2.05	1.27–2.61
5 mm Hg/min	2.46	1.35–3.31

From (52).
AUC for excursions outside SBP range of 85–145 mm Hg pre- and postoperatively and 75–135 mm Hg intraoperatively.

TABLE 2–7. ECLIPSE: BP control predicts 30-day renal dysfunction outcome

Variables	P value	OR	95% CI
Preop serum creatinine ≥1.2 mg/dL	<.0001	5.466	3.506–8.521
Preop Hgb (g/dL)	<.0001	0.785	0.699–0.881
BMI	.0074	1.049	1.013–1.087
Surgery duration (h)	.0077	1.292	1.070–1.559
Age (y)	.0086	1.033	1.008–1.059
BP (4th quartile of AUC)	.0126	1.785	1.132–2.815
Race (African-American)	.0151	2.164	1.161–4.035
Primary CABG + valve	.0165	1.944	1.129–3.348

BMI = body mass index; CABG = coronary artery bypass graft; Hgb = hemoglobin.
Adapted from (114).

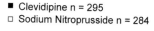

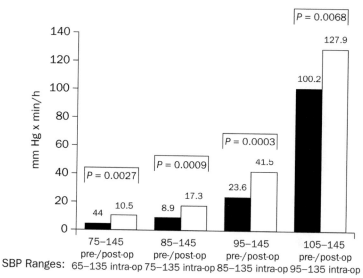

FIGURE 2–22. Perioperative BP control: clevidipine versus sodium nitroprusside (113).

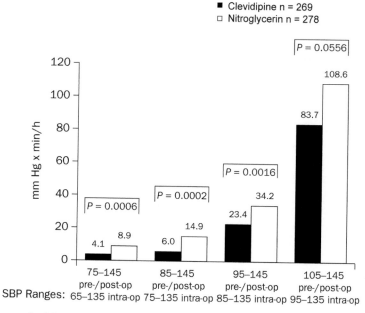

FIGURE 2–23. Perioperative BP control: clevidipine versus nitroglycerin (113).

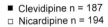

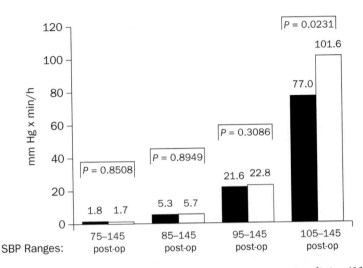

FIGURE 2–24. Postoperative BP control: clevidipine versus nicardipine (113).

Based on data in other clinical settings as well as findings from studies that specifically address the cardiac surgical patient population, a number of approaches to the management of hypertension have been identified. For example, cardiac surgery patients requiring acute BP management before incision have a slightly increased risk of death, and the outcome is significantly influenced by treatment. In a subset analysis of the ECLIPSE trial (83), 282 patients who required treatment for BP control prior to incision were evaluated (Table 2–8). The overall incidence of 30-day mortality was 5%, with a significant difference between treatment groups. The initiation of BP control with SNP or NTG was associated with an increased risk of 30-day mortality (11/145, 8%) compared with CLV (3/137, 2%; $P = .037$). Other factors that increased the risk of 30-day mortality were equal between groups (Table 2–8) (83).

A total of 342 patients from the ECLIPSE trial (Table 2–9) were evaluated to determine if maintaining a defined SBP range during cardiac valve surgery predicted 30-day mortality (115). All patients were treated with intravenous antihypertensive agents (61% operative setting, 39% postoperative setting). BP excursions outside the SBP range of 75–145 mm Hg predicted 30-day mortality, which was more significant as the SBP range was narrowed (105–145 mm Hg) (115).

Continuous BP recordings in patients undergoing cardiac surgery at Duke University (Figure 2–25) showed that the degree and amount

Table 2–8. ECLIPSE: Predictors of 30-day mortality based on BP control prior to incision

	P value	OR	95% CI
Treatment,* SNP/NTG vs. CLV	.0150	7.6	1.5–38.4
Additional procedure	.0071	5.8	1.6–21.2
Preop creatinine >1.2 mg/dL	.0158	4.9	1.3–17.8

From (83).
*Pre-incision treatment for acute hypertension.

TABLE 2–9. ECLIPSE: Predictors of 30-day mortality based on SBP treatment during valve surgery

Variable	P value	OR	95% CI
Screening SBP (mm Hg)	.0012	1.038	1.015–1.061
Preoperative hemoglobin (g/dL)	.0270	0.715	0.531–0.963
AUC (mm Hg × min/h)	.0272	1.004	1.000–1.008

From (115).

of time that BP outside a predefined range is predictive of 30-day mortality (84). This study highlighted the need for defining BP control targets. Data from 7808 consecutive patients undergoing surgical coronary revascularization at Duke between January 1, 1996 and December 31, 2005 were evaluated. SBP instability was assessed by the integrated summation of cumulative BP excursions (defined as magnitude × duration) expressed as AUC (outside SBP range of >135 or <95 mm Hg), similar to the analysis performed for BP control in the ECLIPSE trial. In addition, the number of excursions above and below the predetermined pressure threshold (SBP >135 or <95 mm Hg), the magnitude of the excursion, and the cumulative and mean duration of the excursion (minutes) above and below the threshold, were independently examined. It was observed that the mean duration of intraoperative BP excursions outside the SBP range of 140–100 mm Hg during cardiac surgery was the most predictive BP control variable associated with 30-day mortality. As a result, the careful control of BP within a relatively narrow range should be the goal of perioperative therapy. No single drug or combination of drugs has been demonstrated to be superior to any other pharmacologic regimen. The BP end point seems to be important without regard to how it is achieved.

CONCLUSION

For nearly a century, careful management of arterial BP has been a mainstay of perioperative treatment for patients with a history of hyperten-

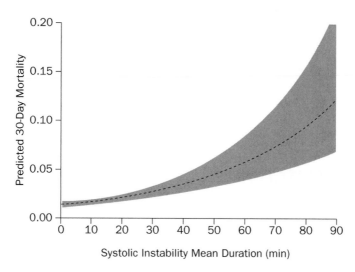

FIGURE 2–25. Duration of blood pressure lability and risk of 30-day mortality (84).

sion. In addition, patients with preoperative poorly controlled or uncontrolled BP have had elective surgery delayed to optimize BP management prior to induction of anesthesia. In surgical patients with preexisting hypertension, acute perioperative BP control may be more challenging, as the therapeutic window of acceptable pressure is both narrowed and shifted to the right. Challenging BP control is particularly true in the elderly hypertensive population requiring surgery and anesthetic management with changes in normal autoregulatory physiology. Despite these approaches to the hypertensive patient and the importance given to closely monitoring BP during and after surgery, little is known about perioperative outcomes associated with abnormal BP targets.

Perioperative hypertension is characterized by acute physiologic perturbation involving the excessive release of catecholamine, reperfusion injury, humoral and cellular inflammatory response, and platelet activation, which can compromise microvascular blood flow. It increases myocardial oxygen consumption and LV end-diastolic pressure, and contributes to subendocardial hypoperfusion and myocardial ischemia. In addition, perioperative hypertension increases the risk of stroke and neurocognitive and renal dysfunction, and contributes to surgical bleeding and anastomotic disruption.

There is now evidence to suggest that poor BP control is a strong predictor of adverse postoperative outcomes in cardiovascular patients. Targeted BP control mitigates this risk. There is much to be learned about integrating these observations into management strategies for individual patients in specific situations. Perhaps nowhere is the assessment, characterization, and management of hypertension more common and more important than during the perioperative period, particularly for the cardiac surgical patient. Clearly the acute and stressful physiologic perturbations including the excessive release of catecholamine, reperfusion injury, humoral and cellular inflammatory response, and platelet activation can compromise microvascular blood flow—a period susceptible to acute hypertension syndrome. The key to management is close attention to these changes, monitors that allow appropriate assessment of BP, a determination of the "sweet spot" for an individual patient, and treatment strategies to maintain the BP within this narrow range. This approach will optimize the perioperative care and reduce the likelihood of an adverse postoperative outcome.

References

1. Ezzati M, Oza S, Danaei G, Murray CJ: Trends and cardiovascular mortality effects of state-level blood pressure and uncontrolled hypertension in the United States. Circulation 2008; 117:905–14
2. Wang TJ, Vasan RS: Epidemiology of uncontrolled hypertension in the United States. Circulation 2005; 112:1651–62
3. Chobanian AV, Bakris GL, Black HR, et al.: The Seventh Report of the Joint National Committee on Prevention, Detection, Evaluation, and Treatment of High Blood Pressure: the JNC 7 report. JAMA 2003; 289:2560–72
4. Fields LE, Burt VL, Cutler JA, Hughes J, Roccella EJ, Sorlie P: The burden of adult hypertension in the United States, 1999 to 2000: a rising tide. Hypertension 2004; 44:398–404
5. National Institutes of Health/National Heart, Lung, and Blood Institute (NIH/NHLBI). Fact Book, Fiscal Year 2007. Washington, DC, NIH/NHLBI, 2008
6. Hajjar I, Kotchen TA: Trends in prevalence, awareness, treatment, and control of hypertension in the United States, 1988–2000. JAMA 2003; 290:199–206
7. Lloyd-Jones D, Adams R, Carnethon M, et al.: Heart disease and stroke statistics—2009 update: a report from the American Heart Association Statistics Committee and Stroke Statistics Subcommittee. Circulation 2009; 119:e21–e181
8. Vasan RS, Beiser A, Seshadri S, et al.: Residual lifetime risk for developing hypertension in middle-aged women and men: the Framingham Heart Study. JAMA 2002; 287:1003–10
9. National Institute on Aging. US Department of Commerce, Economics and Statistics Administration, Bureau of the Census. Aging in

the Americas Into the XXI Century. Washington, DC Pan American Health Organization/World Health Organization, 2009

10. Kearney PM, Whelton M, Reynolds K, Muntner P, Whelton PK, He J: Global burden of hypertension: analysis of worldwide data. Lancet 2005; 365:217–23

11. World Health Organization. Global burden of disease 2004. Part 2: causes of death. Available at: http://www.who.int/healthinfo/global_burden_disease/GBD_report_2004update_part2.pdf. Accessed January 22, 2009

12. Yusuf S, Mehta SR, Chrolavicius S, et al.; Fifth Organization to Assess Strategies in Acute Ischemic Syndromes Investigators. Comparison of fondaparinux and enoxaparin in acute coronary syndromes. N Engl J Med 2006; 354:1464–76

13. Global Use of Strategies to Open Occluded Coronary Arteries (GUSTO) IIb Investigators. A comparison of recombinant hirudin with heparin for the treatment of acute coronary syndromes. N Engl J Med 1996; 335:775–82

14. Fox KA, Steg PG, Eagle KA, et al.: Decline in rates of death and heart failure in acute coronary syndromes, 1999–2006. JAMA 2007; 297:1892–900

15. O'Connor CM, Stough WG, Gallup DS, Hasselblad V, Gheorghiade M: Demographics, clinical characteristics, and outcomes of patients hospitalized for decompensated heart failure: observations from the IMPACT-HF registry. J Card Fail 2005; 11:200–5

16. Menzin J, Wygant G, Hauch O, Jackel J, Friedman M: One-year costs of ischemic heart disease among patients with acute coronary syndromes: findings from a multi-employer claims database. Curr Med Res Opin 2008; 24:461–8

17. Kleinschmidt K, Granger C, Peacock F, et al.; STAT Investigators. Acute severe hypertension—diverse management and high morbidity and mortality: results from STAT. Presented at: the Society of Critical Care Medicine's 37th Critical Care Congress; February 2–6, 2008, Honolulu, HI

18. Centers for Disease Control Diabetes Cost-effectiveness Group. Cost-effectiveness of intensive glycemic control, intensified hypertension control, and serum cholesterol level reduction for type 2 diabetes. JAMA 2002; 287:2542–51

19. Weiser TG, Regenbogen SE, Thompson KD, et al.: An estimation of the global volume of surgery: a modelling strategy based on available data. Lancet 2008; 372:139–44

20. Casadei B, Abuzeid H: Is there a strong rationale for deferring elective surgery in patients with poorly controlled hypertension? J Hypertens 2005; 23:19–22

21. Fischer UM, Weissenberger WK, Warters RD, Geissler HJ, Allen SJ, Mehlhorn U: Impact of cardiopulmonary bypass management on postcardiac surgery renal function. Perfusion 2002; 17:401–6
22. Eagle KA, Berger PB, Calkins H, et al.: ACC/AHA guideline update for perioperative cardiovascular evaluation for noncardiac surgery—executive summary: a report of the American College of Cardiology/American Heart Association Task Force on Practice Guidelines (Committee to Update the 1996 Guidelines on Perioperative Cardiovascular Evaluation for Noncardiac Surgery). J Am Coll Cardiol 2002; 39:542–53
23. Erdogan D, Yildirim I, Ciftci O, et al.: Effects of normal blood pressure, prehypertension, and hypertension on coronary microvascular function. Circulation 2007; 115:593–9
24. Qureshi AI, Suri MF, Kirmani JF, Divani AA, Mohammad Y: Is prehypertension a risk factor for cardiovascular diseases? Stroke 2005; 36:1859–63
25. Lewington S, Clarke R, Qizilbash N, Peto R, Collins R: Age-specific relevance of usual blood pressure to vascular mortality: a meta-analysis of individual data for one million adults in 61 prospective studies. Lancet 2002; 360:1903–13
26. Turnbull F, Neal B, Algert C, Chalmers J, Woodward M, MacMahon S; Blood Pressure Lowering Treatment Trialists' Collaboration: Effects of different blood-pressure-lowering regimens on major cardiovascular events: results of prospectively-designed overviews of randomised trials. Lancet 2003; 362:1527–35
27. Staessen JA, Li Y, Thijs L, Wang JG: Blood pressure reduction and cardiovascular prevention: an update including the 2003–2004 secondary prevention trials. Hypertens Res 2005; 28:385–407
28. Stewart S, MacIntyre K, Capewell S, McMurray JJ: Heart failure and the aging population: an increasing burden in the 21st century? Heart 2003; 89:49–53
29. Aronson S, Boisvert D, Lapp W: Isolated systolic hypertension is associated with adverse outcomes from coronary artery bypass grafting surgery. Anesth Analg 2002; 94:1079–84
30. Aronson S, Fontes ML, Miao Y, Mangano DT: Risk index for perioperative renal dysfunction/failure: critical dependence on pulse pressure hypertension. Circulation 2007; 115:733–42
31. Fontes ML, Aronson S, Mathew JP, et al.: Pulse pressure and risk of adverse outcome in coronary bypass surgery. Anesth Analg 2008; 107:1122–9
32. Lawes CM, Bennett DA, Feigin VL, Rodgers A: Blood pressure and stroke: an overview of published reviews. Stroke 2004; 35:1024–33

33. Roach GW, Kanchuger M, Mangano CM, et al.; Multicenter Study of Perioperative Ischemia Research Group and the Ischemia Research and Education Foundation Investigators. Adverse cerebral outcomes after coronary bypass surgery. N Engl J Med 1996; 335:1857–63

34. Waldstein SR, Rice SC, Thayer JF, Najjar SS, Scuteri A, Zonderman AB: Pulse pressure and pulse wave velocity are related to cognitive decline in the Baltimore Longitudinal Study of Aging. Hypertension 2008; 51:99–104

35. Benetos A, Laurent S, Asmar RG, Lacolley P: Large artery stiffness in hypertension. J Hypertens 1997; 15(Suppl):S89–S97

36. Joint National Committee on Prevention, Detection, Evaluation, and Treatment of High Blood Pressure. The sixth report of the Joint National Committee on Prevention, Detection, Evaluation, and Treatment of High Blood Pressure. Arch Intern Med 1997; 157: 2413–46

37. Systolic Hypertension in the Elderly Program (SHEP) Cooperative Research Group. Prevention of stroke by antihypertensive drug treatment in older persons with isolated systolic hypertension. Final results of the Systolic Hypertension in the Elderly Program. JAMA 1991; 265:3255–64

38. Friday G, Alter M, Lai SM: Control of hypertension and risk of stroke recurrence. Stroke 2002; 33:2652–7

39. Reich DL, Bennett-Guerrero E, Bodian CA, Hossain S, Winfree W, Krol M: Intraoperative tachycardia and hypertension are independently associated with adverse outcome in noncardiac surgery of long duration. Anesth Analg 2002; 95:273–7

40. Benjo A, Thompson RE, Fine D, et al.: Pulse pressure is an age-independent predictor of stroke development after cardiac surgery. Hypertension 2007; 50:630–5

41. Prys-Roberts C, Meloche R, Foex P: Studies of anaesthesia in relation to hypertension. I. Cardiovascular responses of treated and untreated patients. Br J Anaesth 1971; 43:122–37

42. Seshadri S, Wolf PA, Beiser A, et al.: Elevated midlife blood pressure increases stroke risk in elderly persons: the Framingham Study. Arch Intern Med 2001; 161:2343–50

43. Charlson ME, MacKenzie CR, Gold JP, et al.: The preoperative and intraoperative hemodynamic predictors of postoperative myocardial infarction or ischemia in patients undergoing noncardiac surgery. Ann Surg 1989; 210:637–48

44. Charlson ME, MacKenzie CR, Gold JP, Ales KL, Topkins M, Shires GT: Intraoperative blood pressure. What patterns identify patients at risk for postoperative complications? Ann Surg 1990; 212:567–80

45. Gold JP, Charlson ME, Williams-Russo P, et al.: Improvement of outcomes after coronary artery bypass randomized trial comparing intraoperative high versus low mean arterial pressure. J Thorac Cardiovasc Surg 1995; 110:1302–11
46. Gottesman RF, Hillis AE, Grega MA, et al.: Early postoperative cognitive dysfunction and blood pressure during coronary artery bypass graft operation. Arch Neurol 2007; 64:1111–4
47. Hartman GS, Yao FS, Bruefach M III, et al.: Severity of aortic atheromatous disease diagnosed by transesophageal echocardiography predicts stroke and other outcomes associated with coronary artery surgery: a prospective study. Anesth Analg 1996; 83:701–8
48. Gore JM, Katz JN, Varon J, et al.; STAT Investigators. Heterogeneous management of acute severe hypertension is associated with high morbidity and mortality: the STAT registry. Presented at: the Society of Critical Care Medicine's 37th Critical Care Congress; February 2–6, 2008, Honolulu, HI
49. Vuylsteke A, Feneck RO, Jolin-Mellgard A, et al.: Perioperative blood pressure control: a prospective survey of patient management in cardiac surgery. J Cardiothorac Vasc Anesth 2000; 14:269–73
50. O'Rourke MF, Hashimoto J: Mechanical factors in arterial aging: a clinical perspective. J Am Coll Cardiol 2007; 50:1–13
51. Widlansky ME, Gokce N, Keaney JF, Jr., Vita JA: The clinical implications of endothelial dysfunction. J Am Coll Cardiol 2003; 42:1149–60
52. Aronson S, Dyke C, Kereiakes D, et al.: Blood pressure control is an independent predictor of short-term mortality in cardiac surgery patients: analysis from the three randomized ECLIPSE Trials. Presented at the American College of Cardiology 56ᵗʰ Annual Scientific Session, New Orleans, LA, 2007
53. O'Rourke MF, Taylor MG: Input impedance of the systemic circulation. Circ Res 1967; 20:365–80
54. O'Rourke MF, Blazek JV, Morreels CL, Jr., Krovetz LJ: Pressure wave transmission along the human aorta: changes with age and in arterial degenerative disease. Circ Res 1968; 23:567–79
55. Wilkinson IB, Franklin SS, Hall IR, Tyrrell S, Cockcroft JR: Pressure amplification explains why pulse pressure is unrelated to risk in young subjects. Hypertension 2001; 38:1461–6
56. Franklin SS, Gustin W, Wong ND, et al.: Hemodynamic patterns of age-related changes in blood pressure. The Framingham Heart Study. Circulation 1997; 96:308–15
57. Hoffman JI, Buckberg GD: The myocardial supply:demand ratio—a critical review. Am J Cardiol 1978; 41:327–32

58. O'Rourke MF, Safar ME: Relationship between aortic stiffening and microvascular disease in brain and kidney: cause and logic of therapy. Hypertension 2005; 46:200–4

59. Chatzizisis YS, Coskun AU, Jonas M, Edelman ER, Feldman CL, Stone PH: Role of endothelial shear stress in the natural history of coronary atherosclerosis and vascular remodeling: molecular, cellular, and vascular behavior. J Am Coll Cardiol 2007; 49:2379–93

60. Doyle B, Caplice N: Plaque neovascularization and antiangiogenic therapy for atherosclerosis. J Am Coll Cardiol 2007; 49:2073–80

61. Wentzel JJ, Janssen E, Vos J, et al.: Extension of increased atherosclerotic wall thickness into high shear stress regions is associated with loss of compensatory remodeling. Circulation 2003; 108:17–23

62. Li ZY, Gillard JH: Plaque rupture: plaque stress, shear stress, and pressure drop. J Am Coll Cardiol 2008; 52:499–500; author reply 500

63. Fukumoto Y, Hiro T, Fujii T, et al.: Localized elevation of shear stress is related to coronary plaque rupture: a 3-dimensional intravascular ultrasound study with in-vivo color mapping of shear stress distribution. J Am Coll Cardiol 2008; 51:645–50

64. Virmani R, Kolodgie FD, Burke AP, et al.: Atherosclerotic plaque progression and vulnerability to rupture: angiogenesis as a source of intraplaque hemorrhage. Arterioscler Thromb Vasc Biol 2005; 25:2054–61

65. Vasan RS: Biomarkers of cardiovascular disease: molecular basis and practical considerations. Circulation 2006; 113:2335–62

66. Mueller CFH, Laude K, McNally JS, Harrison DG: ATVB in focus: redox mechanisms in blood vessels. Arterioscler Thromb Vasc Biol 2005; 25:274–8

67. Stone PH, Coskun AU, Kinlay S, et al.: Regions of low endothelial shear stress are the sites where coronary plaque progresses and vascular remodelling occurs in humans: an in vivo serial study. Eur Heart J 2007; 28:705–10

68. Richter Y, Edelman ER: Cardiology is flow. Circulation 2006; 113:2679–82

69. Ludmer PL, Selwyn AP, Shook TL, et al.: Paradoxical vasoconstriction induced by acetylcholine in atherosclerotic coronary arteries. N Engl J Med 1986; 315:1046–51

70. Creager MA, Cooke JP, Mendelsohn ME, et al.: Impaired vasodilation of forearm resistance vessels in hypercholesterolemic humans. J Clin Invest 1990; 86:228–34

71. Corretti MC, Anderson TJ, Benjamin EJ, et al.: Guidelines for the ultrasound assessment of endothelial-dependent flow-mediated vasodilation of the brachial artery: a report of the International

Brachial Artery Reactivity Task Force. J Am Coll Cardiol 2002; 39:257–65

72. McGrath BP, Liang YL, Kotsopoulos D, Cameron JD: Impact of physical and physiological factors on arterial function. Clin Exp Pharmacol Physiol 2001; 28:1104–7

73. Wilkinson IB, MacCallum H, Flint L, Cockcroft JR, Newby DE, Webb DJ: The influence of heart rate on augmentation index and central arterial pressure in humans. J Physiol 2000; 525(Pt 1):263–70

74. Cameron JD, McGrath BP, Dart AM: Use of radial artery applanation tonometry and a generalized transfer function to determine aortic pressure augmentation in subjects with treated hypertension. J Am Coll Cardiol 1998; 32:1214–20

75. Bramwell JC, Hill AV: Velocity of transmission of the pulse wave and elasticity of arteries. Lancet 1922; 1:891–2

76. Ridker PM, Hennekens CH, Roitman-Johnson B, Stampfer MJ, Allen J: Plasma concentration of soluble intercellular adhesion molecule 1 and risks of future myocardial infarction in apparently healthy men. Lancet 1998; 351:88–92

77. Thompson SG, Kienast J, Pyke SD, Haverkate F, van de Loo JC; European Concerted Action on Thrombosis and Disabilities Angina Pectoris Study Group. Hemostatic factors and the risk of myocardial infarction or sudden death in patients with angina pectoris. N Engl J Med 1995; 332:635–41

78. Williams B, Lacy PS, Thom SM, et al.; CAFE Investigators, for the Anglo-Scandinavian Cardiac Outcomes Trial (ASCOT) Investigators: Differential impact of blood pressure–lowering drugs on central aortic pressure and clinical outcomes: principal results of the Conduit Artery Function Evaluation (CAFE) study. Circulation 2006; 113:1213–25

79. Cheung AT: Exploring an optimum intra/postoperative management strategy for acute hypertension in the cardiac surgery patient. J Card Surg 2006; 21(Suppl 1):S8–S14

80. Brooks TW, Finch CK, Lobo BL, Deaton PR, Varner CF: Blood pressure management in acute hypertensive emergency. Am J Health Syst Pharm 2007; 64:2579–82

81. Katz JN, Gore JM, Amin A, et al.: Practice patterns, outcomes, and end-organ dysfunction for patients with acute, severe hypertension: results from the STAT (Studying the treatment of acute hypertension) registry. Hypertension Submitted.

82. Dasta JF, Bollinger JE, Gerlach AT: National survey of acute hypertension management. Presented at the Society of Critical Care Medicine's 37th Critical Care Congress, February 4, 2008, Honolulu, HI

83. Aronson S, Levy JH, Lumb PD, et al.; DCRI-GPRO Investigators. Preoperative blood pressure management with sodium nitroprusside or nitroglycerin is associated with and increased risk of 30-day mortality compared with clevidipine: results of the ECLIPSE trials. Presented at the Society of Cardiovascular Anesthesiologists 30th Annual Meeting and Workshops, June 20, 2008, Vancouver, BC, Canada

84. Aronson S, Stafford-Smith M, Phillips-Burke B, Roche A, Newman M: Blood pressure lability as a predictor of mortality in cardiac surgery patients: analysis of the Duke Database. Presented at the Society of Critical Care Medicine's 37th Critical Care Congress, February 4, 2008, Honolulu, HI

85. Bijker JB, van Klei WA, Kappen TH, van Wolfswinkel L, Moons KG, Kalkman CJ: Incidence of intraoperative hypotension as a function of the chosen definition: literature definitions applied to a retrospective cohort using automated data collection. Anesthesiology 2007; 107:213–20

86. Haas CE, LeBlanc JM: Acute postoperative hypertension: a review of therapeutic options. Am J Health Syst Pharm 2004; 61:1661–73

87. Weiss SJ, Longnecker DE: Perioperative hypertension: an overview. Coron Artery Dis 1993; 4:401–6

88. Leslie JB: Incidence and aetiology of perioperative hypertension. Acta Anaesthesiol Scand Suppl 1993; 99:5–9

89. Hennein HA, Ebba H, Rodriguez JL, et al.: Relationship of the proinflammatory cytokines to myocardial ischemia and dysfunction after uncomplicated coronary revascularization. J Thorac Cardiovasc Surg 1994; 108:626–35

90. Wolfsthal SD: Is blood pressure control necessary before surgery? Med Clin North Am 1993; 77:349–63

91. Kobzar G, Mardla V, Rätsep I, Samel N: Platelet activity before and after coronary artery bypass grafting. Platelets 2006; 17:289–91

92. Bolli R, Marban E: Molecular and cellular mechanisms of myocardial stunning. Physiol Rev 1999; 79:609–34

93. Julia PL, Buckberg GD, Acar C, Partington MT, Sherman MP: Studies of controlled reperfusion after ischemia. XXI. Reperfusate composition: superiority of blood cardioplegia over crystalloid cardioplegia in limiting reperfusion damage—importance of endogenous oxygen free radical scavengers in red blood cells. J Thorac Cardiovasc Surg 1991; 101:303–13

94. Herskowitz A, Mangano DT: Inflammatory cascade: a final common pathway for perioperative injury? Anesthesiology 1996; 85:957–60

95. Agmon Y, Khandheria BK, Meissner I, et al.: Independent association of high blood pressure and aortic atherosclerosis: a population-based study. Circulation 2000; 102:2087–93

96. Sen S, Hinderliter A, Sen PK, et al.: Aortic arch atheroma progression and recurrent vascular events in patients with stroke or transient ischemic attack. Circulation 2007; 116:928–35

97. Davila-Roman VG, Kouchoukos NT, Schechtman KB, Barzilai B: Atherosclerosis of the ascending aorta is a predictor of renal dysfunction after cardiac operations. J Thorac Cardiovasc Surg 1999; 117:111–6

98. Ganushchak YM, Fransen EJ, Visser C, De Jong DS, Maessen JG: Neurological complications after coronary artery bypass grafting related to the performance of cardiopulmonary bypass. Chest 2004; 125:2196–205

99. Fleisher LA: Preoperative evaluation of the patient with hypertension. JAMA 2002; 287:2043–6

100. Khattar RS, Swales JD, Dore C, Senior R, Lahiri A: Effect of aging on the prognostic significance of ambulatory systolic, diastolic, and pulse pressure in essential hypertension. Circulation 2001; 104:783–9

101. Benetos A, Thomas F, Bean KE, Guize L: Why cardiovascular mortality is higher in treated hypertensives versus subjects of the same age, in the general population. J Hypertens 2003; 21:1635–40

102. Salomaa V, Riley W, Kark JD, Nardo C, Folsom AR: Non–insulin-dependent diabetes mellitus and fasting glucose and insulin concentrations are associated with arterial stiffness indexes: the ARIC Study. Circulation 1995; 91:1432–43

103. Rajkumar C, Kingwell BA, Cameron JD, et al.: Hormonal therapy increases arterial compliance in postmenopausal women. J Am Coll Cardiol 1997; 30:350–6

104. Madhavan S, Ooi WL, Cohen H, Alderman MH: Relation of pulse pressure and blood pressure reduction to the incidence of myocardial infarction. Hypertension 1994; 23:395–401

105. Dart AM, Kingwell BA: Pulse pressure—a review of mechanisms and clinical relevance. J Am Coll Cardiol 2001; 37:975–84

106. Goldman L, Caldera DL, Nussbaum SR, et al.: Multifactorial index of cardiac risk in noncardiac surgical procedures. N Engl J Med 1977; 297:845–50

107. Goldman L, Caldera DL: Risks of general anesthesia and elective operation in the hypertensive patient. Anesthesiology 1979; 50:285–92

108. Franklin SS, Khan SA, Wong ND, Larson MG, Levy D: Is pulse pressure useful in predicting risk for coronary heart disease? The Framingham Heart Study. Circulation 1999; 100:354–60
109. Somes GW, Pahor M, Shorr RI, Cushman WC, Applegate WB: The role of diastolic blood pressure when treating isolated systolic hypertension. Arch Intern Med 1999; 159:2004–9
110. Glynn RJ, Chae CU, Guralnik JM, Taylor JO, Hennekens CH: Pulse pressure and mortality in older people. Arch Intern Med 2000; 160:2765–72
111. Lee KW, Blann AD, Lip GY: High pulse pressure and nondipping circadian blood pressure in patients with coronary artery disease: relationship to thrombogenesis and endothelial damage/dysfunction. Am J Hypertens 2005; 18:104–15
112. Chobanian AV: Isolated systolic hypertension in the elderly. N Engl J Med 2007; 357:789–96
113. Aronson S, Dyke CA, Stierer KA, et al.: The ECLIPSE trials: comparative studies of clevidipine to nitroglycerin, sodium nitroprusside, and nicardipine for acute hypertension treatment in cardiac surgery patients. Anesth Analg 2008; 107:1110–21
114. Aronson S, Cheung A, Stierer K, Levy JH, Lumb P; DCRI-GPRO Investigators: Perioperative blood pressure control predicts renal dysfunction in cardiac surgery patients. Presented at: the American Society of Anesthesiologists Annual Meeting, October 15, 2007, San Francisco, CA
115. Dyke C, Aronson S, Maier G, Bhatia D, Chen JC: Perioperative blood pressure excursions are an independent predictor of 30-day mortality in patients undergoing valve surgery. Presented at: the American College of Chest Physicians, Chest 2008, October 25–30, 2008, Philadelphia, PA

E. Andrew Ochroch, MD, MSCE
Audrey Oware, MD
John E. Ellis, MD

Carotid Stenosis and Coronary Disease: Understanding the Disease Processes and Defining How to Approach Them

3

INTRODUCTION

In 1972 Victor Bernhard and colleagues (1) published the first evaluation of the role of synchronous or staged carotid endarterectomy (CEA) in patients undergoing coronary artery bypass grafting (CABG). They proposed that stroke after CABG in subjects with known carotid stenosis was caused by flow limitation in the cerebral arteries during cardiopulmonary bypass (CPB). By performing the CEA prior to CABG in a synchronous (same operation) manner, they hoped to reduce the rate of stroke. The concerns these investigators had more than three and one-half decades ago are the same concerns we have today; unfortunately, the perioperative stroke rate after CABG has remained fairly constant over this period of time, ranging between 0.8% and 6% (2,3). In addition to the neurologic deficit associated with post-CABG stroke, the complication has other important risks and costs associated with it. For example, the patient who suffers a stroke after CABG has a mean hospital stay of 25 days and a 21% risk of dying within 30 days of surgery (4). In addition to the obvious deficits associated with a stroke, patients with carotid

Medically Challenging Patients Undergoing Cardiothoracic Surgery, edited by Neal H. Cohen, MD, MPH, MS, Lippincott Williams & Wilkins, Baltimore © 2009.

disease also suffer from more subtle neurologic complications after CABG surgery. When more sensitive neurocognitive testing is used in the perioperative period, neurologic deficits are detected in 1%–37% of patients studied within 2–6 weeks after CABG surgery, depending on which tests are examined (5). These changes have a profound impact on the postoperative course, quality of life, and costs associated with the care they require.

Similar findings are noted when evaluating the risk of myocardial complications after CEA in patients with combined carotid and coronary disease. The risk of myocardial infarction (MI) in patients undergoing CEA who have known coronary artery disease (CAD) ranges from 0.5% to 3% (6–8). The impact and costs associated with a perioperative MI are significant, with perioperative management decisions having a profound impact on outcome (9). Consequently, having a clearly defined plan to address both the carotid and coronary disease is essential. The management must balance the risks associated with MI or stroke against the strategies to optimize cerebral blood flow and myocardial function and perfusion.

To help the reader more fully appreciate the perioperative care of the patient with concomitant carotid and coronary disease, this chapter will review the prevalence of concomitant disease. It will then examine the perioperative risk factors for MI and stroke associated with CABG surgery and the effect on outcome of modification of these risk factors. Similarly, it will explore the risk factors for MI and stroke in patients who undergo CEA and the effects of these management strategies on outcome. The chapter will conclude with recommendations regarding combined procedures and the staging of the carotid and cardiac procedures, as well as consideration of the role of alternative approaches to medical management, including coronary angioplasty, coronary stenting, and carotid angioplasty or stenting.

PREVALENCE OF CONCOMITANT CAROTID AND CORONARY DISEASE

The coprevalence of coronary and carotid disease is quite high. The exact prevalence and the impact of the combined disease processes are dependent on how investigators have categorized the patients and the timing of the initial evaluation for either the CEA or CABG procedure. Salasidis et al. (10) performed a case series of carotid duplex scanning on 395 subjects presenting for CABG. The prevalence of severe carotid disease (stenosis >80%) was 8.5%. These patients were significantly older (65.6 ± 6.5 years vs. 62.5 ± 10.4 years, $P = .02$), had previous CEA (27.3% vs. 2.0%, $P = .00001$), had preoperative neurologic symptoms (21.2% vs. 5.9%, $P = .002$), and had peripheral vascular disease

(PVD) (63.6% vs. 16.9%, $P = .00001$). The incidence of postoperative stroke (temporary or permanent) in patients with severe carotid disease was 18.2% versus 1.7% in patients without severe carotid disease ($P = .001$). The sensitivity associated with the presence of severe carotid disease on the incidence of postoperative stroke was 40% ($n = 4/10$) (specificity 95.1%, positive predictive value 18.2%, negative predictive value 98.3%). Similarly, Berens et al. (11) evaluated 1087 patients 65 years old or older who underwent cardiac surgical procedures (91% had CAD) with carotid duplex ultrasonography. The prevalence of disease was 17.0% for 50% or greater carotid stenosis and 5.9% for 80% or greater stenosis. With use of a stepwise, logistic regression model, female sex, PVD, history of transient ischemic attack (TIA) or stroke, smoking history, and left main (LM) CAD predicted 95% of patients with 80% or greater stenosis and 91% of patients with 50% or greater stenosis.

One subtype of CAD and its relation to carotid disease that deserves special attention is LM CAD. A LM stenosis (>50% occlusion) was more frequently associated with carotid stenosis (>60% occlusion) compared with patients who did not have significant LM disease (31.2% vs. 15.2%, $P < .0001$) (12). Vigneswaran et al. (13) performed a case–control study in which the cases were subjects presenting with LM disease and the controls presented with three-vessel CAD. LM disease was associated with significantly more frequent and severe carotid stenosis. Patients with LM disease also had lower ejection fraction (EF) and more thoracic aortic atheromata. This finding was supported by Kallikazaros et al. (14), who found similar rates of LM disease and decreased EF associated with carotid disease.

Concomitant coronary and carotid disease can also be regarded as a marker of more severe generalized atheromatous disease. Rates of abdominal aortic disease increase in subjects with concomitant disease (15), and PVD is similarly significantly increased (12). Carotid intimal thickening may be a more specific marker of atherosclerotic disease burden, and increasing intima thickness has been correlated with the degree of aortic plaque (16). In a study of more than 12,000 subjects, Chambless et al. (17) developed Cox proportional hazards models (adjusted only for age, race, and medical center), the hazard rate ratio for development of coronary heart disease comparing extreme mean intima-media thickness (≥ 1 mm) to not extreme (<1 mm) was 5.07 for women [95% (confidence interval), 3.08–8.36] and 1.85 for men (95% CI, 1.28–2.69). This relationship of carotid disease as a marker of overall atherosclerotic burden will be examined later in this chapter as it clearly is a factor in perioperative outcomes in subjects undergoing cardiac and vascular surgery.

TABLE 3–1. Risk factors for perioperative stroke

Preoperative (patient-related) factors
Advanced age
Female sex
Hypertension, diabetes mellitus, renal insufficiency (creatinine >2 mg/dL), smoking, chronic obstructive pulmonary disease, peripheral vascular disease, coronary artery disease, arrhythmias, heart failure, left ventricular ejection fraction <40%
History of stroke or transient ischemic attack
Atherosclerosis of the ascending aorta
Abrupt cessation of antithrombotic/anticoagulant medications

Intraoperative (procedure-related) risk factors
Type and nature of surgical procedure
Duration of surgery
Duration of cardiopulmonary bypass
Manipulation of proximal aortic atherosclerotic lesions
Arrhythmias, hyperglycemia, hypotension, or hypertension

Postoperative risk factors
Heart failure, low or decreased left ventricular ejection fraction, myocardial infarction, arrhythmias
Dehydration or blood loss
Hyperglycemia

Reprinted with permission from Selim et al. (18).

PERIOPERATIVE RISK FACTORS FOR STROKE

Patient-Related Risk Factors

Selim's (18) review in the *New England Journal of Medicine* (Table 3–1) indicates that the patient-related risk factors for perioperative stroke for any operation increase with advanced age. Although age itself does not predict stroke, it seems to be a marker for coexisting conditions and potentially for decreased cerebrovascular reserve. A patient's medical history determines a large component of preoperative risk as hypertension, creatinine >2 mg/dL, smoking, chronic obstructive pulmonary disease, PVD, CAD, arrhythmias, heart failure, and left ventricular EF (LVEF) below 40% are part of various regression determined risk models (18–20). Many of these factors also can be judged as predicting the risk of cerebrovascular and/or atherosclerotic disease burden. Similarly, a history of stroke, TIA, carotid stenosis, and aortic atheroma also increase the risk of stroke.

Risk Factors for Stroke from CABG

The incidence of stroke from CABG ranges from 1.4% to 3.8% (18–21). Naylor et al. (22, 23) have focused on the role of asymptomatic carotid stenosis as a risk factor for stroke during CABG. Their reviews indicate that an overall risk of stroke of 2% is increased to 3% among patients with asymptomatic unilateral stenosis of between 50% and 99%. This risk increases to 5% when bilateral stenoses of 50%–99% is present and 7% with carotid occlusion.

Procedure-specific risk factors for stroke during CABG include the duration of CPB, the duration of aortic clamp time, the number of aortic clamping events, and manipulation of proximal aortic atheromata (18–20, 22, 23).

Anesthetic management may impact the risk of stroke as well. Hemodynamic changes including arrhythmia, hypotension, hypertension, and hyperglycemia have been shown to be risk factors for perioperative stroke. These risks continue into the postoperative period as intensive care unit (ICU) management strategies also impact the risk for postoperative stroke. Some of the factors associated with an increased risk of stroke in the postoperative period include the presence of reduced EF, MI, atrial fibrillation, dehydration, blood loss, and hyperglycemia while in the ICU (18).

Risk Factors for Stroke from Percutaneous Coronary Interventions

In a meta-analysis that included 4944 patients undergoing percutaneous coronary interventions (PCI), Bravata et al. (24) found a stroke rate of 0.6%. Similar to CABG surgery, advanced age, a history of TIA or stroke, atrial fibrillation, contralateral carotid occlusion, congestive heart failure, and diabetes are significant independent predictors for stroke.

Risk Factors for Stroke from CEA

The risk of stroke after CEA is 3%; the risk has remained relatively constant for the past 20 years despite increasing attention to addressing carotid perfusion and management of atheroma (25–29). Similar to CABG surgery, a history of TIA or stroke, atrial fibrillation, contralateral carotid occlusion, congestive heart failure, and diabetes are significant independent predictors for stroke (25–30). Anesthetic technique, electroencephalography (EEG), universal carotid artery shunting to optimize cerebral blood flow during cross-clamping, or selective shunting do not appear to impact stroke risk (25–29).

Risk Factors for Stroke from Carotid Artery Stenting

The risk of stroke from carotid artery stenting (CAS) has dramatically changed in the last decade with the introduction of distal thromboembolic capture devices. Currently the risk seems to be approximately that of CEA, ~3%–4%. The BEACH (*B*oston Scientific *E* PI: *A* Carotid Stenting Trial for *H* igh-Risk Surgical Patients) trial, which had CAS in high- risk patients, reported a 4.4% rate of any stroke within 30 days (31). The CArotid Revascularization using Endarterectomy or Stenting Systems (CaRESS) trial reported a 2.1% rate of stroke with a healthier population (32). The Carotid Acculink/Accunet Post-Approval Trial to Uncover Unanticipated or Rare Events (CAPTURE) study (33), which is a large (~3500) case-series utilizing the Acculink/Accunet device reported a 4.8% stroke rate (2% major and 2.9% minor) (33). Overall, similar to CEA, a history of TIA or stroke, atrial fibrillation , contralateral carotid occlusion, congestive heart failure, and diabetes are significant independent predictors for stroke. However, many trials have excluded these high-risk subgroups from inclusion in the study, so the reported rates of stroke may not represent the risk for a broad population of patients with both carotid and coronary disease.

Stroke Risk CEA Versus CAS

CAS has been promoted as a less invasive procedure than CEA for carotid revascularization. CEA has a long history of success with more data to document both the risk and the potential advantages of the procedure, whereas CAS is relatively new and undergoing refinement based on experience and improvements in the available stents. As a result, a comparison of the outcomes requires careful interpretation. Initial problems with CAS have, to some extent, been lessened with the introduction of devices that can prevent, lessen, and/or retrieve embolic materials. The Carotid and Vertebral Artery Transluminal Angioplasty Study (CAVATAS) (34) randomized 504 subjects. Of the 251 angioplasty subjects, 55 (26%) were stented and the remainder only had angioplasty. There were no differences in any category of stroke between the CEA and CAS arms at 30 days (CAVATAS) (34), 1 year (CAVATAS) (34), or 3 years (35). However, because there was a low rate of stenting and there was no distal embolic protection device, these data probably do not represent the current risk of stroke associated with carotid-stenting procedures.

The Stenting and Angioplasty with Protection in Patients at High Risk for Endarterectomy (SAPPHIRE) trial (36) compared the safety and effectiveness of carotid stenting with embolic protection to surgical endarterectomy in the treatment of carotid artery disease in high-risk patients. All patients were treated with aspirin. For those randomized to endovascular treatment, the Cordis PRECISE Nitinol Stent (Cordis Co, Warren, NJ) and the ANGIOGUARD XP Emboli Capture Device (Cordis Co, Warren, NJ) were used, and clopidogrel was taken before and for 30 days after the procedure (but not after CEA). There was no difference in stroke rate for CAS (3.6%) versus CEA (3.1%).

The Stent-protected Percutaneous Angioplasty of the Carotid versus Endarterectomy (SPACE) study (37) analyzed 1183 subjects randomized between CEA and CAS. The rate of stroke from randomization to 30 days after the procedure was 7.5% with CAS and 6.2% with CEA, which were not statistically different. Similar to SAPPHIRE, dual antiplatelet therapy was used after CAS. The stroke rates for both CEA and CAS are higher than usually cited, and this study is open to criticism because many of the physicians performing the procedure were relatively inexperienced as compared to physicians taking part in the SAPPHIRE study.

The Endarterectomy versus Stenting in Patients with Symptomatic Severe Carotid Stenosis (EVA-S3) trial had dramatically different results than other studies. In this study the stroke rates after CAS were approximately 9% versus about 3.5% for CEA (38–40). However, this trial is open to criticism because 17% of subjects were not on dual antiplatelet therapy prior to, and for 30 days following the stenting procedure. Furthermore, many of the physicians performing the procedure were relatively inexperienced as compared to the physicians who participated in the SAPPHIRE study.

Overall, in a high-risk population, CEA and CAS seem to have similar rates of stroke, averaging between 3% and 6%. Obviously, these results rely on optimal perioperative management (as described later in this chapter) and an experienced operative team.

PREOPERATIVE PHARMACOLOGIC PREVENTION OF PERIOPERATIVE STROKE

Antiplatelet Therapy

The value of perioperative antiplatelet therapy in the reduction of stroke risk is best established in perioperative management of CEA. Lindblad et al. (41) performed a double-blind study comparing administration of 75 mg of aspirin a day versus placebo started prior to CEA and continued for 1 year. Perioperative and 30-day stroke rates were reduced in the aspirin group, but overall mortality was not decreased. Despite the apparent advantage of aspirin therapy, the most appropriate dose of aspirin remains controversial. A large trial by Taylor et al. (42) in which 2849 subjects were randomized to receive 81, 325, 650, or 1300 mg of aspirin a day prior to CEA and continued for 3 months reaffirmed the ability of aspirin to reduce perioperative stroke and the risk of stroke and provided some guidance regarding dosing strategy. MI and death were lowest in the groups of patients receiving either 81 or 325 mg per day. This finding is in contrast to a secondary analysis performed as part of the *North American Symptomatic Carotid Endarterectomy Trial* (NASCET)

TABLE 3–2.   Procedural subgroup analysis of the CURE trial (44)

Procedure	Clopiogrel	Placebo	Effect size
PCI	9.6%	13.2%	RR, 0.72; 95% CI, 0.57–0.90
CABG surgery	14.5%	16.2%	RR, 0.89; 95% CI, 0.71–1.11
Medical management	8.1%	10.0%	RR, 0.80; 95% CI, 0.69–0.92

The percentages listed are primary outcome of myocardial infarction, stroke, and/or death. CURE = Clopidogrel in Unstable Angina to Prevent Recurrent Events; RR = relative risk; CI = confidence interval; PCI = percutaneous coronary intervention; CABG = coronary artery bypass graft.

trial (8) that suggested that 650 mg of aspirin was superior to either 81 or 325 mg. However, in that study the doses were not randomly distributed among centers participating in the study, so there could have been significant other "center" effects accounting for the differences.

Similar to the patients undergoing CEA, those undergoing CAS clearly benefit from antiplatelet therapy (43). The recommended therapy consists of dual antiplatelet therapy similar to that employed for bare metal coronary stent thromboprophylaxis: 2–3 weeks of preprocedural and 4 weeks postprocedural aspirin and clopidogrel therapy. As discussed earlier in this chapter, some of the varying stroke rates obtained from the large CAS trials, at least in part, may be caused by the level of adherence of subjects to this dual antiplatelet therapy.

The Clopidogrel in Unstable Angina to Prevent Recurrent Events (CURE) trial (44) randomized subjects who were all receiving aspirin to also receive either clopidogrel or placebo prior to medical management, CABG, or PCI (Table 3–2). In each subgroup, clopidogrel reduced the risk of the primary outcome of MI, stroke, and/or death. The benefits were consistent among persons undergoing PCI [9.6% for clopidogrel, 13.2% for placebo; relative risk (RR), 0.72; 95% CI, 0.57–0.90],CABG surgery (14.5% for clopidogrel, 16.2% for placebo; RR, 0.89; 95% CI, 0.71–1.11), and medical therapy only (8.1% for clopidogrel, 10.0% for placebo; RR, 0.80; 95% CI, 0.69–0.92). For CABG during the initial hospitalization (530 for placebo, 485 for clopidogrel), the frequency of cardiovascular death, MI, or stroke before CABG was 4.7% for placebo and 2.9% for clopidogrel (RR, 0.56; 95% CI, 0.29–1.08) (45).

The role of clopidogrel in CEA for stroke reduction has been examined by Payne et al. (46). In their study, all subjects received 150 mg of aspirin daily and were randomized to receive either 75 mg of clopidogrel or placebo started the night prior to surgery. Although they found a significant decrease in cerebral emboli as measured by transcranial

Doppler, one subject in each group had a stroke. The potential for this management to reduce the embolic load and therefore improve postoperative neurocognitive function deserves further study. However, perioperative use of clopidogrel remains controversial because of the risk of increased bleeding. In the CURE trial (44), there was a 1% excess of major bleeding, but no significant excess of life-threatening bleeding for subjects on clopidogrel. Among patients undergoing CABG, the rates of life-threatening bleeding were 5.6% for clopidogrel and 4.2% for placebo (RR, 1.30; 95% CI, 0.91–1.95) (45). Similarly, although times to closure were longer, there were no increased bleeding incidents for subjects on clopidogrel undergoing CEA (46).

Statin Therapy

Multiple studies have demonstrated that hydroxymethylglutaryl-CoA reductase inhibitors (statins) reduce the risk of stroke after CABG (47–56) surgery. The value of statins is also demonstrated based on adherence to prescribed therapy. Nonadherence and withdrawal from statin therapy prior to CABG surgery has been shown to be a risk factor for stroke (51), possibly because of the stabilizing effect of statins on atheromata (49), although the exact mechanism for this improved outcome remains poorly defined.

There is growing evidence that statins may be especially effective in reducing cardiovascular morbidity and improving outcomes after CEA surgery (57–61). A recent retrospective study performed at Johns Hopkins Hospital demonstrated a threefold reduction in the rate of perioperative stroke ($P < .05$) among 1566 patients undergoing CEA (59). This benefit was confirmed in a series of 3360 CEAs performed at multiple hospitals throughout Western Canada. Statin use was independently associated with a 75% reduction [odds ratio (OR) = 0.25; 95% CI, 0.07–0.90] in the odds of death and 45% reduction (OR = 0.55; 95% CI, 0.32–0.95) in the odds of ischemic stroke or death among patients with symptomatic carotid disease (57). Preliminary work indicates a similar benefit of statin use in reducing neurologic morbidity among patients undergoing carotid angioplasty and stent procedures.

It has become clear in the last decade that the efficacy of statins in reducing stroke and MI may not relate to absolute cholesterol levels. In the following section, "Biomarkers of Atheromatous Instability," the pleiotropic effects of statins in reducing inflammatory mediators (62, 63) are examined. This may very well be the mechanism of protection by statins.

Biomarkers of Atheromatous Instability

Inflammation in the arterial vessels plays an essential role in plaque development, growth, destabilization, rupture, and embolization (64).

Pathologic studies consistently find abundant inflammatory cells including monocyte-derived macrophages and T lymphocytes at sites of plaque rupture. These invasive cells secrete cytokines, chemokines, growth factors, and disintegrins and lead to a proliferation of smooth muscle cells, lesion progression, and an eventual weakening of plaque matrix (65). Biomarkers of plaque destabilization have been shown to predict arterial events, and their measurement carry important prognostic information independent of traditional risk markers (64,66).

The most actively studied clinically useful marker of at-risk plaque inflammation is C-reactive protein (CRP). CRP is a robust clinical marker because of its analytical stability, and scientific reproducibility; its sensitive assays are available commercially (67). CRP is produced in hepatocytes and vascular endothelium under transcriptional control of several cytokines, with interleukin-6 (IL-6) being a primary factor. Along with being a marker of inflammation, CRP also has direct pro-inflammatory effects (68). A meta-analysis (69) of 22 studies with 7086 subjects showed a vascular risk OR of 1.45 for elevated CRP levels. Although CRP levels are probably not useful for general population screening, in high-risk populations (such as patients who are being considered for staged or combined CEA and CABG), CRP is probably an independent risk factor for MI (70,71) and may also indicate risk of stroke as an independent predictor (70,72). Using this assay as a guide to both diagnosis and therapy is probably useful, particularly with respect to the potential administration of statins in the perioperative period. Multiple studies have documented the ability of statins to dramatically reduce CRP and the risk of postoperative vascular events (70,72,73).

Other well-studied biomarkers of inflammation that predict atheromatous plaque instability include the cytokines, of which IL-6 is the best studied. IL-6 both increases plaque instability by stimulating CRP production and macrophage activity and is a procoagulant (64,66,74). Its most important function may be the amplification of the inflammation cascade. Increased levels of IL-6 have been associated with increased hospital mortality (75), and patients with higher levels of IL-6 benefit from earlier vascular intervention (76). Unlike the use of CRP as a guide to perioperative management for patients with severe vascular disease, whereas several longitudinal studies indicate an increased risk from vascular disease in subjects with high IL-6 levels (64,66), there have been no perioperative trials to indicate its clinical usefulness as a predictive tool. Statins have been shown to reduce IL-6 levels (62,63), but there has been no direct link to perioperative stroke or MI reduction, perhaps in large part because the multitude of statin studies have focused on cholesterol and only recently has inflammation become a key focus. Further investigation of the role of statins and the potential value of IL-6 measurement in the perioperative period should be of value in defining optimal management strategies.

Angiotensin-Converting Enzyme Inhibitors/ Angiotensin Receptor Blockers

Angiotensin-converting enzyme (ACE) inhibitors and angiotensin receptor blockers (ARBs) have been shown to be effective in reducing ischemic events associated with atherosclerotic disease. Although they were originally developed for their vasodilator properties, recent studies have demonstrated that a major effect of ACE inhibitors is prevention of angiotensin II–mediated cardiac and vascular tissue remodeling (77–81). ACE inhibitors may act through multiple mechanisms. By reducing angiotensin II–mediated vasoconstriction, ACE inhibitors reduce systemic vascular resistance in patients with LV systolic failure and thus improve cardiac output. In addition to this effect on circulating angiotensin II, ACE inhibitors cause a decrease in the metabolism (breakdown) of bradykinin that stimulates the release of nitric oxide, prostaglandins, and other endothelium-dependent vasodilators, thereby acting to improve endothelial function. Because of the high concentration of renin–angiotensin systems in vascular endothelium and myocardium, ACE inhibitors act to prevent vascular and myocardial tissue remodeling. These effects may be the predominant mechanism by which ACE inhibitors achieve their beneficial outcomes in patients with atherosclerotic vascular disease (77–81).

The vast majority of the data on ACE inhibitors and ARBs come from trials designed to identify ways to reduce stroke. For instance, the ongoing Prevention Regimen for Effectively Avoiding Second Strokes (PRoFESS) trial is designed to evaluate whether extended-release dipyridamole plus aspirin compared with clopidogrel, and whether telmisartan in addition to usual care, in individuals after a stroke, will reduce the risk of further strokes (77). Such data need to be closely evaluated to determine if they have any ramifications for the perioperative management of high-risk patients undergoing cardiac and/or carotid surgery.

STROKE PREVENTION BY CEA

The Asymptomatic Carotid Atherosclerosis Study (ACAS) (82) enrolled subjects with 60% or greater carotid stenosis. Medical management included administration of aspirin and control of comorbidities. After initiation of optimal medical management, subjects were then randomly assigned either to undergo CEA or to continue medical management. "After a median follow-up of 2.7 years, with 4657 patient-years of observation, the aggregate risk over 5 years for ipsilateral stroke and any perioperative stroke or death was estimated to be 5.1% for surgical patients and 11.0% for patients treated medically" (82). Similarly, the NASCET (83) also ensured aspirin therapy and aggressive comorbidity management. For patients with severe stenosis of 70%–99%, the trial reported a "cumulative risk of any ipsilateral stroke at two years of 26 percent in the 331 medical patients and 9 percent in the 328 surgical patients—an absolute risk reduction ($\pm$ SE) 17 ± 3.5 percent. For a major or fatal ipsilateral stroke, the corresponding estimates were 13.1 percent and 2.5 percent."

The European Carotid Stenosis Trial (ECST) randomized 3018 patients to medical versus surgical management and followed them up for a mean of 73 months. Surgery reduced the 5-year risk of any stroke or surgical death by 5.7% (95% CI, 0–11.6) in patients with 50%–69% stenosis ($n = 646$, $P = .05$) and by 21.2% (95% CI, 12.9–29.4) in patients with 70%–99% stenosis without "near occlusion" ($n = 429$, $P < .0001$). These benefits were maintained at the 10-year follow-up. However, surgery was of no benefit in patients ($n = 125$) with near occlusion. The effect of surgery in this group was highly significantly different from that in patients with 70%–99% stenosis without near occlusion ($P = .002$). Surgery was harmful in patients with <30% stenosis ($n = 1321$, $P = .007$) and of no benefit in patients with 30%–49% stenosis ($n = 478$, $P = .6$)" (84,85).

RISK OF MI AFTER CEA

As discussed earlier in this chapter in the section "Prevalence of Concomitant Carotid and Coronary Disease," many patients presenting for CEA have significant CAD that may or may not be known. Hertzer and Lees (86) reported in 1981 that a series of 335 CEA patients had a 1.8% rate of fatal MI. This accounted for 60% of the early postoperative deaths. Ten years later, McCrory et al. (87) studied 1100 patients randomly selected from 10 medical centers and found a rate of nonfatal MI of 2.1%. It should be noted that, although some large trials have reported perioperative MI rates as low as 0.9% (depending on criteria for MI; CKMB vs troponin $\pm$ EKG) (82,83,85), these trials have excluded the highest risk patients (recent MI and unstable angina), and nonfatal MI post-CEA for all patients seems to occur approximately 2% of the time.

RISK OF MI AFTER CAS

CAS might seem to incur less risk of MI than CEA does. It has been difficult to show an advantage in the immediate perioperative period because of the low rate of MI post-CEA. The CAVATAS trial included

251 CAS and 253 CEA subjects. There were no perioperative MIs in the CAS and three in the CEA group. There was no statistical significance between the two groups. Data from the vast majority of stenting trials (31–33, 36, 38, 88–90) indicate that, 30 days after the procedure and beyond, the rate of MI from CAS seems to be the same as that from CEA—1.5%–2.5% MI. This rate is probably more related to the risk strata of the patients than to the risk of procedure, but perioperative instability may contribute to postoperative MIs. For example, instances of prolonged postoperative hypotension and bradycardia, typically vagally mediated, can clearly be a cause of postoperative MI.

RISK OF MI AFTER CABG OR PCI

The risk of perioperative MI (2%), 30 day MI (2%–3%), or long-term MI (5%–6%) after PCI or CABG has remained stable over the past few years (91–94). There seems to be an advantage to left internal mammary artery grafts for preserving LV systolic function and decreasing long-term MI. Similarly, diabetics, who typically have more microvascular disease, tend to fare better after CABG than after PCI, as they have higher rates of needing revascularization after PCI (91–94).

PCIS VERSUS CABG

There is significant controversy as to the optimal route of coronary revascularization for patients with multivessel coronary disease. Multiple meta-analyses and reviews (91–95) indicated that, when patients were randomized between complete PCI and CABG, there were no significant differences in perioperative MI or stroke. At 1 year, repeat revascularization procedures occurred more frequently after PCI than after CABG. The percentage of patients who were free from angina was slightly lower after PCI associated with multiple stents than after CABG surgery. There was no survival difference over a multiyear follow-up period.

SURGICAL APPROACHES TO COMBINED CAROTID AND CORONARY DISEASE

Patients who have concomitant coronary and carotid artery disease represent a very high-risk population whose optimal management remains controversial. The best surgical timing to these comorbid illnesses is not well defined, with the sequencing of carotid revascularization in relation to coronary surgery being the key variable. Different approaches include 1) staged approach (CEA followed by CABG at a second operation days or weeks later), 2) reverse staged (CABG preceding CEA), or 3) synchronous procedures (simultaneous CEA and CABG during the same period of anesthesia). As importantly, controversy exists as to whether the two interventions should be performed as a combined approach or staged. The risks of each approach also vary, including the overall length of hospital stay and the incidence of events such as stroke, myocardial dysfunction, and death. Multiple studies have been undertaken over the last few decades to address these issues. However, randomized controlled trials examining the different surgical approaches are limited. In addition, problems with the study designs (such as selection bias and confounding variables) compromise the validity of many of the studies or make comparisons difficult. As a result, it is not possible to define the management strategy. (Please see Table 3–3 for a summary of combined carotid and CABG surgery articles.)

Despite the lack of clarity about the best approach to the patient with carotid and coronary disease, often the decision as to whether to proceed with coronary or carotid revascularization is primarily dictated by the condition of the heart. In patients with LM disease, diffuse multivessel CAD, unstable angina, or severe LV dysfunction (or combinations of these 4), the perioperative cardiac risk associated with a staged approach of initial CEA followed by CABG is often felt to be too great. In these cases, synchronous carotid and coronary revascularization procedures are preferred. In contrast, those patients with stable angina may be better able to tolerate CEA as a stand-alone procedure or as the initial procedure followed immediately by CABG with a low risk of myocardial complications. Das et al. (20) found the staged procedure to be suitable for patients with minimal cardiac disease, minor or no LM disease, and patients with triple-vessel disease with good LV function as the delay in coronary intervention did not add significant risk. The degree of carotid artery stenosis also plays an important role; patients with high grade carotid stenosis with preserved LV function or single-vessel CAD may be considered for a preceding carotid revascularization to decrease the risk of stroke with the ensuing CABG.

Determining the risk factors for postoperative complications is critical in deciding how to approach surgical decision making. Akins et al. (96) reviewed the records of 200 consecutive patients who underwent combined CEA–CABG. They found that multivariate predictors of hospital death included postoperative stroke, failure to use internal mammary arterial graft, and the need for intraoperative intraaortic balloon pump (IABP). Predictors of postoperative stroke were PVD and unstable angina, and predictors of prolonged hospital stay were postoperative stroke, advanced age, and nonelective operation. In a meta-analysis by Das et al. (20) 33 different risk factors were identified for perioperative stroke during CABG, including aortic atheromatous disease, emergent procedures, impaired LV function, and PVD. Higher grade carotid artery stenosis (50% vs. 80%, P = .009) resulted in an increased risk of stroke with CABG. One may argue that the above factors in this high-risk population of patients may contribute to perioperative complications regardless of the surgical strategy chosen, and that many cannot either be controlled or predicted preoperatively.

Many studies have focused on the potential value of the combined procedure. Combined procedures have the benefit of exposing the patient to only one anesthetic and the potential for a shorter hospital stay. This decreased anesthetic exposure and shorter hospital stay may result in significant cost-saving and could reduce the risk of nosocomial infections or other hospital-associated complications. Also synchronous procedures may result in greater patient satisfaction as patients would most certainly prefer to undergo just one surgical "event" rather than two separate operations. Other arguments for combined CEA–CABG include protecting the carotid circulation from stroke during CABG (whether the etiology is embolism or a state of hypoperfusion) although, as noted above, the data do not clearly document the value of specific sequencing of the procedures.

Overall Morbidity and Mortality of Combined Approaches

Despite the potential advantages of a single anesthetic and surgical procedure for patients requiring both CABG and CEA, the combined procedure has not been definitively shown to be safer or less risky than a staged procedure. Many studies have been unable to demonstrate any advantage regarding the treatment of the carotid artery stenosis during simultaneous procedures over a staged approach. In a meta-analysis (20), a significant reduction in stroke was found for the staged procedure versus the combined procedure (1.5% vs. 3.9%, P = .007), however with a slightly, although not statistically significant, higher mortality (5.9% vs. 4.5%, P = .1, not significant). Interestingly, the stroke rate in the staged procedure was significantly lower than the stroke rate for CABG alone (see "Risk Factors for Stroke from CABG" section, earlier in this chapter). However, when total risks were analyzed (mean stroke rate and mean mortality rate), similar results were found between the groups; staged = 7.4%, reverse staged = 7.2%, combined = 8.4%, and isolated CABG in patients with carotid artery stenosis >50%–11.5%. This finding suggests that, overall, there is no significant advantage in a staged versus combined procedure in terms of stroke and death. Gaudino et al. (97) found similar in-hospital outcomes for either a staged or simultaneous repair of severe monolateral asymptomatic carotid artery stenosis (SMACS) at the time of CABG versus no carotid intervention. Specifically, outcomes such as in-hospital mortality and stroke were similar between the two

TABLE 3–3.   Summary of combined carotid–CABG studies

Year	First author	Title	What was studied
1995	Akins (96)	Safety and Efficacy of Concomitant Carotid and Coronary Artery Operations	Safety of concurrent CEA/CABG
1998	Allie (110)	Rapid-staged Strategy for Concomitant Critical Carotid and LM Coronary Disease with LV Dysfunction: IABP Use	IABP use in high-risk pts with concomitant critical carotid (>90% stenosis), LM coronary disease (>70% stenosis), and LV dysfunction (EF < 30%)
1998	Darling (114)	Combined Carotid Endarterectomy and Coronary Artery Bypass Grafting Does not Increase the Risk of Perioperative Stroke	Prospective collection of data was performed in pts undergoing combined CEA and CABG
2000	Das (20)	Continuing Controversy in the Management of Concomitant Coronary and Carotid Disease: An Overview	Meta-analysis Four strategies were analyzed: CABG in the presence of carotid artery stenosis, combined (CEA + CABG), reverse (CABG + CEA > 3 mo), prior staged (CEA + CABG < 3 mo) Outcome assessed by 30-day permanent MSR and MMR

. of pts	Outcomes	Conclusions
200	• Predictors of hospital death: postop stroke, failure to use IMA graft, intraop IABP, nonelective operations • Predictors of postop stroke: PVD, unstable angina • Predictors of prolonged hospital stay: postop stroke, advanced age, nonelective operation	Concomitant CEA + CABG has acceptably low operative risk and long-term freedom from coronary and neurologic events
20	• 18 pts extubated on DOS (after CABG) • 16 pts transferred from ICU within 48 h • Total hospital stay ranged from 6 to 12 days (mean = 8) • No 30-day postop deaths, MI, neurologic, vascular, or bleeding complications • At mean 30-mo follow-up, 2 noncardiac deaths and no neurologic events	Rapid-staged procedure with IABP is safe/effective and is an option to decrease risks of staged CEA and CABG
420	• Operative mortality was 10/420 pts (2.4%); 9 of those 10 pts died from cardiac complications postop; 1 ptt died of a stroke • Permanent neurological deficits occurred in 5 pts (1%); 6 pts (1.7%) had a transient neurological deficit that improved prior to discharge	Simultaneous CEA + CABG can be performed with an acceptable mortality and morbidity and does not place the ptt at a higher risk than when either procedure is performed alone
	• 33 different risk factors for stroke at CABG, including: ascending aortic atheroma, emergent procedures, severe LV dysfunction, and PVD • Risk of stroke at CABG increased with higher grade carotid artery stenosis (50% vs. 80%, $P = .009$) • Significant reduction in stroke for staged vs. combined (1.5% vs. 3.9%, $P = .007$) with a higher mortality (5.9% vs. 4.5%, $P = .1$, NS) • Stroke rate in staged group significantly lower vs. unprotected CABG • Analysis of total risks (MSR and MMR) showed similar results between the groups: staged 7.4%, reverse staged 7.2%, combined 8.4%, unprotected CABG w/>50% carotid stenosis 11.5%	• Stroke at CABG caused by multiple risk factors, one of which is high-grade carotid stenosis • Embolism appears to be the primary mechanism (not flow limitation) • No significant difference in overall stroke and mortality risk between various strategies • Analysis suggests that pts do better by staging • In pts with severe cardiac disease (i.e., unstable angina, triple-vessel disease with poor LV function, and LM disease) prior staging should not be considered • Pts w/o severe cardiac disease should be considered for staging and the rest for combined procedure or reverse staged

— *continued next page*

TABLE 3–3. (continued)

Year	First author	Title	What was studied
2001	Farooq (115)	Combined Carotid Endarterectomy and Coronary Bypass: A Decade Experience at UCLA	Combined procedures (CEA and CABG)
2001	Gaudino (97)	Should Severe Monolateral Asymptomatic Carotid Artery Stenosis Be Treated at the Time of Coronary Artery Bypass Operation?	• Pts w/SMACS >80% • CABG ($n = 73$) vs. CEA + CABG ($n = 66$) • CEA/CABG pts divided into two groups: (1) Staged (CEA then CABG, pts w/stable angina, $n = 20$) (2) Concurrent (same operating room visit, CEA before sternotomy, pts w/unstable angina $n = 46$)
2001	Hamulu (98)	Coronary Artery Bypass and Carotid Endarterectomy	Combined approach vs. isolated CABG • 88 pts w/coronary artery and carotid artery disease underwent combined coronary artery surgery and CEA • Demographics and perioperative variables of the study pts undergoing combined procedures were compared with those of 266 pts undergoing isolated coronary artery surgery

. of pts	Outcomes	Conclusions
43	• 34 pts (79%) with asymptomatic carotid stenosis • Neurological events occurred in 5 postop pts (11.5%) • TIA occurred in 2 pts, both from the asymptomatic carotid group (4.6%) • Stroke occurred in 3 pts (6.9%): 1 from the asymptomatic CEA (2.9%) and 2 from the symptomatic group stroke (22%) • In-hospital death occurred in 3 pts (6.9%) • No stroke-related deaths • Hospital stay averaged 16 days, (range 4–80) • Combined stroke and death rate was 13.8% • Stroke-free and cumulative survival were 82% and 89%, respectively, at 36 mo using life-table analysis	• The incidence of stroke is increased after CABG in pts with known high-grade carotid stenoses Performance of the combined procedure in pts with asymptomatic carotid stenosis can be reserved for those considered at excessive cardiac risk for an isolated procedure • Contralateral high-grade or occluded internal carotid arteries support more aggressive treatment with a combined procedure Long-term benefit from the combined procedure can be achieved in these pts
139	• Similar postop incidence of neurological events between the CABG-only group and CEA groups • Two in-hospital deaths occurred among the 139 pts (one in each group; $P = $ NS), both noncardiac or -cerebral related • No significant difference between the two groups found in terms of the incidence of major postoperative cx (MI, ARF, bleeding) and the mean ICU or hospital stay • Dyslipidemia and hypertension strongly associated w/the occurrence of stroke and TIA during follow-up in pts in whom the carotid lesion was left untouched	Concomitant treatment (either staged or simultaneous) of SMACS at the time of CABG does not influence the in-hospital results, but confers significant neurological protection during the years after the operation • Prophylactic benefit of carotid surgery is particularly evident in hypertensive and dyslipidemic cases • Logistic and economic considerations favor the performance of the carotid operation during the same hospitalization • CABG pts with SMACS who are hypertensive and/or dyslipidemic represent a particular subgroup of cases at very high cerebrovascular risk
88	• Pts in the combined CABG/CEA group were elderly pts ($P = .0001$) w/higher prevalence of women ($P = .0001$), LV dysfunction ($P = .006$), LM CAD ($P = .033$), triple-vessel CAD ($P = .002$), unstable angina pectoris ($P = .004$), and w/o prior neurologic events ($P = .0001$) • Three (3.4%) pts in the combined group and 5 (1.9%) pts in the CABG group ($P = .317$) developed periop MI • Two (2.3%) pts in the combined group developed a permanent postop neuro event • Hospital mortality was 5.7% (5 pts) in the combined CABG/CEA and 1.5% (4 pts) in the CABG group ($P = .046$)	• This study supports the performance of concomitant CEA and CABG in this high-risk population with severe coexistent disease • This strategy reduces the short-term risk of treatment of either disease alone and the cost of subsequent hospitalization required for a second operation

— *continued next page*

TABLE 3–3. (continued)

Year	First author	Title	What was studied
2002	Antunes (116)	Staged Carotid and Coronary Surgery for Concomitant Carotid and Coronary Artery Disease	Staged CEA + CABG • 77 (2.1%) of 3633 consecutive pts who were referred for isolated coronary surgery were found to have significant carotid disease (>70%) and underwent staged CEA and CABG • The mean age was 65.2 ± 5.9 years, and 66 (85.7%) were men • 84.4% had triple vessel and 19.4% had LM disease • Carotid disease was unilateral 71 pts (92.2%) and bilateral in 6 (7.8%), and 57 (74.0%) were asymptomatic
2003	Dworschak (113)	The Impact of Asymptomatic Carotid Artery Disease on the Intraoperative Course of Coronary Artery Bypass Surgery	Whether routinely determined carotid duplex results, beyond detecting high-risk pts, additionally influence intraoperative course 50% cut-off for the definition of significant carotid artery stenosis No stenosis (n = 89) Stenosis (n = 19)
2003	Vitali (117)	Combined Surgical Approach to Coexistent Carotid and Coronary Artery Disease: Early and Late Results	Retrospective review of the records and follow-up data of 139 consecutive pts undergoing simultaneous CABG and CEA
2004	Guibaud (108)	Extracorporeal Circulation as an Additional Method for Cerebral Protection in Simultaneous Carotid Endarterectomy and Coronary Artery Surgical Revascularization	Retrospective review of 124 pts undergoing simultaneous CEA + CABG between January 1994 and December 2001 Group 1: CEA was performed prior to ECC in 65 pts (mean age: 70.4 y; sex ratio: 49 men/16 women) Group 2: CEA performed under ECC, prior to CABG in 59 pts (mean age: 69.9 y; sex ratio: 46 men/13 women)

). of pts	Outcomes	Conclusions
77	83 isolated CEAs were performed: • no deaths • two strokes (2.4%) • three (3.6%) MIs • mean admission time was 6.0 ± 3.5 days For coronary surgery: • 1 pt (1.3%) died, two cases (2.6%) of MI, and three strokes (3.9%) Hence, overall rates: • Periop mortality = 1.3% • MI = 6.3% • Stroke = 6.3% • Mean admission time was 8.3 ± 6 days	Staging of CEA + CABG resulted in low global periop morbidity and mortality
108	Higher incidence of prior cerebrovascular events and peripheral artery disease in carotid artery stenosis pts ($P < .05$) • Pulsatile flow was used more frequently in this group ($P < .05$) • Avoided severe hyperventilation, hyperglycemia, hemodilution, hyperthermia, and lactic acidosis • Labile hemodynamics of carotid artery stenosis pts required more interventions ($P < .05$) and there was tendency toward greater mortality • Stroke and TIA occurred in two pts w/o carotid artery stenosis	Carotid artery stenosis may be indicative of a compromised cardiovascular control system and could result in increased in-hospital mortality
139	• Early mortality was 2.1% • Perioperative MI and stroke rates were 2.8% and 1.4%, respectively • Survival at 7 years was 74.7 ± 5.1%, and event-free survival at 7 years was 67.9 ± 5.6%	Combined surgical approach is effective and safe, allowing the treatment of both diseases in a single operative procedure
124	• Overall hospital mortality was 7.3% (9/124): cardiac-related in 5 pts, stroke in 2 pts • Univariate analysis demonstrated overweight status, unstable angina, and emergency to be significant risk factors • Bilateral carotid stenosis was a significant risk factor of neurologic event when CEA performed prior to ECC ($P < .05$) • In Group 1, mortality was 9.2% (6/65), and the incidence of neurologic events was 10.7% (7/65) and was responsible for two of the early deaths in pts with bilateral carotid stenosis	Hospital mortality in pts undergoing simultaneous CEA and CABGs was mainly cardiac-related The combined approach appears to be mandatory, when carotid stenosis, even asymptomatic, was hemodynamically significant, or with ulcerative lesions likely to be responsible for embolism CEA, first performed under ECC, appears to be a safe procedure, combining, in terms of cerebral protection, the benefits previously called up

— *continued next page*

TABLE 3–3. (continued)

Year	First author	Title	What was studied
2004 (cont.)	Guibaud (108) (cont.)		
2004	Mishra (107)	Concomitant Carotid Endarterectomy and Coronary Bypass Surgery: Outcome of On-Pump and Off-Pump Techniques	Reviewed results of CABG using conventional cardiopulmonary bypass (CPB) or off-pump techniques and CEA done as a combined procedure 166 pts (Group 1) had off-pump CABG whereas in 192 pts (Group 2) the procedure was done using conventional CPB CEA performed before CABG in both groups
2005	Akins (118)	Late Results of Combined Carotid and Coronary Surgery Using Actual vs. Actuarial Methodology	Concomitant CEA + CABG
2005	Chiappini (119)	Simultaneous Carotid and Coronary Arteries Disease: Staged or Combined Surgical Approach?	Staged vs. Combined surgical approach Group 1 (140 pts) CABG and CEA were performed simultaneously Group 2 (62 pts) CABG and CEA were performed as two-staged procedures

. of pts	Outcomes	Conclusions
	In Group 2, mortality was 5.1% (3/59) but never related to CEA, and the neurologic morbidity was 1.7% (1 TIA)	ECC, because of full heparinization, hemodilution, pulsatile flow, and hypothermia, could provide better cerebral protection during CEA
358	• 2 deaths (1.2%) in Group 1 and 3 deaths (1.6%) in Group 2 ($P = .870$) • No ptt from Group 1 and 1 patient (0.5%) from Group 2 had postop stroke ($P = .941$) • Mean hospital stay was 9.0 ± 1.2 days in Group 1 and 11.2 ± 1.7days in Group 2 ($P < .001$) • At mean follow-up of 2.8 ± 0.9 years in Group 1, 2 pts (1.2%) had late death caused by cardiac failure and contralateral CEA was done in 2 pts (1.2%) Group 2 had mean follow-up of 2.4 ± 0.6 years, during which 4 pts (2.1%) had late death, and contralateral CEA was done in 3 pts (1.6%) • Late stroke was seen in 1 ptt (0.6%) from Group 1 and 2 pts (1.0%) from Group 2	No difference seen between on- and off-pump CABG Concomitant CEA and CABG is a safe and effective procedure in pts with significant coronary and carotid artery disease Equally good results can be reproduced using CPB or off-pump techniques for coronary artery surgery, with low morbidity, mortality, and good long-term results
500	Hospital mortality = 3.6% • Predictors of hospital death: preop TIA, MI, nonelective operation Periop stroke = 4.6% • Predictors: PVD, use RIMA for CABG TIA = 1.6% Periop MI = 2% • Predictors: operative IABP, previous CABG, preop stroke Mean hospital stay = 11 days • Predictors of prolonged hospital stay: failure to use LIMA, periop stroke, advanced age	Concomitant carotid and coronary artery surgery is safe and effective, particularly in preventing ipsilateral stroke, and neutralizes the impact of unilateral carotid stenosis on early and late stroke
202	• Rate of postop stroke was 6.4% in Group 1 (9/140) vs. 4.8% in Group 2 (3/62) • Significant univariate predictors of MI were smoking history and previous MI • Significant univariate predictors for stroke were age >70 y and a smoking history • Significant univariate predictors of death were the operative approach, the low EF, smoking history, ARF, and PVD The hospital mortality was 6.4% in Group 1 vs. 12.9% in Group 2	Management of these pts needs careful pre-, intra-, and postoperative assessment and timing aimed at reducing the ischemic injuries, both cerebral and cardiac

TABLE 3–3. (continued)

Year	First author	Title	What was studied
2007	Dubinsky (99)	Mortality from Combined Carotid Endarterectomy and Coronary Artery Bypass Surgery in the US	Combined CEA + CABG vs. isolated CABG Same-day CEA + CABG ($n = 1230$) Staged CEA–CABG ($n = 5807$) Isolated CABG ($n = 471,881$) Isolated CEA ($n = 178,959$)
2008	Timaran (111)	Trends and Outcomes of Concurrent Carotid Revascularization and Coronary Bypass	Concurrent carotid (either CEA or carotid artery stenting) and coronary revascularization procedures

IMA = internal mammary artery; DOS = day of surgery; MSR = mean stroke rate; MMR = mean m
left internal mammary artery

o. of pts	Outcomes	Conclusions
657, 877	• 15.6% w/postop stroke died • OR for the combined outcomes of postop stroke or death for same-day CEA–CABG compared w/CABG was 2.16 (95% CI, 1.78–2.62, $P < .0001$) OR for combined outcome of postop stroke or death for all combined CEA–CABG was 2.25 (95% CI, 2.08 –2.44, $P < .0001$) • no change over time in the rate of postop stroke or death in combined CEA–CABG group • adjusted OR for CEA–CABG combined, age >65 y, urban, nonteaching hospital, and Charlson index were all >1, indicating that these factors were associated with higher in-hospital mortality and postop stroke • female sex was associated w/lower in-hospital mortality	38% greater chance of death or postop stroke with combined CEA–CABG Note that residual confounders, such as the degree of carotid stenosis or severity or previous stroke, could account for the increased risk The largest contributions by individual comorbidities were age <65 y and previous stroke Being female was slightly protective
27, 084	27,084 concurrent carotid revascularizations and CABG were done • 96.7% (26,197 pts) underwent CEA–CABG • 3.3% (887 pts) had carotid stenting–CABG Pts undergoing carotid stenting–CABG had fewer major adverse events than those undergoing CEA–CABG • Carotid stenting–CABG pts had lower incidence of postop stroke (2.4% vs. 3.9%) • Lower incidence of combined stroke and death (6.9% vs. 8.6%) than the combined CEA–CABG group ($P < .001$) • In-hospital death rates were similar (5.2% vs. 5.4%) • After risk stratification, CEA–CABG pts had a 62% increased risk of postop stroke compared w/pts undergoing carotid stenting before CABG • No differences in the risk of combined stroke and death were observed (OR, 1.26; 95% CI, 0.9–1.6, P = NS)	Pts who undergo carotid stenting–CABG have significantly decreased in-hospital stroke rates compared with pts undergoing CEA–CABG but similar in-hospital mortality Carotid stenting may provide a safer carotid revascularization option for pts who require CABG

NS = not significant; ARF = acute renal failure; RIMA = Right internal mammary artery; LIMA =

groups. However, there was a considerable degree of long-term neurological protection conferred by the carotid surgery, especially in patients who were hypertensive and dyslipidemic. This protection is similar to that seen in the ACAS (82) and similar trials of CEA for asymptomatic stenosis (see "Stroke Prevention by CEA" section earlier in this chapter).

The combined procedure is associated with some downsides. For example, the combined procedure may result in significant "stress" on the both the cerebrovascular and cardiovascular systems. While Hamulu et al. (98) found that combined CABG and CEA was associated with a lower risk of neurologic complications, there was also a higher risk of death and perioperative MI than in isolated coronary artery surgery. Dubinsky and Lai (99) examined mortality in patients undergoing isolated CABG versus those undergoing the staged CEA–CABG or combined CEA–CABG. They found a 38% greater chance of death or postoperative stroke in patients having both procedures as opposed to isolated CABG. However, they argued that residual confounders, such as the degree of carotid stenosis or severity of previous stroke, could account for the increased risk. They found that the largest contributors to mortality and perioperative stroke to be age >65 years and previous stroke. Review of a large series of patients ($n = 702$) who underwent synchronous CEA and CABG for hemodynamically significant (>70%) asymptomatic carotid artery stenosis and CAD studied for 25 years provides some interesting insights. Seven (1%) permanent nonfatal neurologic deficits occurred in this series (one woman, six men). The combined stroke/mortality was 4.3%. This results compares to a 30-day stroke/mortality of 6.1% in 132 symptomatic combined CEA–CABG patients (100).

Many studies highlight the fact that combined CABG and CEA are performed in higher-risk populations, with many patients having multiple coexisting comorbidities such as poorly controlled hypertension, diabetes mellitus, renal insufficiency, and peripheral occlusive vascular disease, which further complicate surgical and medical management (99–104). Although combined procedures are sometimes criticized for increased morbidity and mortality, these procedures are often reserved for urgent cases in the sickest patients with bilateral or symptomatic carotid artery stenosis. These procedures are often performed in patients with unstable angina or poor cardiac markers, poor LV function or LM disease. Therefore, this selection bias may influence the incidence of preoperative complications using the combined technique.

An additional source of significant bias stemming from the often urgent presentation of patients selected for combined CEA–CABG surgery is the inadequacy of preoperative medical management. For example, antiplatelet therapy and statin therapy can profoundly reduce the risk of periprocedural stroke and MI if there is time to initiate the therapy before proceeding with surgery. In urgent and emergent situations, this preoperative management may not be possible.

Strategies to Reduce Stroke in Combined Procedures

Because of the potential increase in risk of stroke, MI, prolonged hospital stay, or death using the combined technique, a more careful identification of possible perioperative risk factors is critical to our understanding. Examining factors such as significant ascending aortic atheromatous disease or mural thrombus resulting in carotid artery embolism may help to identify patients at increased risk. Atheromatous disease of the ascending aorta is an important contributor to the risk of perioperative stroke and may be detected intraoperatively by transesophageal echocardiography (TEE) or epiaortic scanning (105). Of note, epiaortic imaging has been found to be superior to TEE and palpation as a means of assessing ascending aortic atheromatous disease (106). This assessment may lead to the identification of high-risk patients and provide the opportunity to revise the surgical approach to minimize the risk of postoperative stroke from CABG. The alternative techniques include femoral arterial cannulation, proximal anastomoses during cardioplegic arrest, or performing off-pump procedures in selected patients.

There are many studies examining different surgical techniques to improve the perioperative outcome during combined CEA–CABG. Mishra et al. (107) examined 358 patients undergoing concurrent CEA and CABG using CPB versus the off-pump technique. Using stroke, mean hospital stay, and death as endpoints, they found no difference between on- and off-pump techniques. However whether the off-pump technique may prove to be more favorable in terms of perioperative complications needs a larger cohort for further evaluation.

In 2004, Guibaud et al. (108) considered that extracorporeal circulation (ECC) could provide better cerebral protection during carotid revascularization due to hypothermia, heparinization, hemodilution, and the pulsatile flow of the CPB circuit. They postulated that hypothermia ≤28°C during the period of carotid clamping time would be the optimal method for cerebral protection when cerebrovascular blood flow supply is reduced because of significant carotid occlusive disease. They found that both mortality and neurologic morbidity was reduced in patients who underwent concurrent CEA–CABG with the CEA performed during ECC as opposed to before ECC. In the group that underwent CEA during ECC, mortality was 5.1% (and interestingly not related to CEA), whereas the neurologic morbidity was 1.7% (one patient had a TIA). In the group that underwent CEA prior to ECC, mortality was

9.2%, and the incidence of neurologic events was 10.7% (one patient had a TIA, and five others had a stroke). Both the decreased incidence of neurologic morbidity and mortality with CEA performed under ECC were found to be statistically significant. However, this study was retrospective, consisted of only 124 subjects, and covered a 7-year period (1994–2001) when perioperative therapy dramatically changed. Consequently, a larger randomized trial with strict preoperative medical management is needed to confirm the decreased stroke risk of CEA done during CPB with cooling.

Risk Reduction in Combined Carotid and LM Disease

As described above, patients with carotid and LM disease are at significant perioperative risk. Patients with severe carotid disease may also have severe atherosclerotic disease in other vascular systems, such as the coronary arterial system and LM disease. The outcome of undiagnosed LM disease in patients undergoing carotid revascularization can be devastating as evidenced in a case study of a cardiovascular collapse during an elective CEA (109). The exact incidence of coexisting carotid artery stenosis and LM disease is unclear. In a study by Doonan et al. (12), 2099 patients underwent coronary angiograms and carotid artery ultrasounds. Of this group, there were 186 patients found to have LM disease and 1913 patients without LM disease. Patients with significant LM disease were found to have significant carotid stenosis (defined as >60%) more frequently as compared with patients without LM disease (31.2% vs. 15.2%, $P < .0001$).

To address this unique cohort, Allie et al. (110) examined the perioperative use of IABP during staged CEA–CABG as an option to decrease the risks and increase the safety of the staged CEA–CABG procedure in subjects with LM disease. An IABP was placed 1 day prior to CEA and, less than 24 hours later, coronary revascularization was performed on cardiopulmonary bypass and the IABP was removed afterward with a total IABP duration of approximately 36 hours. They found no 30-day postoperative MI, neurologic, vascular, or other major complication or deaths, but they had a cohort of only 20 patients. The specific population for which the insertion of the IABP may be of benefit requires further evaluation.

Combined CABG and Carotid Stenting

Although many of the studies examine carotid revascularization by surgical endarterectomy, the role of CAS also requires careful examination. It may provide a safe alternative when used as part of combined therapy. Timaran et al. (111) performed a large population-based, retrospective study examining outcomes of patients who underwent simultaneous carotid artery revascularizations and CABG (n = 27,084): 26,197 patients or 96.7% underwent combined CEA and CABG, whereas 887 patients or 3.3% underwent CAS prior to CABG. The study found that patients undergoing CAS–CABG had fewer major adverse events than those undergoing CEA–CABG. Patients who underwent CAS–CABG were also found to have a lower incidence of postoperative stroke (2.4% vs. 3.9%) and a lower incidence of combined stroke and death than the combined CEA–CABG group (6.9% vs. 8.6%, $P < .001$). After risk-stratification, the CEA–CABG patients had a 62% greater risk of postoperative stroke than the patients who underwent CAS–CABG. The in-hospital death rates were found to be similar (5.2% vs. 5.4%), and no differences in the overall risk of combined stroke and death were observed (OR, 1.26, P = not significant). As a result, CAS may provide an alternative option for carotid revascularization in patients who require CABG and have associated significant carotid artery disease. However, because there was no randomization as part of this study design, it could be biased because the patients with more difficult carotid anatomy were assigned to CEA. Coronary angioplasty and stenting of multivessel CAD and even LM disease is increasing, and may represent an alternative to CABG in high-risk patients (112). However, additional studies will be needed to determine whether and when to elect to perform PCI of carotid and/or coronary lesions in these complex clinical situations.

An additional concern must be recognized by the anesthesiologist caring for the patient with combined carotid stenosis and coronary disease. Whether the patient undergoes staged procedures or has isolated cardiac surgery, the patient with severe carotid disease is at risk for significant hemodynamic instability *as a result of the carotid disease alone*. Patients with carotid artery stenosis have lability in heart rate, blood pressure, and perfusion for a number of reasons, including impact of the carotid disease on baroreceptor responsiveness. Dworschak et al. (113) examined the records of 108 consecutive patients who underwent elective or urgent CABG surgery. All of these patients had preoperative carotid ultrasonography performed and were without new signs of an impaired cerebral circulation. The researchers found that labile hemodynamics of patients with carotid artery stenosis required more corrective interventions ($P < 0.05$), and also there was a tendency toward greater mortality. The mere presence of asymptomatic carotid artery disease has been associated with intraoperative hemodynamic instability and coexisting vascular disease, which may complicate surgery. Carotid artery stenosis may also be a marker of a compromised cardiovascular system, which may result in increased perioperative complications and increased in-hospital mortality.

CONCLUSION

The approach to coexisting CAD and carotid artery disease should focus on protecting both the cerebrovascular and cardiovascular systems. The surgical options vary from a simultaneous (same anesthetic) procedures to a staged procedure, where carotid revascularization, usually endarterectomy, is performed prior to coronary revascularization, or a reverse staged approach in which CABG precedes the CEA. Each of these methods has advantages and disadvantages, which can be defined based on the incidence of stroke, MI, and death but require careful analysis of the data to determine the relevance of published studies to individual clinical practice decisions. High-grade (>70%) unilateral carotid stenosis or bilateral carotid stenosis supports aggressive treatment with a combined procedure to decrease the risk of stroke. Staged techniques may be reserved for patients with severe carotid stenosis with single-vessel CAD or preserved LV function. The role of CAS is also an important consideration and will require further study to document both its value and the clinical implications in management of patients with carotid artery disease and CAD. The overall goal of any of these approaches is to decrease the risk of both cerebral and coronary ischemic injuries and death. The lack of randomized trials makes it difficult to draw firm conclusions regarding the best management strategy. Ultimately, the surgical technique should be individualized for each patient by careful consideration of each patient's cardiovascular and cerebrovascular status and other existing comorbidities that may contribute to their perioperative and long-term outcome.

REFERENCES

1. Bernhard VM, Johnson WD, Peterson JJ: Carotid artery stenosis. Association with surgery for coronary artery disease. Arch Surg 1972; 105:837–40
2. Gardner TJ, Horneffer PJ, Manolio TA, et al.: Stroke following coronary artery bypass grafting: a ten-year study. Ann Thorac Surg 1985; 40:574–81
3. John R, Choudhri AF, Weinberg AD, et al.: Multicenter review of preoperative risk factors for stroke after coronary artery bypass grafting.[see comment]. Ann Thorac Surg 2000; 69:30–5; discussion 5–6
4. Roach GW, Kanchuger M, Mangano CM, et al.: Adverse cerebral outcomes after coronary bypass surgery. Multicenter Study of Perioperative Ischemia Research Group and the Ischemia Research

and Education Foundation Investigators [see comment]. N Engl J Med 1996; 335:1857–63

5. Selnes OA, McKhann GM: Neurocognitive complications after coronary artery bypass surgery. Ann Neurol 2005; 57:615–21

6. Coward LJ, Featherstone RL, Brown MM: Safety and efficacy of endovascular treatment of carotid artery stenosis compared with carotid endarterectomy: a Cochrane systematic review of the randomized evidence [see comment]. Stroke 2005; 36:905–11

7. Rajamani K, Chaturvedi S: Surgery insight: carotid endarterectomy—which patients to treat and when? Nat Clin Pract Cardiovasc Med 2007; 4:621–9

8. Ferguson GG, Eliasziw M, Barr HW, et al.: The North American Symptomatic Carotid Endarterectomy Trial: surgical results in 1415 patients [see comment]. Stroke 1999; 30:1751–8

9. Eagle KA, Berger PB, Calkins H, et al.: ACC/AHA guideline update for perioperative cardiovascular evaluation for noncardiac surgery—executive summary: a report of the American College of Cardiology/American Heart Association Task Force on Practice Guidelines (Committee to Update the 1996 Guidelines on Perioperative Cardiovascular Evaluation for Noncardiac Surgery) [erratum appears in J Am Coll Cardiol 2006 Jun 6; 47(11):2356]. J Am Coll Cardiol 2002; 39:542–53

10. Salasidis GC, Latter DA, Steinmetz OK, et al.: Carotid artery duplex scanning in preoperative assessment for coronary artery revascularization: the association between peripheral vascular disease, carotid artery stenosis, and stroke. J Vasc Surg 1995; 21:154–60; discussion 61–2

11. Berens ES, Kouchoukos NT, Murphy SF, Wareing TH: Preoperative carotid artery screening in elderly patients undergoing cardiac surgery. J Vasc Surg 1992; 15:313–21; discussion 22–3

12. Doonan AL, Karha J, Carrigan TP, et al.: Presence of carotid and peripheral arterial disease in patients with left main disease. Am J Cardiol 2007; 100:1087–9

13. Vigneswaran WT, Sapsford RN, Stanbridge RD: Disease of the left main coronary artery: early surgical results and their association with carotid artery stenosis. Br Heart J 1993; 70:342–5

14. Kallikazaros I, Tsioufis C, Sideris S, et al.: Carotid artery disease as a marker for the presence of severe coronary artery disease in patients evaluated for chest pain [see comment]. Stroke 1999; 30: 1002–7

15. Fusari M, Parolari A, Agostinelli A, et al.: Coronary and major vascular disease: aggressive screening and priority-based therapy. Cardiovasc Surg 2000; 8:22–30

16. Kallikazaros IE, Tsioufis CP, Stefanadis CI, et al.: Closed relation between carotid and ascending aortic atherosclerosis in cardiac patients. Circulation 2000; 102:III263–8
17. Chambless LE, Heiss G, Folsom AR, et al.: Association of coronary heart disease incidence with carotid arterial wall thickness and major risk factors: the Atherosclerosis Risk in Communities (ARIC) Study, 1987–1993. Am J Epidemiol 1997; 146:483–94
18. Selim M: Perioperative stroke [see comment]. N Engl J Med 2007; 356:706–13
19. Gottesman RF, Wityk RJ: Brain injury from cardiac bypass procedures. Semin Neurol 2006; 26:432–9
20. Das SK, Brow TD, Pepper J: Continuing controversy in the management of concomitant coronary and carotid disease: an overview. Int J Cardiol 2000; 74:47–65
21. Bronster DJ: Neurologic complications of cardiac surgery: current concepts and recent advances. Curr Cardiol Rep 2006; 8:9–16
22. Naylor AR: A critical review of the role of carotid disease and the outcomes of staged and synchronous carotid surgery. Semin Cardiothorac Vasc Anesth 2004; 8:37–42
23. Naylor AR, Mehta Z, Rothwell PM, Bell PRF: Carotid artery disease and stroke during coronary artery bypass: a critical review of the literature. Eur J Vasc Endovasc Surg 2002; 23:283–94
24. Bravata DM, Gienger AL, McDonald KM, et al.: Systematic review: the comparative effectiveness of percutaneous coronary interventions and coronary artery bypass graft surgery [see comment]. Ann Intern Med 2007; 147:703–16
25. Holt PJE, Poloniecki JD, Loftus IM, Thompson MM: Meta-analysis and systematic review of the relationship between hospital volume and outcome following carotid endarterectomy. Eur J Vasc Endovasc Surg 2007; 33:645–51
26. Chambers BR, Donnan GA: Carotid endarterectomy for asymptomatic carotid stenosis [update of Cochrane Database Syst Rev 2000;(2):CD001923; PMID: 10796451]. Cochrane Database of Syst Rev 2005:CD001923
27. Bond R, Rerkasem K, Cuffe R, Rothwell PM: A systematic review of the associations between age and sex and the operative risks of carotid endarterectomy. Cerebrovasc Dis 2005; 20:69–77
28. Bond R, Rerkasem K, Shearman CP, Rothwell PM: Time trends in the published risks of stroke and death due to endarterectomy for symptomatic carotid stenosis. Cerebrovasc Dis 2004; 18:37–46
29. Bond R, Rerkasem K, Rothwell PM: Systematic review of the risks of carotid endarterectomy in relation to the clinical indication for and timing of surgery [see comment]. Stroke 2003; 34:2290–301

30. Tu JV, Wang H, Bowyer B, et al.: Risk factors for death or stroke after carotid endarterectomy: observations from the Ontario Carotid Endarterectomy Registry [see comment]. Stroke 2003; 34:2568–73

31. White CJ, Iyer SS, Hopkins LN, et al.: Carotid stenting with distal protection in high surgical risk patients: the BEACH trial 30 day results. Catheter Cardiovasc Interv 2006; 67:503–12

32. CaRESS Steering Committee. Carotid revascularization using endarterectomy or stenting systems (CaRESS) phase I clinical trial: 1-year results. J Vasc Surg 2005; 42:213–9

33. Gray WA, Yadav JS, Verta P, et al.: The CAPTURE registry: predictors of outcomes in carotid artery stenting with embolic protection for high surgical risk patients in the early post-approval setting. Catheter Cardiovasc Interv 2007; 70:1025–33

34. Endovascular versus surgical treatment in patients with carotid stenosis in the Carotid and Vertebral Artery Transluminal Angioplasty Study (CAVATAS): a randomised trial [see comment]. Lancet 2001; 357:1729–37

35. Gurm HS, Yadav JS, Fayad P, et al.: Long-term results of carotid stenting versus endarterectomy in high-risk patients. N Engl J Med 2008; 358:1572–9

36. Yadav JS, Wholey MH, Kuntz RE, et al.: Protected carotid-artery stenting versus endarterectomy in high-risk patients [see comment]. N Engl J Med 2004; 351:1493–501

37. Group SC, Ringleb PA, Allenberg J, et al.: 30 day results from the SPACE trial of stent-protected angioplasty versus carotid endarterectomy in symptomatic patients: a randomised non-inferiority trial [see comment] [erratum appears in Lancet 2006 Oct 7; 368(9543):1238]. Lancet 2006; 368:1239–47

38. Mas J-L, Chatellier G, Beyssen B, et al.: Endarterectomy versus stenting in patients with symptomatic severe carotid stenosis [see comment]. N Engl J Med 2006; 355:1660–71

39. Investigators E-S. Endarterectomy vs. Angioplasty in Patients with Symptomatic Severe Carotid Stenosis (EVA-3S) Trial. Cerebrovasc Dis 2004; 18:62–5.

40. Mas JL, Chatellier G, Beyssen B, Investigators E-S: Carotid angioplasty and stenting with and without cerebral protection: clinical alert from the Endarterectomy Versus Angioplasty in Patients With Symptomatic Severe Carotid Stenosis (EVA-3S) trial [see comment]. Stroke 2004; 35:e18–20

41. Lindblad B, Persson NH, Takolander R, Bergqvist D: Does low-dose acetylsalicylic acid prevent stroke after carotid surgery? A double-blind, placebo-controlled randomized trial. Stroke 1993; 24:1125–8

42. Taylor DW, Barnett HJ, Haynes RB, et al.: Low-dose and high-dose acetylsalicylic acid for patients undergoing carotid endarterectomy: a randomised controlled trial. ASA and Carotid Endarterectomy (ACE) Trial Collaborators [see comment]. Lancet 1999; 353:2179–84

43. Chaturvedi S, Yadav JS: The role of antiplatelet therapy in carotid stenting for ischemic stroke prevention [see comment]. Stroke 2006; 37:1572–7

44. Yusuf S, Zhao F, Mehta SR, et al.: Effects of clopidogrel in addition to aspirin in patients with acute coronary syndromes without ST-segment elevation [see comment] [erratum appears in N Engl J Med 2001 Dec 6; 345(23):1716]. N Engl J Med 2001; 345:494–502

45. Fox KAA, Mehta SR, Peters R, et al.: Benefits and risks of the combination of clopidogrel and aspirin in patients undergoing surgical revascularization for non-ST-elevation acute coronary syndrome: the Clopidogrel in Unstable angina to prevent Recurrent ischemic Events (CURE) Trial. Circulation 2004; 110:1202–8

46. Payne DA, Jones CI, Hayes PD, et al.: Beneficial effects of clopidogrel combined with aspirin in reducing cerebral emboli in patients undergoing carotid endarterectomy [see comment]. Circulation 2004; 109:1476–81

47. Anselmino M, Malmberg K, Ohrvik J, et al.: Evidence-based medication and revascularization: powerful tools in the management of patients with diabetes and coronary artery disease: a report from the Euro Heart Survey on diabetes and the heart. Eur J Cardiovasc Prev Rehabil 2008; 15:216–23

48. Khanal S, Obeidat O, Hudson MP, et al.: Active Lipid Management In Coronary Artery Disease (ALMICAD) study. Am J Med 2007; 120:734.e11–7

49. Djaiani GN: Aortic arch atheroma: stroke reduction in cardiac surgical patients. Semin Cardiothorac Vasc Anesth 2006; 10:143–57

50. Aboyans V, Labrousse L, Lacroix P, et al.: Predictive factors of stroke in patients undergoing coronary bypass grafting: statins are protective. Eur J Cardiothorac Surg 2006; 30:300–4

51. Blackburn DF, Dobson RT, Blackburn JL, Wilson TW: Cardiovascular morbidity associated with nonadherence to statin therapy. Pharmacotherapy 2005; 25:1035–43

52. Ali IS, Buth KJ: Preoperative statin use and in-hospital outcomes following heart surgery in patients with unstable angina. Eur J Cardiothorac Surg 2005; 27:1051–6

53. Pan W, Pintar T, Anton J, et al.: Statins are associated with a reduced incidence of perioperative mortality after coronary artery bypass graft surgery. Circulation 2004; 110:II45–9

54. Lazar HL: Role of statin therapy in the coronary bypass patient. Ann Thorac Surg 2004; 78:730–40
55. Anselmino M, Malmberg K, Ohrvik J, et al.: Evidence-based medication and revascularization: powerful tools in the management of patients with diabetes and coronary artery disease: a report from the Euro Heart Survey on diabetes and the heart. Eur J Cardiovasc Prev Rehabil 2008; 15:216–23
56. Dotani MI, Elnicki DM, Jain AC, Gibson CM: Effect of preoperative statin therapy and cardiac outcomes after coronary artery bypass grafting. Am J Cardiol 2000; 86:1128–30
57. Perler BA: The effect of statin medications on perioperative and long-term outcomes following carotid endarterectomy or stenting. Semin Vasc Surg 2007; 20:252–8
58. Perler BA: Should statins be given routinely before carotid endarterectomy? [see comment]. Perspect Vasc Surg Endovasc Ther 2007; 19:240–5
59. McGirt MJ, Perler BA, Brooke BS, et al.: 3-hydroxy-3-methylglutaryl coenzyme A reductase inhibitors reduce the risk of perioperative stroke and mortality after carotid endarterectomy [see comment]. J Vasc Surg 2005; 42:829–36; discussion 36–7
60. Kennedy J, Quan H, Buchan AM, et al.: Statins are associated with better outcomes after carotid endarterectomy in symptomatic patients [see comment]. Stroke 2005; 36:2072–6
61. Kent DM: Improved perioperative outcomes from carotid endarterectomy: yet another statin side effect? [comment]. Stroke 2005; 36:2058–9
62. Ikonomidis I, Stamatelopoulos K, Lekakis J, et al.: Inflammatory and non-invasive vascular markers: the multimarker approach for risk stratification in coronary artery disease. Atherosclerosis 2008; 199:3–11
63. Ky B, Rader DJ: The effects of statin therapy on plasma markers of inflammation in patients without vascular disease. Clin Cardiol 2005; 28:67–70
64. Koenig W, Khuseyinova N: Biomarkers of atherosclerotic plaque instability and rupture. Arterioscler Thromb Vasc Biol 2007; 27:15–26
65. Shah PK: Mechanisms of plaque vulnerability and rupture. J Am Coll Cardiol 2003; 41:15S–22S
66. Emerging Risk Factors Collaberation, Danesh J, Erqou S, et al.: The Emerging Risk Factors Collaboration: analysis of individual data on lipid, inflammatory and other markers in over 1.1 million participants in 104 prospective studies of cardiovascular diseases. Eur J Epidemiol 2007; 22:839–69

67. Scirica BM, Morrow DA: Is C-reactive protein an innocent by-stander or proatherogenic culprit? The verdict is still out [see comment]. Circulation 2006; 113:2128–34; discussion 51.

68. Verma S, Devaraj S, Jialal I: Is C-reactive protein an innocent bystander or proatherogenic culprit? C-reactive protein promotes atherothrombosis [comment]. Circulation 2006; 113:2135–50; discussion 50

69. Danesh J, Wheeler JG, Hirschfield GM, et al.: C-reactive protein and other circulating markers of inflammation in the prediction of coronary heart disease [see comment]. N Engl J Med 2004; 350:1387–97

70. Ridker PM: Inflammatory biomarkers and risks of myocardial infarction, stroke, diabetes, and total mortality: implications for longevity. Nutr Rev 2007; 65:S253–9

71. Osman R, L'Allier PL, Elgharib N, Tardif J-C: Critical appraisal of C-reactive protein throughout the spectrum of cardiovascular disease. Vasc Health Risk Manag 2006; 2:221–37

72. Krupinski J, Turu MM, Slevin M, Martinez-Gonzalez J: Carotid plaque, stroke pathogenesis, and CRP: treatment of ischemic stroke. Curr Cardiol Rep 2008; 10:25–30

73. Patel TN, Shishehbor MH, Bhatt DL: A review of high-dose statin therapy: targeting cholesterol and inflammation in atherosclerosis. Eur Heart J 2007; 28:664–72

74. Kerr R, Stirling D, Ludlam CA. Interleukin 6 and haemostasis. Br J Haematol 2001; 115:3–12

75. Biasucci LM, Liuzzo G, Fantuzzi G, et al.: Increasing levels of interleukin (IL)-1Ra and IL-6 during the first 2 days of hospitalization in unstable angina are associated with increased risk of in-hospital coronary events. Circulation 1999; 99:2079–84

76. Lindmark E, Diderholm E, Wallentin L, Siegbahn A: Relationship between interleukin 6 and mortality in patients with unstable coronary artery disease: effects of an early invasive or noninvasive strategy [see comment]. JAMA 2001; 286:2107–13

77. Diener H-C: The PRoFESS trial: future impact on secondary stroke prevention. Expert Rev Neurother 2007; 7:1085–91

78. Dahlof B: Prevention of stroke in patients with hypertension. Am J Cardiol 2007; 100:17J–24J

79. Chrysant SG: The pathophysiologic role of the brain renin-angiotensin system in stroke protection: clinical implications. J Clin Hypertens 2007; 9:454–9

80. Fletcher GF, Bufalino V, Costa F, et al.: Efficacy of drug therapy in the secondary prevention of cardiovascular disease and stroke. Am J Cardiol 2007; 99:1E–35E

81. Volpe M, Tocci G: Antihypertensive therapy and cerebrovascular protection. Curr Opin Nephrol Hypertens 2006; 15:498–504
82. Endarterectomy for asymptomatic carotid artery stenosis. Executive Committee for the Asymptomatic Carotid Atherosclerosis Study [see comment]. JAMA 1995; 273:1421–8
83. Beneficial effect of carotid endarterectomy in symptomatic patients with high-grade carotid stenosis. North American Symptomatic Carotid Endarterectomy Trial Collaborators [see comment]. N Engl J Med 1991; 325:445–53
84. Rothwell PM, Gutnikov SA, Warlow CP, European Carotid Surgery Trialist's Collaberation. Reanalysis of the final results of the European Carotid Surgery Trial. Stroke 2003; 34:514–23
85. Randomised trial of endarterectomy for recently symptomatic carotid stenosis: final results of the MRC European Carotid Surgery Trial (ECST) [see comment]. Lancet 1998; 351:1379–87
86. Hertzer NR, Lees CD: Fatal myocardial infarction following carotid endarterectomy: three hundred thirty-five patients followed 6–11 years after operation. Ann Surg 1981; 194:212–8
87. McCrory DC, Goldstein LB, Samsa GP, et al.: Predicting complications of carotid endarterectomy. Stroke 1993; 24:1285–91
88. Waigand J, Gross CM, Uhlich F, et al.: Elective stenting of carotid artery stenosis in patients with severe coronary artery disease [see comment]. Eur Heart J 1998; 19:1365–70
89. Gray WA, Yadav JS, Verta P, et al.: The CAPTURE registry: results of carotid stenting with embolic protection in the post approval setting. Catheter Cardiovasc Interv 2007; 69:341–8
90. Sugita J, Cremonesi A, Van Elst F, et al.: European carotid PROCAR Trial: prospective multicenter trial to evaluate the safety and performance of the ev3 Protege stent in the treatment of carotid artery stenosis—1- and 6-month follow-up. J Interv Cardiol 2006; 19:215–21
91. Hlatky MA, Bravata DM: Stents or surgery? New data on the comparative outcomes of percutaneous coronary intervention and coronary artery bypass graft surgery [comment]. Circulation 2008; 118:325–7
92. Wong SH, Wan S, Underwood MJ: Myocardial revascularization: surgery or stenting? Asian Cardiovasc Thorac Ann 2007; 15:264–9
93. Onuma Y, Daemen J, Kukreja N, Serruys P: Revascularization in the high-risk patient: multivessel disease. Minerva Cardioangiol 2007; 55:579–92
94. Taggart DP: Coronary artery bypass graft vs. percutaneous coronary angioplasty: CABG on the rebound? Curr Opin Cardiol 2007; 22:517–23

95. Mercado N, Wijns W, Serruys PW, et al.: One-year outcomes of coronary artery bypass graft surgery versus percutaneous coronary intervention with multiple stenting for multisystem disease: a meta-analysis of individual patient data from randomized clinical trials. J Thorac Cardiovasc Surg 2005; 130:512–9

96. Akins CW, Moncure AC, Daggett WM, et al.: Safety and efficacy of concomitant carotid and coronary artery operations. Ann Thorac Surg 1995; 60:311–7; discussion 8

97. Gaudino M, Glieca F, Luciani N, et al.: Should severe monolateral asymptomatic carotid artery stenosis be treated at the time of coronary artery bypass operation? Eur J Cardiothorac Surg 2001; 19:619–26

98. Hamulu A, Yagdi T, Atay Y, et al.: Coronary artery bypass and carotid endarterectomy: combined approach. Jpn Heart J 2001; 42:539–52

99. Dubinsky RM, Lai SM: Mortality from combined carotid endarterectomy and coronary artery bypass surgery in the US [see comment]. Neurology 2007; 68:195–7

100. Byrne J, Darling RC, 3rd, Roddy SP, et al.: Combined carotid endarterectomy and coronary artery bypass grafting in patients with asymptomatic high-grade stenoses: an analysis of 758 procedures. J Vasc Surg 2006; 44:67–72

101. Bulat C, Alfirevic I, Korda ZA, et al.: Combined surgical approach to carotid and coronary artery disease. Coll Antropol 2008; 32:209–16

102. Giorgetti PL, Odero A, Jr., Poletto GL, Franciosi E: Combined carotid endarterectomy and coronary artery bypass: a still-feasible procedure? [comment]. Stroke 2007; 38:e51

103. Chakravarthy M, Jawali V, Manohar MV, et al.: Combined carotid endarterectomy and off-pump coronary artery bypass surgery under thoracic epidural anesthesia without endotracheal general anesthesia. J Cardiothorac Vasc Anesth 2006; 20:850–2

104. Goksel OS: Combined carotid and coronary surgery: early and late results [comment]. Ann Thorac Surg 2006; 82:1571–2; author reply 2

105. Eagle KA, Guyton RA, Davidoff R, et al.: ACC/AHA 2004 guideline update for coronary artery bypass graft surgery: a report of the American College of Cardiology/American Heart Association Task Force on Practice Guidelines (Committee to Update the 1999 Guidelines for Coronary Artery Bypass Graft Surgery) [see comment] [erratum appears in Circulation 2005 Apr 19; 111(15):2014]. Circulation 2004; 110:e340–437

106. Sylivris S, Calafiore P, Matalanis G, et al.: The intraoperative assessment of ascending aortic atheroma: epiaortic imaging is superior

to both transesophageal echocardiography and direct palpation. J Cardiothorac Vasc Anesth 1997; 11:704–7

107. Mishra Y, Wasir H, Kohli V, et al.: Concomitant carotid endarterectomy and coronary bypass surgery: outcome of on-pump and off-pump techniques. Ann Thorac Surg 2004; 78:2037–42; discussion 42–3

108. Guibaud JP, Roques X, Laborde N, et al.: Extracorporeal circulation as an additional method for cerebral protection in simultaneous carotid endarterectomy and coronary artery surgical revascularization. J Card Surg 2004; 19:415–9

109. Hecker JG, Laslett L, Campbell E, et al.: Case 2–2006: catastrophic cardiovascular collapse during carotid endarterectomy. J Cardiothorac Vasc Anesth 2006; 20:259–68

110. Allie DE, Lirtzman M, Malik AP, et al.: Rapid-staged strategy for concomitant critical carotid and left main coronary disease with left ventricular dysfunction: IABP use. Ann Thorac Surg 1998; 66:1230–5

111. Timaran CH, Rosero EB, Smith ST, et al.: Trends and outcomes of concurrent carotid revascularization and coronary bypass. J Vasc Surg 2008; 48:355–60; discussion 60–1

112. Buszman PE, Kiesz SR, Bochenek A, et al.: Acute and late outcomes of unprotected left main stenting in comparison with surgical revascularization. J Am Coll Cardiol 2008; 51:538–45

113. Dworschak M, Czerny M, Grimm M, et al.: The impact of asymptomatic carotid artery disease on the intraoperative course of coronary artery bypass surgery. Perfusion 2003; 18:15–8

114. Darling RC, 3rd, Dylewski M, Chang BB, et al.: Combined carotid endarterectomy and coronary artery bypass grafting does not increase the risk of perioperative stroke [see comment]. Cardiovasc Surg 1998; 6:448–52

115. Farooq MM, Reil TD, Gelabert HA, et al.: Combined carotid endarterectomy and coronary bypass: a decade experience at UCLA. Cardiovasc Surg 2001; 9:339–44

116. Antunes PE, Anacleto G, de Oliveira JMF, et al.: Staged carotid and coronary surgery for concomitant carotid and coronary artery disease [see comment]. Eur J Cardiothorac Surg 2002; 21:181–6

117. Vitali E, Lanfranconi M, Bruschi G, et al.: Combined surgical approach to coexistent carotid and coronary artery disease: early and late results. Cardiovasc Surg 2003; 11:113–9

118. Akins CW, Hilgenberg AD, Vlahakes GJ, et al.: Late results of combined carotid and coronary surgery using actual versus actuarial methodology [see comment]. Ann Thorac Surg 2005; 80:2091–7

119. Chiappini B, Dell' Amore A, Di Marco L, et al.: Simultaneous carotid and coronary arteries disease: staged or combined surgical approach? J Card Surg 2005; 20:234–40

Kevin W. Hatton, MD
Brenda G. Fahy, MD, FCCM

Glucose Control for the Diabetic Patient Requiring Cardio-thoracic Surgery:

4 | Does It Matter?

INTRODUCTION

Glucose control is an important aspect of the management of the patient undergoing cardiothoracic surgery and has a significant impact on postoperative outcome. Although many of the patients who develop hyperglycemia during or after cardiac surgery have diabetes mellitus (DM), hyperglycemia is a risk for any patient undergoing any major surgical procedure, particularly those procedures associated with cardiopulmonary bypass (CPB).

The anesthesiologist who cares for the cardiothoracic surgical patient should have an understanding of the incidence and clinical manifestations of hyperglycemia and DM to define a management strategy that minimizes the likelihood of complications. DM is characterized principally by hyperglycemia resulting from either inadequate insulin secretion or insulin receptor insensitivity in peripheral tissues. The American Diabetes Association reports DM in about 6% of the general population in the United States representing approximately 18.2 million people (1). The prevalence of DM is increasing worldwide because of multiple environmental and socioeconomic factors (2). DM is associated with significant short-term and chronic morbidity. Regardless of the underlying etiology, DM produces, among many other complications, a two- to four-fold increase in the incidence of cardiovascular diseases and, in fact, the prevalence of DM among patients requiring cardiac surgery has been reported to be as high as 28% (3–6). In addition, as demonstrated in a

Medically Challenging Patients Undergoing Cardiothoracic Surgery, edited by Neal H. Cohen, MD, MPH, MS, Lippincott Williams & Wilkins, Baltimore © 2009.

recent prospective analysis of more than 7000 patients, approximately 5.2% of patients who undergo cardiac surgery may have undiagnosed diabetes prior to surgery (6). As a result, in the United States alone, as many as 166,000 patients with either diagnosed or undiagnosed diabetes undergo cardiac surgery every year (7, 8).

In numerous clinical studies, the diagnosis of DM preoperatively has been shown to be a significant independent risk factor for both increased short-term and long-term morbidity and mortality following cardiac surgery (5, 9–13). Historically, a significant part of this increased morbidity and mortality has been attributed to the associated preoperative comorbid conditions such as obesity, peripheral arterial disease, chronic renal insufficiency, systemic hypertension, and extensive small-vessel atherosclerosis (14). However, the management of perioperative hyperglycemia may also play a role in the outcome after cardiac surgery. Although most of the patients for whom glucose control is important have underlying or previously unrecognized DM, hyperglycemia in the nondiabetic patient also requires careful management. This chapter provides an overview of the incidence of hyperglycemia in the perioperative period, its impact on morbidity and mortality, and a strategy for managing glucose during cardiac surgical procedures.

MORBIDITY AND MORTALITY ASSOCIATED WITH HYPERGLYCEMIA

Morbidity and mortality after cardiac surgery are increased in patients with DM, as well as in nondiabetic patients who develop hyperglycemia in the perioperative period (8, 15–19). A number of studies of varying population groups and glucose management strategies have demonstrated a consistent increase in morbidity and mortality associated with hyperglycemia both intraoperatively and postoperatively in patients who undergo cardiac surgery with or without CPB. A recent retrospective study examined the influence of maximum intraoperative blood glucose levels on mortality after cardiac surgery in both diabetic ($n = 1579$) and nondiabetic ($n = 4701$) patients (15). Hyperglycemia (as defined as blood glucose >270 mg/dL) during CPB was treated with insulin administered by bolus without a standard insulin protocol. Intraoperative hyperglycemia was an independent predictor of in-hospital mortality and morbidity for both diabetic and nondiabetic patients. For each 18 mg/dL (1 mmol/L) increase in blood glucose, the respective odds ratio for in-hospital mortality was 1.20 ($P = .005$) for diabetic and 1.12 ($P < .001$) for nondiabetic patients and for all adverse events was 1.04 ($P = .038$) and 1.06 ($P < .001$) for diabetic and nondiabetic patients, respectively (15).

In a prospective observational study of 200 consecutive diabetic patients undergoing cardiac surgery with CPB, a perioperative insulin protocol was used to optimize glucose control. The insulin infusion was titrated to maintain the glucose below 180 mg/dL intraoperatively and below 140 mg/dL in the intensive care unit (ICU). Patients with poor intraoperative glycemic control (as defined by four consecutive intraoperative blood glucose measurements >200 mg/dL) demonstrated increased in-hospital mortality (11.7% vs. 2.4%, $P < .05$), prolonged ICU length of stay ($P = .001$), and increased rate of severe morbidities compared to patients without intraoperative hyperglycemia (16).

Another observational study that included 409 consecutive cardiac surgery patients, 22.5% of whom had a history of DM ($n = 92$) demonstrated that the mean and maximal intraoperative glucose levels were independent predictors of morbidity and mortality within 30 days after surgery (8). It is important to note, however, that in this study postoperative intensive insulin therapy was not initiated. Nonetheless, the mean intraoperative glucose was a significant predictor for mortality ($P < .01$) as well as pulmonary and renal complications ($P < .01$). Logistic regression analyses revealed that a 20 mg/dL increase in mean intraoperative blood glucose increased (more than 30%) the likelihood of an adverse event (odds ratio, 1.34). This trend continued despite adjustment for confounding variables including postoperative blood glucose. The authors concluded that preoperative diagnosis with DM alone was a significant risk factor for morbidity and mortality ($P = .01$). Finally, the Portland Diabetic Project, which includes a large database of diabetic patients, has identified that hyperglycemia within the first 3 days of cardiac surgery in diabetic patients is independently predictive of increased mortality ($P < .0001$), increased risk of deep sternal wound infection (DSWI) ($P = .0001$), and increased length of hospital stay ($P < .002$) (17). Each of these studies documents that intraoperative hyperglycemia alone is a risk factor for perioperative morbidity and mortality. Although no specific glucose endpoint has been clearly defined, control of hyperglycemia (maintaining glucose at least at a level <200 mg/dL) does reduce the incidence of complications.

POTENTIAL CAUSES FOR INTRAOPERATIVE HYPERGLYCEMIA

Significant intraoperative hyperglycemia can occur both in diabetic and nondiabetic patients undergoing cardiac surgery with or without CPB, particularly when exogenous insulin is not administered (20). The cause for the hyperglycemia is multifactorial. Hyperglycemia is known to occur under hypothermic conditions and as a result of administration of glucose-containing solutions, including those in the CPB prime solution (21). Contact with the lengthy CPB circuit may cause endogenous insulin to bind with the plastic, reducing circulating insulin levels. In addition, a severe systemic inflammatory response initiated by the surgical stress, blood contact with the CPB circuit as well as the ischemia, and subsequent reperfusion associated with the procedure itself may contribute to intraoperative hyperglycemia (22–26). Patients with preexisting DM, reduced left ventricular function, and prolonged CPB exposure seem to have an even greater stress response compared to other cardiac surgery patients (27, 28). Even though CPB is commonly considered the most important stimulus for inflammation, significant inflammation has also been documented in patients who undergo off-pump coronary artery bypass grafting, signifying the importance of the general surgical stress response as a potential cause for hyperglycemia (29). The inflammatory response results in hyperglycemia through a number of pathways. The release of pro-inflammatory cytokines and hormones— including cortisol, glucagon, growth hormone, and various catecholamines (epinephrine and norepinephrine)—causes an increase in hepatic gluconeogenesis, cellular glycogenolysis, and relative peripheral insulin resistance (28, 30).

COMPLICATIONS ASSOCIATED WITH HYPERGLYCEMIA

Hyperglycemia is associated with many potential complications. The change in osmolality associated with elevated glucose creates fluid shifts and may impact cellular function. The most notable impact of hyperglycemia is its influence on perioperative infections. Multiple studies have demonstrated that patients who develop hyperglycemia following cardiac surgery have an increased risk of serious infection, including not only those directly related to the surgical procedure, such as DSWI and other surgical site infections, but also urinary tract infections (28). Patients with preexisting DM appear to be particularly prone to these complications. They have a fourfold increase in infectious risk of DSWI (3.5% incidence in diabetic patients compared to 0.8% in nondiabetic patients) following cardiac surgery (31, 32). The actual reason for this increased rate of infection is not known, although it may be related to chronic comorbid conditions such as chronic hyperglycemia-induced immune dysfunction and small-vessel vasculopathy with local tissue hypoxia (31).

A number of other studies have demonstrated that patients with postoperative hyperglycemia are at significantly increased risk compared to "euglycemic" patients of surgical site infections (33, 34). These infectious complications are presumed to develop based on an acute,

reversible immunologic dysfunction, including reduced polymorphonuclear leukocyte phagocytic function and bactericidal activity (35). The
administration of a continuous insulin infusion following surgery and
continued for 24 hours postoperatively restores polymorphonuclear
leukocyte activity to baseline levels (28, 35). Hyperglycemia following
cardiac surgery also has been demonstrated to reduce polymorphonuclear leukocyte chemotaxis, opsonization, and generalized antioxidant
defense (32). Many of these changes in immune function can be reversed
with the administration of insulin, although the optimal dose and timing remain unclear (28, 36, 37).

PERIOPERATIVE GLUCOSE CONTROL STRATEGIES

As a result of the documented complications associated with hyperglycemia in patients who undergo cardiac surgery, a number of
approaches have been recommended to provide intensive glucose control both intraoperatively and in the postoperative period. The Portland
Diabetic Project probably has the largest database and experience with
glucose management in this patient population. This prospective nonrandomized study includes 5534 diabetic patients who had cardiac surgery. The management strategies used for the patients enrolled in the
study have been modified based on regular reviews of their findings.
Based on their findings, not only have clinical protocols been adjusted,
but the target glucose levels also have been narrowed. In 1992, the target blood glucose level was 150–200 mg/dL and hyperglycemia was
aggressively managed only when the patients were in the ICU after surgery (17). In 1995, these management strategies were modified to include
the intraoperative period. Target glucose levels were intermittently lowered from 125–174 mg/dL (1999–2000), to 100–150 mg/dL (2001–2004),
and (currently) to 70–110 mg/dL (17).

As a result of the changing management strategies, the study provides some insights into the optimal management of glucose in the perioperative period for diabetic patients undergoing cardiac surgery.
Although the study has many limitations, it has provided some interesting data on the impact of glucose management strategies on outcome
after cardiac surgery (14, 33, 38). For example, data from patients who
were treated with continuous insulin infusion were compared with the
outcomes associated with historical controls who received subcutaneous
insulin alone (14). In the analysis of 3554 patients, continuous insulin
infusion independently predicted improved in-hospital survival with a
mortality rate of 2.5% compared to 5.3% for those patients treated with
subcutaneous insulin ($P = .001$) (14). The observed hospital mortality
for the group treated with continuous insulin infusion was lower than

the expected mortality based on the Society of Thoracic Surgeons multivariable risk factor analysis model (14).

Intraoperative Glucose Control

The optimal approach to intraoperative glucose control remains unclear. In a recent prospective randomized controlled trial designed to evaluate whether *intraoperative* tight glycemic control in patients with and without DM could improve outcome, 400 patients (20% of whom were diabetic) undergoing elective cardiac surgery with CPB were evaluated (39). Patients were randomized to receive either intensive insulin therapy titrated to maintain blood glucose levels 80–100 mg/dL or conventional treatment (instituted when blood glucose ≥200 mg/dL) during surgery. Postoperatively all patients received intensive insulin therapy to maintain blood glucose levels 80–100 mg/dL. In the group managed with tight glucose control, there was a trend toward *increased* mortality ($n = 4$ vs. 1, $p = .061$) and a statistically significant increase in stroke incidence ($n = 8$ vs. 1, $p = .020$) (39). This increased morbidity is obviously concerning and warrants further investigation. When the data were analyzed for the diabetic patients alone, intraoperative intensive insulin did not improve either hospital or ICU length of stay ($p = .36$) (39). Based on their findings, the authors concluded that institution of tight glycemic control intraoperatively conferred no significant benefit over tight glycemic control postoperatively—and it may have deleterious effects. Based on limited data and lack of specific protocols for intraoperative management of glucose during cardiac surgery, the optimal approach is not obvious. Because hypoglycemia remains a concern (particularly in anesthetized patients with vascular disease), tight glucose control may impose greater risk than benefit. In contrast, as noted, intraoperative hyperglycemia has associated risks. As a result, attention should be paid to glucose levels during cardiac surgery and CPB, and glucose levels above some threshold (perhaps >150 mg/dL) should be treated. The optimal method for insulin administration is not clear. Additional studies are needed to define the optimal intraoperative target for glucose control and the best method for achieving the target.

Postoperative Glucose Control

In 2001, Van den Berghe and colleagues (40) performed the first prospective randomized controlled trial of intensive insulin therapy in critically ill patients. In this study, 1548 surgical ICU patients were randomized to receive either an "intensive insulin treatment" or "conventional therapy." Interestingly, the majority of these patients (63%) were critically ill following cardiac surgery. Patients received insulin infusions to maintain glucose between 80 and 110 mg/dL in the intensive insulin therapy group; the control group received insulin when glucose exceeded 215 mg/dL in an attempt to keep the glucose between 180 and 200 mg/dL (40). Intensive insulin therapy was associated with reductions in both 12-month mortality (4.6% vs. 8.0%, $P < .04$) and in-hospital hospital mortality (7.2% vs. 10.9%, $P = .01$) (40). In subgroup analysis, patients who stayed in the ICU for more than 5 days had the greatest improvement in mortality with intensive insulin therapy (10.6% vs. 20.2%, $P = .01$) (40). In addition to the survival benefit, intensive insulin therapy reduced morbidity from bloodstream infections by 46%, from acute renal failure requiring dialysis or hemofiltration by 41%, from the mean number of blood transfusions by 50%, and from critical illness polyneuropathy by 44%. Study results may have been impacted by the overall surgical mortality rate; in fact, the control group had an overall mortality rate of 8.0% with the mortality rate for the subgroup of patients who stayed in the ICU more than 5 days greater than 20% (40). Other potential factors that may have impacted the results included a continuous feeding regimen initiated on ICU admission of 200–300 grams of intravenous dextrose followed the next day by enteral, parenteral, or a combined enteral and parenteral nutrition. This study and subsequent studies completed by this research group are commonly referred to as the "Leuven" studies, named for the city in which the primary research hospital is located. Despite these limitations, the outcome of this study has had significant impact on glucose control strategies for both surgical and medical patients requiring ICU care.

Following the success of this initial study in surgical ICU patients, a similar study design was repeated in the medical ICU of the same hospital (41). Intensive insulin therapy in this population (in whom about 17% had DM) resulted in a reduction in mortality for patients who stayed in the ICU for 3 or more days from 52.5% to 43% ($P = .009$) compared to conventional therapy. On day 3, intensive insulin compared to conventional therapy had a nonsignificant trend toward increased mortality in the ICU (3.9% vs. 2.8%, $P = .31$) and in-hospital mortality (4.0% vs. 3.6%, $P = .72$).

Subsequent to the completion of these studies, the same investigator performed a pooled analysis of their data with intense subgroup analysis (42). In the pooled data analysis, intensive insulin therapy reduced overall mortality from 23.6% to 20.4% ($P = .04$). Analysis of diabetic patients alone, however, failed to show a decrease in ICU or in-hospital mortality with intensive insulin therapy. In-hospital mortality did not differ between patients with a mean blood glucose 110–150 mg/dL and patients with a mean blood glucose >150 mg/dL (21.2% vs. 21.6%, $P = .9$); in patients with mean glucose level <100 mg/dL, there was a trend toward increased in-hospital mortality compared to patients with mean glucose level 110–150 mg/dL (26.2% vs. 21.6%, $P = .4$) (42). There was a trend toward reduced morbidity with intensive insulin compared to conventional therapy, in the diabetic patients, including a significant decrease in the incidence of new kidney injury (11 vs. 14 cases) and critical illness polyneuropathy (14 vs. 25 cases). All other large diagnostic subgroups (including cardiovascular disease, respiratory disease, gastrointestinal or hepatic disease, sepsis, and "active malignancy") evaluated in this study demonstrated improved morbidity and mortality with intensive insulin therapy compared to conventional treatment (42). Based on this additional analysis of their data, the investigators concluded that inherent adaptive mechanisms in diabetic patients may limit the positive benefit of intensive insulin therapy and that rapid lowering of glucose levels in diabetic patients with preadmission hyperglycemia might be deleterious. The investigators suggested that, until more data are available, it is prudent to target blood glucose concentration to achieve levels consistent with those maintained by the patient chronically.

In a focused follow-up analysis of the cardiac surgery patients from the original Leuven study, 941 patients (from the original 970 patients), of whom approximately 16.6% had DM (insulin-dependent DM was 5.4%; oral or diet-controlled DM was 11.2%), were assessed for 4-year outcome (43). Patients who received intensive insulin therapy for at least 3 days had reduced 4-year mortality compared to the conventional therapy group (23% vs. 36%, $P = .03$) (43). Interestingly, patients in the intensive insulin therapy group with ICU length of stay of at least 3 days reported a perceived decreased quality of life even though they did not require more medical care after discharge than did those in the control group.

In another retrospective analysis, data for 8727 adult patients who underwent cardiac surgery over an 8-year period were analyzed to determine the highest blood glucose level recorded over the first 60 hours postoperatively to determine the effect of a standardized insulin infusion protocol on glucose control (44). All diabetic patients received an insulin infusion postoperatively with a glucose concentration target of 90–144 mg/dL (5–8 mmol/L). Nondiabetic patients also received insulin infusion by protocol if they developed either one glucose concentration >144 mg/dL (8 mmol/L) or two consecutive glucose concentrations >126 mg/dL (7 mmol/L). The highest blood glucose was used to prospectively classify patients by blood glucose control with "good" (<200 mg/dL), "moderate" (200–250 mg/dL), or "poor" (>250 mg/dL) glycemic control. Increased hospital mortality was associated with both the "moderate" and "poor" blood glucose control groups. The observed mortality rate was 1.8% for the "good" control group, compared to 4.2% for the "moderate" control group (95% confidence interval [CI], 1.25–2.25) and

9.6% for the "poor" control group (95% CI, 2.47–6.15) (44). Poor glucose control was associated with postoperative myocardial infarction (95% CI, 1.74–4.26) and pulmonary and renal complications (95% CI, 1.65–3.12).

A meta-analysis of 34 randomized controlled trials that utilized perioperative insulin infusions (with or without glucose targets) and measured perioperative outcome (during hospitalization or within 30 days of surgery) was recently published (45). In this meta-analysis, treatment groups could receive a variety of intravenous insulin protocols; control groups could receive insulin via an infusion or subcutaneous administration as long as the treatment glucose threshold was greater than the threshold used to initiate intensive therapy. Thirty-four trials met inclusion criteria; the majority included cardiac surgery patients (23 trials). Few trials included patients with a history of diabetes (9 trials). Most trials initiated an insulin infusion during surgery and continued these infusions for a variable length postoperatively. This pooled analysis of 14 trials ($n = 4355$) demonstrated that hospital mortality was reduced with intensive insulin infusion compared to standard treatment regimens (4.5% to 3.1%, 95% CI, 0.51–0.94).

Another meta-analysis of randomized controlled trials evaluated studies in which adult ICU patients were randomly assigned to either a tight glucose control (blood glucose <150 mg/dL using an insulin infusion) or conventional therapy (46). Primary or secondary endpoints for study inclusion were hospital or short-term mortality, septicemia, new need for dialysis, or hypoglycemia. Twenty-nine trials with a total of 8432 patients were included in the analysis. There was no difference in hospital mortality between tight glucose control and traditional care (21.5% vs. 23.5%, 95% CI, 0.85–1.03). No significant difference in mortality could be detected when patients were stratified by type of ICU (surgical, medical, or mixed) or by glucose goal of either very tight control (≤110 mg/dL) or moderately tight glucose control (<150 mg/dL) (46). Tight glucose control was, however, associated with a significantly decreased risk of septicemia compared to conventional therapy (10.9% vs. 13.4%, 95% CI, 0.59–97) although there was no reduction in the need for dialysis (11.2% vs. 12.1%, 95%, CI 0.76–1.20).

Although these studies evaluate somewhat different endpoints, they illustrate a number of potential advantages of intensive insulin therapy in the postoperative period. Subgroup analysis may further delineate specific target populations who might receive the greatest potential positive effects; however, further study to elucidate the optimal (if any) glucose control strategy is still required.

HYPOGLYCEMIA: A RISK OF TIGHT GLYCEMIC CONTROL

One of the major potential complications associated with tight glucose control is hypoglycemia. In addition to the immediate concerns about hypoglycemia, it may also be a significant contributor to mortality and morbidity in these critically ill populations. Because the signs and symptoms associated with hypoglycemia may be masked in the anesthetized or critically ill patient, careful monitoring of glucose is critical when a narrow glucose range is the goal. A number of studies have identified hypoglycemia as a risk and have defined ways to minimize it (47).

A number of studies have documented that the risk of hypoglycemia is increased with the use of intensive insulin therapy in the ICU. In the reported data from the original Leuven protocol (surgical ICU population), the incidence of hypoglycemia (defined as a glucose concentration ≤40 mg/dL) was significantly increased in the intensive insulin therapy group compared to the control [n = 39 (5.1%) versus n = 6 (0.76%)] (40). In the second Leuven protocol, which included medical ICU patients, the incidence of hypoglycemia (also defined as a glucose concentration ≤40 mg/dL) was also significantly higher in the intensive insulin group compared to the conventional therapy group (18.7% vs. 2.8%, $P < .001$) (41). Additionally, the incidence of repeated hypoglycemic episodes was higher in the intensive insulin therapy group compared to the conventional treatment group (3.9% vs. 0.8%, $P < .001$) (41). In a separate, but related, randomized controlled trial of intensive insulin therapy in a mixed medical–surgical unit (utilizing the published protocol and endpoints from the Leuven studies), the incidence of hypoglycemia (defined as a blood glucose ≤40 mg/dL) was also significantly increased to 28.1% in the intensive insulin therapy group versus 3.2% in the control group ($P = .0001$) (48).

Recent randomized controlled trials also have demonstrated that the hypoglycemia has a significant impact on outcome. Mortality is increased when hypoglycemia occurs during intensive insulin therapy (41, 48). Two randomized controlled trials were halted because of hypoglycemia-related safety concerns (including increased mortality) in intensive insulin therapy groups (49, 50). The Glucontrol trial was stopped because of increased mortality associated with hypoglycemia (49). The Efficacy of Volume Substitution and Insulin Therapy in Severe Sepsis trial was also terminated early because of futility (no significant improvement in mean organ failure scale or mortality in septic ICU patients at 28 days) with an increased incidence of overall serious adverse events (10.9% vs. 5.2%, $P = .01$) and hypoglycemia in the intensive insulin therapy group (17.9% vs. 4.1%, $P < .001$) (50).

Two recently published meta-analyses have confirmed that intensive glucose control is associated with a high incidence of hypoglycemia. In the first study, 20 of the 34 eligible trials reported data related to patients undergoing surgery with perioperative intensive insulin therapy and hypoglycemia incidence data (defined as blood glucose low enough to require treatment) (45). The pooled analysis demonstrated an overall increased risk of hypoglycemia in the intensive insulin therapy groups [approximately 8% of the total patients treated with intensive insulin therapy ($n = 1470$) compared to approximately 3% of control groups ($n = 1475$); relative risk, 2.07; 95% CI, 1.29–3.52] (45). A second meta-analysis evaluated 29 randomized controlled trials of critically ill medical and surgical patients and specifically targeted studies that randomly assigned patients to either an intensive insulin therapy treatment group or a control group (defined as usual care). In this analysis, the incidence of hypoglycemia (defined as a blood glucose ≤40 mg/dL) was reported in 15 trials. From these data, the incidence of hypoglycemia was 13.7% in the intensive insulin therapy group versus 2.5% in the control group (relative risk, 5.13; 95% CI, 4.09–6.43) (46). These studies document that hypoglycemia is a risk and that it has long-term consequences that must be balanced against the risks associated with hyperglycemia. As a result of these analyses, insulin management protocols have been modified to reduce the likelihood of hypoglycemia and have resulted in redefining the "optimal" goal for glucose control when initiating intensive insulin therapy.

PERIOPERATIVE INTENSIVE INSULIN THERAPY PROTOCOLS

Based on the outcomes of the previously cited studies and an understanding of the risks associated with hyper- and hypoglycemia, a number of insulin protocols have been proposed for use in the perioperative management of the cardiac surgical patient. Although some of the data are derived from outcomes in other patient populations, there is consensus that careful monitoring of glucose levels and optimizing them has some value. The initial Leuven study (40) was the first large randomized controlled trial to provide guidelines for blood glucose management in a general surgical ICU population. The Portland Diabetic Project provided the first detailed protocol specifically for diabetic cardiac surgery patients. These initial protocols have served as the basis for development of insulin strategies for the cardiac surgical patient population.

One of the challenges in defining the optimal protocol relates to the diversity of patients and management strategies in the various trials reported in the literature—and extrapolating the findings to the cardiac surgery patient population. Wilson and colleagues (51) reviewed protocols from 12 trials in the critically ill ICU patients, including 3 studies in cardiothoracic surgery patients (Tables 4–1 and 4–2). They found tremendous variability among the protocols, including differences in target blood glucose levels, in initiation procedures (insulin load and/or insulin infusion), in the required calculations for adjustment of insulin doses,

TABLE 4–1. Comparison of insulin recommendations in all ICU patients except following cardiac surgery from the American Diabetes Association

First Author	Bolus (units)	Initial Infusion Rate (units/h)	Insulin infused with blood glucose >200 mg/dL (units)	% of insulin infused with blood glucose >200 mg/dL	Highest hourly dose (units)	Total Insulin dose (units)
Bode (52)	0[α]	8	41	90%	11	45
Boord (53)	0	1	14.3	53%	4.3	26.9
Chant (54)	0	6	42	66%	15	63.5
Davidson (55)	0	8	52.3	79%	12.3	66.3
Goldberg (56)	4.5	4.5	26	81%	9	32
Kanji (57)	3	3	41	53%	12	77
Krinsley (58)	0	10	40	91%	10	44
Marks (59)	0	1	54	50%	18	107
Watts (60)	0	1.5	36.5	74%	10.5	49

Adapted from (51). Copyright © 2007 American Diabetes Association.

and in methods of insulin protocol adjustments. Additionally, some of the published studies have provided only treatment guidelines for implementing and improving glycemic control in the cardiothoracic ICU, whereas others studies have provided detailed protocols for the treatment of hyperglycemia (61, 62). In one of the studies that used a specific protocol, the goals were successfully achieved in most patients with minimal risk of hypoglycemia. The study documented five instances (0.2%) in which the glucose fell below 60 mg/dL; each episode responded rapidly to intravenous dextrose and the patients had no sequelae (62).

For cardiothoracic surgery patients, a detailed protocol targeting blood glucose between 80 and 150 mg/dL was recently published. The investigators used historical controls to compare the outcome associated with the use of an aggressive insulin infusion protocol. In this study, the target glucose level was between 80 and 150 mg/dL (61). After the insulin infusion protocol was initiated, patients had improved glycemic control ($P = .001$) and a significant decrease in hyperglycemia (defined as a glucose level >150 mg/dL) during the first 24 hours ($P = .001$). The incidence of hypoglycemia (blood glucose <65 mg/dL) was increased in the intensive insulin therapy compared to the historical control group (16.7% vs. 9.8%, $P = .098$).

Although these studies document that intensive glucose control is possible and that, with careful monitoring, the incidence of hypoglycemia

TABLE 4–2.   Comparison of insulin recommendations
in ICU patients following cardiac surgery

First Author	Bolus (units)	Initial Infusion Rate (units/h)	Insulin infused with blood glucose >200 mg/dL (units)	% of insulin infused with blood glucose >200 mg/dL	Highest hourly dose (units)	Total Insulin dose (units)
Furnary (34)	12	6.5	59.5	76%	18.5	78
Van den Berghe (40)	0	4	40	41%	15	98.5
Zimmerman (61)	10	4	88	77%	21	115

Adapted from (51). Copyright © 2007 American Diabetes Association.

is minimal, none of the studies provide a specific protocol that can be applied in every clinical situation. In most cases patients are treated with glucose-containing intravenous solutions and glucose is controlled using an insulin infusion. The infusion rate is adjusted to maintain the glucose level within a predefined range. For many studies, that range has been modified to reduce the risk of hypoglycemia—with common recommendations for glucose ranging between 100 and 150 mg/dL. To achieve the goals, glucose must be monitored closely, often requiring bedside glucose measurements hourly, both in the operating room and in the ICU. The monitoring and adjustments in insulin infusions are labor intensive, particularly when tight glucose control is the goal of therapy. As a result, the specific glucose goal should be defined and the protocol modified to achieve it while limiting the risk of hypoglycemia.

Further advances in the care of the hyperglycemic patient, both in the operating room and the ICU, will require new technologies and more effective ways to both continuously monitor glucose levels and automatically adjust insulin infusions based on the data. A recent randomized controlled trial evaluated the ability of a computer-controlled algorithm to optimize glucose control in patients scheduled for elective cardiac surgery (63). The algorithm provided better glucose control (mean glucose was 112 mg/dL ± 20) than did a control management strategy (130 ± 20) with $P < .05$ (63). In the study there were no episodes of severe hypoglycemia (glucose <50 mg/dL) in either group. As the technology improves, biofeedback approaches to glucose control will provide better clinical management while also reducing the labor costs associated with tight glucose control.

PERIOPERATIVE GLUCOSE CONTROL AS A QUALITY MEASURE

As a result of the large number of studies documenting the value of glucose control on outcomes, perioperative glucose management has become an important quality indicator for many regulatory agencies. Blood glucose control after cardiac surgery is included in quality measures by The Joint Commission (64) and by the Surgical Care Improvement Project (SCIP) of the Centers for Medicare and Medicaid (65). The specific SCIP performance measure in cardiac surgery is a blood glucose concentration on postoperative day 1 and 2 at 6 a.m. of 200 mg/dL or less (See Table 4–3). Recent initiatives may be increasingly apt to link these quality measures to pay for performance concepts (67). Anesthesiologists should be aware of these quality measures, participate in protocol development to define appropriate glucose targets and insulin infusion regimens, and monitor performance.

Table 4–3. Surgical Care Improvement Project (SCIP) infection improvement measures

Measure	Details
SCIP INF 1	Prophylactic antibiotic received within one hour prior to surgical incision
SCIP INF 2	Prophylactic antibiotic selection for surgical patients
SCIP INF 3	Prophylactic antibiotics discontinued within 24 hours after surgery end time (48 hours for cardiac patients)
SCIP INF 4	Cardiac surgery patients with controlled 6 a.m. postoperative serum glucose on postoperative day one (POD 1) and postoperative day two (POD 2) with surgery ending date being postoperative day zero (POD 0)
SCIP INF 5	Postoperative wound infection diagnosed during index hospitalization
SCIP INF 6	Surgery patients with appropriate hair removal
SCIP INF 7	Colorectal surgery patients with immediate postoperative normothermia

Adapted from (66).

CONCLUSIONS

Hyperglycemia commonly develops during the perioperative period following cardiac surgery, in patients with or without preexisting DM. Hyperglycemia is associated with worse outcomes, particularly in diabetic patients. Although multiple studies have demonstrated the deleterious effects of both intraoperative and postoperative hyperglycemia, the optimal target range glucose control and treatment regimen remains unclear in cardiac surgery patients.

Recommendations from affiliated organizations have been published recently that may help define management strategies and goals of therapy for hyperglycemia. The American College of Endocrinology recently published a position paper on the care of hospitalized patients with DM. The report recommends treatment to maintain a maximum glucose concentration of 110 mg/dL for patients in the ICU and 180 mg/dL for patients in other inpatient settings. This statement was cosponsored by the American Society of Anesthesiologists (68). The American College of Cardiology and the American Heart Association (and supported by the Society of Cardiovascular Anesthesiologists) have also recently published guidelines with specific recommendations about glucose management. Their 2007 Guidelines on Perioperative Evaluation and Care for Noncardiac Surgery recommend that the glucose concentration be controlled during the perioperative period in patients with DM or acute hyperglycemia who are at high risk for myocardial ischemia or who are undergoing vascular and/or major noncardiac (e.g., thoracic) surgical procedures with anticipated ICU admission (a Class IIa recommendation) (69).

Based on the published data and the risks and benefits associated with glucose control, we recommend that blood glucose in cardiac surgery patients be targeted to a range between 120 and 150 mg/dL. This range will probably effectively minimize the risks of major morbidity and mortality that occur with severe intraoperative and postoperative hyperglycemia while reducing the risk of hypoglycemia. There are no comparison studies to evaluate the most effective strategy or protocol to achieve this target glucose control, so each institution should develop a protocol that defines the goals of therapy, uses an insulin infusion to achieve it, and, at the same time, takes into account the clinical setting and monitoring requirements. No matter what protocol is used, each patient will require close observation and frequent laboratory analysis to diagnose hypoglycemia (especially when the symptoms may be masked by anesthetic agents). The recommendations regarding optimal management are likely to change as technological advances such as continuous and reliable glucose monitoring become available. At that point, tighter glucose control may be possible with minimal risk.

References

1. American Diabetes Association, Expert Committee on the Diagnosis and Classification of Diabetes Mellitus: Report of the expert committee on the diagnosis and classification of diabetes mellitus. Diabetes Care 2003; 26: S5–20
2. Burke JP, Williams K, Gaskill SP, Hazuda HP, Haffner SM, Stern MP: Rapid rise in the incidence of type 2 diabetes from 1987 to 1996: results from the San Antonio heart study. Arch Intern Med 1999; 159:1450–6
3. Slaughter TF: Hemostasis and glycemic control in the cardiac surgical patient. Semin Cardiothorac Vasc Anesth 2006; 10:176–9

124 | Hatton and Fahy

4. Kannel WB, McGee DL: Diabetes and cardiovascular risk factors: the Framingham Study. Circulation 1979; 59:8–13
5. Edwards FH, Grover FL, Shroyer AL, Schwartz M, Bero J: The Society of Thoracic Surgeons National Cardiac Surgery Database: current risk assessment. Ann Thorac Surg 1997; 63:903–8
6. Lauruschkat AH, Arnrich B, Albert AA, et al.: Prevalence and risks of undiagnosed diabetes mellitus in patients undergoing coronary artery bypass grafting. Circulation 2005; 112:2397–402
7. DeFrances CJ, Hall MJ. 2005 National hospital discharge survey. Adv Data 2007; 385:1–19.
8. Gandhi GY, Nuttall GA, Abel MD, et al.: Intraoperative hyperglycemia and perioperative outcomes in cardiac surgery patients. Mayo Clin Proc 2005; 80:862–6
9. Herlitz J, Wognsen GB, Emanuelsson H, et al.: Mortality and morbidity in diabetic and nondiabetic patients during a 2-year period after coronary artery bypass grafting. Diabetes Care 1996; 19:698–703
10. Shroyer AL, Plomondon ME, Grover FL, Edwards FH: The 1996 coronary artery bypass risk model: the Society of Thoracic Surgeons Adult Cardiac National Database. Ann Thorac Surg 1999; 67:1205–8
11. Thourani VH, Weintraub WS, Stein B, et al.: Influence of diabetes mellitus on early and late outcome after coronary artery bypass grafting. Ann Thorac Surg 1999; 67:1045–52
12. Morricone L, Ranucci M, Denti S, et al.: Diabetes and complications after cardiac surgery: comparison with a non-diabetic population. Acta Diabetol 1999; 36:77–84
13. Guvener M, Pasaoglu I, Demircin M, Oc M: Perioperative hyperglycemia is a strong correlate of postoperative infection in type II diabetic patients after coronary artery bypass grafting. Endocrinology J 2002; 49:531–7
14. Furnary AP, Gao G, Grunkemeier GL, et al.: Continuous insulin infusion reduces mortality in patients with diabetes undergoing coronary artery bypass grafting. J Thorac Cardiovasc Surg 2003; 125: 1007–21
15. Doenst T, Wijeysundera D, Karkouti K, et al.: Hyperglycemia during cardiopulmonary bypass is an independent risk factor for mortality in patients undergoing cardiac surgery. J Thorac Cardiovasc Surg 2005; 130:1144–50
16. Ouattara A, Lecomte P, Le Manach Y, et al.: Poor intraoperative blood glucose control is associated with a worsened hospital outcome after cardiac surgery in diabetic patients. Anesthesiology 2005; 103:687–94
17. Furnary AP, Wu Y: Clinical effects of hyperglycemia in the cardiac surgery population: the Portland Diabetic Project. Endocr Pract 2006; 12(Suppl 3):22–6

18. Jones KW, Cain AS, Mitchell JH, et al.: Hyperglycemia predicts mortality after CABG: postoperative hyperglycemia predicts dramatic increases in mortality after coronary artery bypass graft surgery. J Diabetes Complicat 2008; 22:365–70

19. Egi M, Bellomo R, Stachowski E, et al.: Blood glucose concentration and outcome of critical illness: the impact of diabetes. Crit Care Med 2008; 36:2249–55

20. Carvalho G, Moore A, Qizilbash B, Lachapelle K, Schricker T: Maintenance of normoglycemia during cardiac surgery. Anesth Analg 2004; 99:319–24

21. Grocott HP: Glucose and outcome after cardiac surgery: what are the issues? J Extra Corpor Technol 2006; 38:65–7

22. Lehot JJ, Piriz H, Villard J, Cohen R, Guidollet J. Glucose homeostasis: Comparison between hypothermic and normothermic cardiopulmonary bypass. *Chest* 1992; 102:106–11.

23. Wan S, LeClerc JL, Vincent JL: Inflammatory response to cardiopulmonary bypass: mechanisms involved and possible therapeutic strategies. Chest 1997; 112:676–92

24. Papparella D, Yau TM, Young E: Cardiopulmonary bypass induced inflammation: pathophysiology and treatment. An update. Eur J Cardiothorac Surg 2002; 21(2):233–44

25. Doenst T, Bugger H, Schwarzer M, et al.: Three good reasons for heart surgeons to understand cardiac metabolism. Eur J Cardiothorac Surg 2008; 33:862–71

26. Donatelli F, Cavagna P, Di Dedda G, et al.: Correlation between pre-operative metabolic syndrome and persistent blood glucose elevation during cardiac surgery in non-diabetic patients. Acta Anaesthesiol Scand 2008; 52:1103–10

27. Kilger E, Weis F, Briegel J, et al.: Stress doses of hydrocortisone reduce severe systemic inflammatory response syndrome and improve early outcome in a risk group of patients after cardiac surgery. Crit Care Med 2003; 31:1068–74

28. Rassias AJ: Intraoperative management of hyperglycemia in the cardiac surgical patient. Semin Thorac Cardiovasc Surg 2006; 18:330–8

29. Anderson RE, Brismar K, Barr G, Ivert T: Effects of cardiopulmonary bypass on glucose homeostasis after coronary artery bypass surgery. Eur J Cardiothorac Surg 2005; 28:425–30

30. Van den Berghe G: How does blood glucose control with insulin save lives in intensive care? J Clin Invest 2004; 114(9):1187–95

31. Talbot TR: Diabetes mellitus and cardiothoracic surgical site infections. Am J Infect Control 2005; 33:353–9

32. Streeter NB: Considerations in prevention of surgical site infections following cardiac surgery. J Cardiovasc Nurs 2006; 21:E14–20

33. Zerr KJ, Furnary AP, Grunkemeier GL, Bookin S, Kanhere V, Starr A: Glucose control lowers the risk of wound infection in diabetics after open-heart operations. Ann Thorac Surg 1997; 63:356–61
34. Furnary AP, Wu Y, Bookin SO: Effect of hyperglycemia and continuous intravenous insulin infusions on outcomes of cardiac surgical procedures: the Portland Diabetic Project. Endocr Pract 2004; 10(Suppl 2):21–33
35. Rassias AJ, Marrin CA, Arruda J, Whalen PK, Beach M, Yeager MP: Insulin infusion improves neutrophil function in diabetic cardiac surgery patients. Anesth Analg 1999; 88:1011–6
36. Oldenborg PA, Sehlin J: Hyperglycemia in vitro attenuates insulin-stimulated chemokinesis in normal human neutrophils. Role of protein kinase C activation. J Leukoc Biol 1999; 65:635–40
37. Hansen TK, Thiel S, Wouters PJ: Intensive insulin therapy exerts anti-inflammatory effects in critically ill patients and counteracts the adverse effect of low mannose-binding lectin levels. J Clin Endocrinol Metab 2003; 88:1082–8
38. Furnary AP, Cheek DB, Holmes SC, Howell WL, Kelly SP: Achieving tight glycemic control in the operating room: lessons learned from 12 years in the trenches of a paradigm shift in anesthetic care. Semin Thorac Cardiovasc Surg 2006; 18:339–45
39. Gandhi GY, Nuttall GA, Abel MD, et al.: Intensive intraoperative insulin therapy versus conventional glucose management during cardiac surgery: a randomized trial. Ann Intern Med 2007; 146:233–43
40. Van den Berghe G, Wouters P, Weekers F, et al.: Intensive insulin therapy in the critically ill patients. N Engl J Med 2001; 345:1359–67
41. Van den Berghe G, Wilmer A, Hermans G, et al.: Intensive insulin therapy in the medical ICU. N Engl J Med 2006; 354:449–61
42. Van den Berghe G, Wilmer A, Milants I, et al.: Intensive insulin therapy in mixed medical/surgical intensive care units: benefit versus harm. Diabetes 2006; 55:3151–9
43. Ingels C, Debaveye Y, Milants I, et al.: Strict blood glucose control with insulin during intensive care after cardiac surgery: impact on 4-years survival, dependency on medical care, and quality-of-life. Eur Heart J 2006; 27:2716–24
44. Ascione R, Rogers CA, Rajakaruna C, Angelini GD: Inadequate blood glucose control is associated with in-hospital mortality and morbidity in diabetic and nondiabetic patients undergoing cardiac surgery. Circulation 2008; 118:113–23
45. Gandhi GY, Murad MH, Flynn DN, et al.: The effect of perioperative insulin infusion of surgical morbidity and mortality: a systematic review and meta-analysis of randomized trials. Mayo Clin Proc 2008; 83:418–30

46. Soylemez-Wiener R, Wiener DC, Larson RJ: Benefits and risks of tight glucose control in critically ill adults: a meta-analysis. JAMA 2008; 300:933–44

47. Fahy BG, Coursin DB: Critical glucose control: the devil is in the details. Mayo Clin Proc 2008; 83:394–7

48. Arabi YM, Dabbagh OC, Tamim HM, et al.: Intensive versus conventional insulin therapy: a randomized controlled trial in medical and surgical critically ill patients. Crit Care Med 2008; 36:3190–7

49. Devos P, Preiser JC: Current controversies around tight glucose control in critically ill patients. Intensive versus conventional insulin therapy: a randomized controlled trial in medical and surgical critically ill patients. Curr Opin Clin Nutr Metab Care 2007; 10(2):206–9

50. Brunkhorst FM, Engel C, Bloos F, et al.: German Competence Network Sepsis (SepNet). Intensive insulin therapy and pentastarch resuscitation in severe sepsis. N Engl J Med 2008; 358:125–39

51. Wilson M, Weinreb J, Hoo GW: Intensive insulin therapy in critical care: a review of 12 protocols. Diabetes Care 2007; 30:1005–11

52. Bode BW, Braithwaite SS, Steed RD, Davidson PC: Intravenous insulin infusion therapy: indications, methods, and transition to subcutaneous insulin therapy. Endocr Pract 2004; 2:71–80

53. Boord JB, Graber AL, Christman JW, Powers AC: Practical management of diabetes in critically ill patients. Am J Respir Crit Care Med 2001; 164:1763–7

54. Chant C, Wilson G, Friedrich JO: Validation of an insulin infusion nomogram for intensive glucose control in critically ill patients. Pharmacotherapy 2005; 25:352–9

55. Davidson PC, Steed RD, Bode BW: Glucommander: a computer-directed intravenous insulin system shown to be safe, simple, and effective in 120,618 h of operation. Diabetes Care 2005; 28:2418–23

56. Goldberg PA, Siegel MD, Sherwin RS, et al.: Implementation of a safe and effective insulin infusion protocol in a medical intensive care unit. Diabetes Care 2004; 27:461–7

57. Kanji S, Singh A, Tierney M, Meggison H, McIntyre L, Hebert PC: Standardization of intravenous insulin therapy improves the efficiency and safety of blood glucose control in critically ill adults. Intensive Care Med 2004; 30:804–10

58. Krinsley JS: Effect of an intensive glucose management protocol on the mortality of critically ill adult patients. Mayo Clin Proc 2004; 79:992–1000

59. Marks JB: Perioperative management of diabetes. Am Fam Physician 2003; 67:93–100

60. Watts NB, Gebhart SS, Clark RV, Phillips LS: Postoperative management of diabetes mellitus: steady-state glucose control with bedside algorithm for insulin adjustment. Diabetes Care 1987; 10:722–8

61. Zimmerman CR, Mlynarek ME, Jordan JA, Rajda CA, Horst HM: An insulin infusion protocol in critically ill cardiothoracic surgery patients. Ann Pharmacother 2004; 38:1123–9

62. Goldberg PA, Sakharova OV, Barrett PW, et al.: Improving glycemic control in the cardiothoracic intensive care unit: clinical experience in two hospital settings. J Cardiothorac Vasc Anesth 2004; 18:690–7

63. Hovorka R, Kremen J, Blaha J, et al.: Blood glucose control by a model predictive control algorithm with variable sampling rate versus a routine glucose management protocol in cardiac surgery patients: a randomized controlled trial. J Clin Endocrinol Metab 2007; 92:2960–4

64. The Joint Commission. Performance Measurement Initiatives, Current Specification Manual for National Hospital Quality Measures. Available at: http://www.jointcommission.org/PerformanceMeasurement/PerformanceMeasurement/Current+NHQM+Manual.htmedition; accessed November 13, 2008

65. Centers for Medicare & Medicaid Services, MedQIC, SCIP Project Information. Available at: http://medqic.org/dcs/ContentServer?cid=1122904930422&pagename=Medqic/Content/ParentShellTemplate&parentName=Topic&c=MQParentsedition Accessed November 13, 2008

66. Premier, Surgical Care Improvement Project. Available at: http://www.premierinc.com/safety/topics/scip/downloads/scip-final-10–14–05.pdf; accessed December 11, 2008

67. Fink AS, Itani KM, Campbell DC: Assessing the quality of surgical care. Surg Clin N Am 2007; 87:837–52

68. Garber AJ, Moghissi ES, Bransome ED, Jr., et al.; American College of Endocrinology Task Force on Inpatient Diabetes Metabolic Control: American College of Endocrinology position statement on inpatient diabetes and metabolic control. Endocr Pract 2004; 10:77–82

69. Fleisher LA, Beckman JA, Brown KA, et al.: ACC/AHA 2007 Guidelines on Perioperative Cardiovascular Evaluation and Care for Noncardiac Surgery: Executive Summary: A Report of the American College of Cardiology/American Heart Association Task Force on Practice Guidelines (Writing Committee to Revise the 2002 Guidelines on Perioperative Cardiovascular Evaluation for Noncardiac Surgery) Developed in Collaboration With the American Society of Echocardiography, American Society of Nuclear Cardiology, Heart Rhythm Society, Society of Cardiovascular Anesthesiologists, Society for Cardiovascular Angiography and Interventions, Society for Vascular Medicine and Biology, and Society for Vascular Surgery. J Am Coll Cardiol 2007; 50:1707–32

Pedram Fatehi, MD
Kathleen D. Liu, MD
Neal H. Cohen, MD, MPH, MS

Perioperative Management of the Patient with Dialysis-Dependent Renal Failure Requiring

5 | Cardiac Surgery

INTRODUCTION

End-stage renal disease (ESRD) has significant impact on the perioperative management of the patient requiring cardiac surgery. Patients with ESRD are at higher risk for perioperative morbidity and mortality compared to the general population. In a retrospective study of 115 hemodialysis patients undergoing cardiac surgery, overall 30-day mortality in this group was 18.3%. Patients receiving either combined valve and coronary bypass or multiple valve surgery had more than twice the mortality rate (39%) of patients with isolated coronary bypass or isolated valve replacement (13%) (1). Similarly, in an observational study of patients undergoing cardiac surgery, dialysis-dependent patients had higher hospital mortality and an increased risk of postoperative sepsis and respiratory failure compared to patients not requiring dialysis. In addition, peripheral vascular disease in the patient with ESRD is an independent predictor of hospital mortality (2).

For reasons that are not entirely clear, the incidence of ESRD is on the rise. Many of the underlying causes for ESRD, such as hypertension and diabetes mellitus also contribute to coronary artery disease. As a

Medically Challenging Patients Undergoing Cardiothoracic Surgery, edited by Neal H. Cohen, MD, MPH, MS, Lippincott Williams & Wilkins, Baltimore © 2009.

result, patients with renal insufficiency associated with these underlying clinical problems frequently require cardiac surgery. Because renal insufficiency and associated medical conditions affect clinical decision making and outcome, the anesthesiologist must understand the implications of renal disease on perioperative care. This chapter reviews the epidemiology of renal disease and the physiologic complications associated with ESRD and provides recommendations for management strategies. The chapter includes a discussion of the different dialysis modalities available to patients in either the acute or chronic setting and their potential application in the perioperative period. Finally, it addresses specific issues of concern to the anesthesiologist, including management of the patient's volume status, electrolyte abnormalities, acid–base disturbances, and hematological disturbances and recommendations regarding vascular access and medication dosing.

EPIDEMIOLOGY OF ESRD

Scope of the Problem

The prevalence of chronic kidney disease (CKD) in the developed world has increased over the past several years, associated with the increasing incidence of diabetes mellitus and hypertension (3). Patients who present with renal insufficiency are at risk of developing ESRD with or without intensive therapy. However, as our understanding of intraglomerular hemodynamics has improved and preventative measures, such as angiotensin-converting enzyme (ACE) inhibitors and angiotensin-2 receptor blockers (ARBs) have been initiated, the pace of progression from renal insufficiency to ESRD has slowed for many patients (4–7). Despite the improved clinical options for patients with renal insufficiency, the number of patients with ESRD is growing out of proportion to the number of patients with CKD. The reasons for this increase in ESRD is probably multifactorial, but is partially accounted for by more rapid transition to dialysis and earlier transplantation to minimize the complications of renal insufficiency and improve quality of life, particularly in patients with associated medical conditions or in frail elderly patients (8). As a result, the number of Americans with dialysis-dependent ESRD is substantial and rising. In 2006, 506,256 individuals in the United States had ESRD, of whom 354,754 were treated with chronic hemodialysis (9). The remaining ESRD patients underwent kidney transplantation; although these patients are considered to have ESRD, their management is outside the scope of this chapter.

TABLE 5–1. Stages of chronic kidney disease*

Stage	Description	GFR (mL/min/1.73m^2)
1	Kidney damage** with normal GFR	>90
2	Mild decrease in GFR	60–89
3	Moderate decrease in GFR	30–59
4	Severe decrease in GFR	15–29
5	Kidney failure/ESRD	<15

From (10).
* By this definition of CKD, the threshold values must be demonstrated for >3 months.
** Kidney damage is defined as pathologic abnormalities in blood or urine test results or imaging studies.

CKD: A Prelude to ESRD

ESRD is the final manifestation of CKD. CKD is classified into 5 stages based on estimated glomerular filtration rate (eGFR) (Table 5–1) in the Kidney Disease Outcome Quality Initiative (K/DOQI) clinical practice guidelines of the National Kidney Foundation (10). Although perioperative management of the patient with early CKD (i.e., non-ESRD) is outside the scope of this review, a few points are worth making. First, recognition of CKD is important to prevent further renal injury in the perioperative setting. The patient with CKD is at higher risk of superimposed acute kidney injury in the perioperative period; when it develops, the patient is at high risk for developing ESRD. Second, because creatinine is produced by muscle tissue, the absolute value for serum creatinine must be interpreted carefully, taking into account age, muscle mass, and nutritional status. Creatinine is considered an insensitive marker of renal insufficiency; eGFR or creatinine clearance is more useful in clinical practice. Although the anesthesiologist does not commonly consider these alternative methods for assessing underlying renal function, such measures should be considered in patients with risk factors consistent with renal impairment. The most commonly used methods of estimating creatinine clearance and GFR are the Cockcroft–Gault equation (11) and the Modified Diet in Renal Disease (MDRD) equation (12, 13), respectively. The Cockcroft–Gault equation uses age, weight, sex, and serum creatinine to estimate creatinine clearance: Creatinine Clearance = (140 − age in years) × (weight in kg) × (0.85 if female) / (72 × Cr). The MDRD equation was derived from a multiethnic cohort of patients with CKD. There are several different versions of the equation; the simplified versions use age, sex, race, and serum creatinine to estimate GFR. Of note, the equation has recently been reexpressed for laboratories that use isotope dilution mass spectrometry (IDMS)-calibrated creatinine measurements (13), which is increasingly common in clinical practice. The primary goal of IDMS-calibrated creatinine measurements is to standardize measurements across clinical laboratories.

In an effort to heighten awareness of patients with CKD for whom serum creatinine levels are within the "normal" range, many laboratories now automatically report the MDRD-based eGFR with the creatinine measurement. Because this equation was derived in a racially diverse cohort, two GFRs are presented, one for patients of African descent and one for patients of other ethnicities. On average, eGFR is higher in African American patients at any given level of serum creatinine because of increased muscle mass. The MDRD equation is imprecise above an eGFR of 60 mL/min, so some laboratories will report that the upper limit as above 60 mL/min rather than report an absolute number. Unfortunately, these estimating equations are not useful in patients with ESRD, as the serum creatinine will vary based on the timing of the last dialysis session. Patients with ESRD may have residual renal function, but a timed urine collection is required to estimate endogenous creatinine clearance based on urinary creatinine excretion. In patients with CKD, timed urine collections are not routinely performed because these collections are often inaccurate (e.g., too much or too little urine is collected); the estimating equations are sufficient for clinical decision making.

The Uremic Syndrome

Essentially all organ systems are affected by the accumulation in the body of organic waste normally cleared by the kidneys. Signs and symptoms associated with a decline in GFR characterize the syndrome of uremia. Although the urea molecule itself causes some cellular dysfunction, its most important role is as a marker for other less understood uremic solutes. Historically, blood urea nitrogen (BUN) level >90 mg/dL has been used as a threshold for uremia (14). There are, however, no absolute values of BUN or creatinine that demarcate the beginning of the uremic syndrome. The findings associated with the uremic syndrome include weakness, fatigue, neuropathy and asterixis, confusion, insomnia, seizures, abnormal calcium–phosphate metabolism, increased muscle catabolism, serositis (including pericarditis), anemia, lymphocyte/granulocyte dysfunction, and abnormal hemostasis (15). As GFR progressively declines, maintenance dialysis is initiated to alleviate these symptoms of uremia. Many of these symptoms are discussed in further detail later in this chapter.

EXTRACORPOREAL SUPPORT OF PATIENTS WITH ESRD

While chronic dialytic therapy is beyond the scope of this chapter, the anesthesiologist must understand the goals of dialysis, how it works, and the implications for perioperative management of the patient undergoing cardiac surgery. In many cases, patients with ESRD will undergo dialysis immediately prior to surgery; under this circumstance the therapy has significant implications for assessment and management of fluids and electrolytes during the surgical procedure. For patients whose fluid status or electrolytes become unstable in the perioperative period, urgent dialysis may be required in the early postoperative period. Finally, some patients with severe myocardial dysfunction may require continuous renal replacement therapy (CRRT) in the perioperative period, and, in the most complicated cases, during cardiac surgery.

Maintenance dialytic treatment options for patients with ESRD include hemodialysis and peritoneal dialysis (PD) (16, 17). In the United States, the majority (>90%) of ESRD patients receive hemodialysis, although there is substantial geographic variation in the selection of dialytic therapy. The benefits of one mode over another for chronic dialysis have not been well studied. Observational data suggest that patient outcomes with the two therapies are similar, although there are no large-scale randomized clinical trials comparing hemodialysis to PD. There are some patients for whom one mode of dialysis is more appropriate than another and some situations in which either hemodialysis or PD is contraindicated. For example, the patient with recent peritonitis or abdominal surgery may not be a good candidate for PD. Under most circumstances in the United States, however, the decision about which modality to use (hemodialysis or PD) for chronic dialysis support is typically based on patient choice, with input from the physician.

Hemodialysis relies on the principles of solute diffusion across a semipermeable membrane (the dialyzer) (18). Movement of metabolic waste products takes place down a concentration (electrochemical) gradient from the circulation into the dialysate. Generally, larger molecules will diffuse more slowly across the membrane. A small molecule such as potassium (39 Da), for example, undergoes significant clearance, whereas a larger molecule such as creatinine (113 Da) is cleared less efficiently. In addition to diffusive clearance, solutes are removed along with water across the semipermeable dialysis membrane by ultrafiltration. This is called "convective clearance."

There are four main components required for hemodialysis: the vascular access, the dialyzer, the dialysate, and the dialysis machine. Options for vascular access include arteriovenous fistulas (AVFs), arteriovenous grafts (AVGs), and tunneled and nontunneled central venous catheters. Because of the risk of infection, AVFs are preferred to AVGs, and AVGs are in turn preferable to catheters for chronic dialysis. The dialyzer consists of a semipermeable synthetic membrane across which both diffusion and ultrafiltration allow for solute clearance. The dialysate is a balanced salt solution that allows for diffusion of uremic toxins and electrolytes (e.g., potassium) down a concentration gradient. Based on the results of the patient's laboratory studies, the nephrologist prescribes the composition of the dialysate. Intermittent hemodialysis (IHD) is generally performed in ambulatory dialysis centers; the majority of hemodialysis patients receive therapy three times a week at a center near their home. Treatments typically last 3–4 hours. In selected cases, IHD is performed more frequently and/or in the patient's home.

When using PD, 1.5–3 liters of a dextrose-containing solution is infused into the peritoneal cavity and allowed to dwell for a set period of time. Access to the peritoneal cavity is achieved with a soft, cuffed silicone catheter. As with hemodialysis, toxic materials are removed through a combination of convective clearance generated through ultrafiltration and diffusive clearance down a concentration gradient. Solute and water clearance occurs across the peritoneal membrane itself via the peritoneal capillary circulation and via peritoneal lymphatics into the lymphatic circulation. The rate of solute transport varies from patient to patient; it is affected by the presence of infection (peritonitis), drugs, and physical factors such as position and exercise.

PD may be carried out as continuous ambulatory PD (CAPD), continuous cyclic PD (CCPD), or a combination of both. In CAPD, the dialysis solution is manually exchanged three to five times daily, using gravity to remove fluid from the peritoneal cavity. In CCPD, exchanges are performed using an automated cycler, usually at night while the patient sleeps. The number and volume of exchange cycles required to optimize solute clearance varies by the peritoneal membrane characteristics and must be tailored to the individual patient.

In the acute setting, additional modalities of therapy are available for the extracorporeal support of ESRD patients. These modalities include plasma ultrafiltration (PUF), in which fluid and solutes are removed via convective clearance across a dialyzer. Fluid removal can be accomplished more rapidly with PUF than with dialysis because there is no diffusive clearance, and therefore no solute flux. In addition, multiple modalities of CRRT are available. The original continuous dialysis modalities relied on systemic (arterial) perfusion pressure to *drive* blood through the circuit and therefore required access to a large central artery. Currently, peristaltic pumps are more commonly used to facilitate blood flow, so that venous access with a dual port system can be used. This change has reduced the potential risk of stroke or limb ischemia associated with placement of large arterial catheters.

The three modalities of venovenous therapies that are available are continuous venovenous hemofiltration (CVVH), continuous venovenous hemodialysis (CVVHD), and continuous venovenous hemodiafiltration

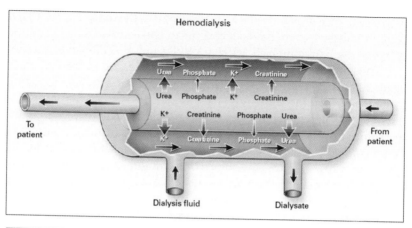

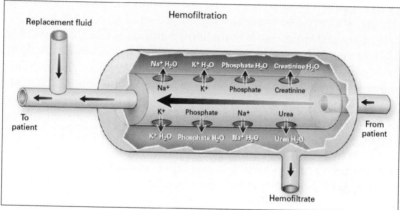

5–1. Principles of hemodialysis (diffusive clearance) and hemofiltration (convective clearance). In hemodialysis, blood and dialysis fluid run countercurrent to one another, resulting in diffusion of solutes down a concentration gradient. Thus, clearance of small molecules (potassium, urea) is more efficient than clearance of larger molecules (creatinine, phosphate). In hemofiltration, ultrafiltrate is removed from the blood via convective clearance across the semipermeable membrane. A balanced salt solution (replacement fluid) is administered to the patient to replace the fluid removed by ultrafiltration. The difference in concentration of solutes in the blood and this replacement fluid leads to net clearance of solutes from the patient. Reproduced with permission from (19).

(CVVHDF). CVVH relies purely on convective clearance; in this modality, fluid is removed from the patient via PUF, and a "replacement" fluid is administered to the patient (Figure 5–1).

This replacement fluid is a physiologic crystalloid solution containing sodium, potassium, chloride, and a base equivalent (bicarbonate, lactate, and acetate have all been used). CVVHD relies primarily on diffusive clearance as blood runs countercurrent to the dialysate. CVVHDF combines these two methods of clearance. There are no data in support of one of these modalities (CVVH, CVVHD, or CVVHDF) over another.

The continuous dialysis modalities for fluid and electrolyte management are frequently used in critically ill patients with hemodynamic instability, including those who have undergone cardiac surgery or in the setting of large obligate fluid intake associated with medications and nutrition; however, it should be noted that no studies to date have demonstrated a survival benefit with CRRT in the setting of acute kidney injury (20–22). Thus, the choice of technique is currently based on the specific needs of the patient, the resources available within the institution to manage the continuous therapy, and the preference and expertise of the physician. Of note, the dialysis machines used for IHD and CRRT are different, so a CRRT program requires significant institutional resources, above and beyond what are required to provide in-patient hemodialysis. Despite these limitations, continuous therapies have been used successfully both in the operating room and postoperatively for those patients who are hemodynamically unstable with significant fluid and/or electrolyte abnormalities. In most cases, the patients have significant underlying renal dysfunction, although CRRT can also be a useful method to address volume overload and its consequences when renal impairment is less severe.

In patients in whom hemodynamic stability is a primary consideration and who cannot tolerate more rapid fluid shifts associated with traditional IHD, sustained low-efficiency hemodialysis (SLED), a relatively new hybrid mode of dialysis, is an excellent alternative. SLED is performed daily over 6–12 hours (compared to 3–4 hours for IHD or continuously for CRRT) with slower blood and dialysate flow rates than IHD. SLED can be performed with a standard IHD machine with a software modification, so no new equipment is needed for this therapy, as opposed to any of the modes of continuous therapy.

PHYSIOLOGY AND COMPLICATIONS OF RENAL FAILURE

In the first three stages of CKD, the ability of the kidneys to maintain homeostasis of the extracellular fluid compartment generally remains intact. As GFR decreases, the kidneys' capacity to control the "internal environment" becomes increasingly limited (23). Dialysis-dependent patients are at particularly high risk of complications including volume overload, electrolyte abnormalities, acid–base disturbances, and the uremic syndrome, including uremic coagulopathy and bleeding.

In the intraoperative setting, dialysis may occasionally be required for volume management or control of hyperkalemia or acidosis. In these circumstances, intermittent or continuous therapy may be performed; the choice of modality will be dictated by the hemodynamic stability of the patient and the resources available in the operating room (including physical plant characteristics and staff to perform therapy). These decisions should be made based on close communication and coordination among the surgeon, anesthesiologist, and nephrologist. As anesthesiologists become comfortable with the equipment and management strategies associated with continuous therapy, intraoperative CRRT use is anticipated to increase in the patients with severe cardiovascular disease and hemodynamic compromise.

Volume Status

Fluid management in the patient with ESRD requires a careful analysis of intake and output and interventions to improve fluid removal. Because most patients with ESRD (particularly those undergoing cardiac surgery) will require hemodialysis to manage fluid and electrolytes in the perioperative period, the anesthesiologist must be aware of the ramifications of dialysis on volume status and hemodynamics. The majority of ESRD patients for whom hemodialysis is initiated will become anuric even if they had some urine output prior to dialysis. In such patients, the administration of fluids required to manage them during the surgical procedure will likely lead to volume overload; for some patients, urgent hemodialysis will be required. Anuric patients will rarely have an adequate, if any, response to administration of diuretics.

Although less common, some renal diseases result in nonoliguric ESRD. Patients with this type of renal dysfunction continue to produce some urine both before and after initiation of dialysis, although clearance of uremic toxins will be poor and most patients will have electrolyte and acid–base abnormalities that require treatment. PD patients also often retain some residual renal function and continue to produce some urine. In contrast to anuric patients, ESRD patients who produce urine may respond to diuretic therapy with improved urine output. Loop diuretics, such as furosemide or bumetanide, can be useful for this subset of patients to facilitate fluid management between dialysis treatments. When administered it is important to provide large enough doses for the drug to reach the target of action in the thick ascending limb of the loop of Henle. The serum concentrations of the loop diuretics must be high enough to be filtered and achieve an effective concentration *within* the renal tubules. Thiazide diuretics, such as metolazone or chlorothiazide, may be given in combination with loop diuretics to block sequential segments of sodium reabsorption along the nephron and achieve more effective diuresis.

The most expedient and efficient way to achieve volume removal in a chronic hemodialysis patient is through the use of hemodialysis or PUF. With ultrafiltration, a plasma ultrafiltrate is removed across the dialysis membrane, but there is no dialysis component. Hemodynamics are usually more stable with this treatment because of the absence of solute flux. Depending on the level of the patient's hemodynamic stability, ultrafiltration can facilitate removal of as much as 2–3 liters of fluid over 1–2 hours. Because there is no diffusive clearance, plasma electrolyte levels will remain essentially unchanged, and medication dosing adjustments are not required.

For the patient receiving PD perioperatively, fluid removal via dialysis can be accomplished by increasing the solute (dextrose) concentration in the dialysate. This process is relatively slow and will allow for volume removal over hours, not minutes. Thus, early recognition of volume overload with appropriate adjustment of the dialysis prescription is important to avoid complications of volume overload, including heart failure exacerbations and respiratory distress. In some cases, if the patient's volume status becomes problematic, the patient may require initiation of hemodialysis during the period of instability to facilitate more rapid control of the volume overload.

Blood Pressure

Although some ESRD patients, particularly those with severe congestive heart failure or cirrhosis, have low blood pressure, most dialysis-dependent patients are hypertensive. Sodium and fluid retention lead to the expansion of extracellular fluid compartment. Chronic volume overload has detrimental effects on the cardiovascular system, including left ventricular hypertrophy (24) and arterial stiffness (25), both of which are associated with increased mortality. In addition to volume-mediated hypertension, vasoconstrictive mechanisms contribute to hypertension in ESRD patients. Dysregulated activation of the renin–angiotensin and sympathetic nervous systems is inappropriate relative to the volume-overloaded state of these patients.

Treatment of volume overload with appropriate fluid removal is critical for blood-pressure control in ESRD patients. In the chronic setting, nephrologists reassess volume status on an ongoing basis; during each dialysis session, fluid is removed to achieve the patient's "dry" weight. Furthermore, most patients have a pattern of intradialytic weight gain (depending on the ability of the patient to comply with fluid restrictions and the patient's size, this may vary from 1 to 6 kg). If the dry weight is not reassessed and the patient loses muscle mass, patients may become fluid overloaded over time, making it more difficult to control their hypertension. In the acute setting, nephrologists must tailor volume removal to obligate intake (medications and infusions) and oral intake. If the cardiac surgical patient receives contrast for a radiologic study, the fluid management must take into account the fluid shifts associated with the high osmolality of the contrast to prevent worsening intravascular volume overload.

Most patients with ESRD require multiple antihypertensive agents to control their blood pressure. Rarely is adequate control achieved with a single agent. ACE inhibitors and ARBs are not contraindicated in the anuric ESRD population despite their effect on electrolytes, particularly potassium. Serum potassium levels are controlled by dialysis, not by urinary potassium excretion. Depending on the patient's surgical and anesthetic course, in most cases the preoperative antihypertensive medications can be restarted postoperatively after the patient's volume, electrolytes, and acid–base status have stabilized. However, because many of these patients have improved hemodynamics and cardiovascular function after surgery, the medication regimen may have to be modified. For most patients, the safest approach is to use intravenous agents to achieve blood-pressure control as needed and then carefully reintroduce one medication at a time until the optimal combination of agents is determined.

Sodium and Tonicity

Patients with advanced CKD have limited diluting and concentrating ability. Anuric patients have no such ability and are at particular risk of developing hyper- or hyponatremia. The serum sodium concentration of the patient with ESRD, as is true for any other patient, is contingent upon intake and losses of free water. The patient with ESRD cannot regulate plasma tonicity via solute excretion. For example, prior to dialysis treatments the ESRD patient who receives hemodialysis often has mild hyponatremia caused by higher free water intake relative to sodium intake. As a result, it is critical to consider the tonicity of intravenous fluids used intraoperatively and for resuscitation.

Hypernatremia is an intense stimulus for thirst, so if the patient has access to free water, the hypernatremia usually will be self-correcting. The same is obviously not true for the critically ill patient. For the intubated patient receiving hyperosmolar tube feedings, free water may have to be provided through the feeding tube to maintain a normal serum sodium concentration. The amount of free water must be carefully monitored to avoid fluid overload for the dialysis-dependent patient. For this group of patients, however, it might be easiest to correct both hyper- and hyponatremia with dialysis, because sodium is freely diffusible across the dialysis membrane and will reequilibrate in either direction, depending on the direction of the concentration gradient. When dialysis is used to normalize serum sodium, caution must be used to prevent overcorrection of the sodium. The sodium concentration of the dialysis bath is usually set between 135 and 145 mmol/L; this concentration may be adjusted in the setting of severe, long-standing hyponatremia, but has to be done cautiously to avoid complications of rapid correction or overcorrection (e.g., central pontine myelinolysis). The same is true when intravenous hypertonic saline is used to correct severe symptomatic hyponatremia. Although the hypertonic solution will correct the serum sodium, it may also contribute to volume overload and hypertension. CRRT may be the safest way to slowly correct sodium (rather than using intermittent dialysis), although this will depend on the dialysis solutions available for CRRT; with intermittent dialysis, the dialysate sodium can be varied considerably.

Potassium

Total-body balance of potassium (mostly stored in cells of skeletal muscle, along with red blood cells, hepatocytes, and within bone) and its distribution between intracellular and extracellular compartments determine the serum potassium concentration (26). ESRD patients are at risk of developing hyperkalemia because of an impaired ability to excrete potassium and as a result of multiple factors that may contribute to shifting of potassium from the intracellular to extracellular compartments (27). Unlike patients with normal renal function, ESRD patients cannot increase potassium excretion in the face of increased intake of potassium, either because of dietary indiscretion or iatrogenic potassium administration, increasing the risk for hyperkalemia and its consequences. The most dangerous complications associated with hyperkalemia are well known to the anesthesiologist and include cardiac conduction abnormalities, which may manifest as electrocardiographic changes and arrhythmias and result in death if not recognized and treated.

The kidneys and, to a lesser extent, the intestines regulate total-body potassium homeostasis. Thus, a large dietary or parenteral potassium load will put the patient with ESRD at high risk for hyperkalemia. Parenteral sources of potassium in the perioperative period include transfusion of blood products, intravenous administration of fluids containing potassium, and cardioplegic solutions, all of which can cause hyperkalemia in the patient with ESRD. Transfused blood products (whole blood, packed red blood cells, platelets) have high concentrations of potassium because of intracellular-to-extracellular shift as a result of cell breakdown. Washing of these blood products will reduce the potassium load and can be useful for the patient with ESRD, particularly when massive transfusion is anticipated. Crystalloid solutions also can contribute to hyperkalemia. Both Lactated Ringer's solution and PLASMA-LYTE (Baxter, Deerfield, IL) contain potassium (4 and 5 mmol/L, respectively); large volume infusions of these fluids should be avoided, unless the patient has documented massive potassium losses via the gastrointestinal tract.

Another exogenous source of potassium during cardiac surgery with cardiopulmonary bypass is the cardioplegia solution. Cardioplegia solutions usually contain between 10 and 30 mmol/L of potassium. Even with this additional potassium, with careful preoperative and intraoperative management of intravenous fluids and monitoring of electrolytes, the majority of patients with ESRD who undergo elective cardiac surgery will not require urgent or emergent postoperative dialysis for hyperkalemia. In most cases, the patient's potassium (and fluid status as well as that of other electrolytes) can be maintained by providing dialysis on the day prior to or the day of surgery preoperatively and postoperative dialysis on the first postoperative day. If hyperkalemia develops intraoperatively or in the early postoperative period, alternative therapies, including normalizing the pH and administering glucose and insulin may be needed. If these are ineffective at controlling the potassium, either emergent dialysis or CRRT may be required.

Because the intracellular concentration of potassium is so high (150 mmol/L) compared with the extracellular concentration (4 mmol/L), small shifts between these compartments can cause significant changes in serum potassium levels. A number of mechanisms have been implicated in such shifts, including the sodium–potassium pump on cell membranes. This pump's activity is stimulated by β-agonists and insulin.

Nonselective β-blockade (such as with propranolol and nadolol) or absorption of topical beta blockers such as timolol eye drops may contribute to hyperkalemia. Labetalol, a nonselective beta blocker, has been associated with severe hyperkalemia when administered to ESRD patients for treatment of severe hypertension (28, 29). Thus, more selective beta blockers (e.g., metoprolol) may be preferable in this population. Deficiency of endogenous insulin production, as occurs in diabetic ketoacidosis, and blockade of insulin release, as with somatostatin, affect potassium homeostasis by this mechanism. The fasting state (especially if longer than 8 hours) perioperatively may also cause hypoinsulinemia and contribute to hyperkalemia.

Succinylcholine has been shown to cause hyperkalemia, particularly when administered to patients with paralysis, prolonged immobilization, burn injury, and/or other processes that lead to denervated muscle tissue. Acetylcholine receptors are upregulated and redistributed in denervated muscle. Depolarization of the denervated muscle tissue causes an exaggerated efflux of potassium from the cells into extracellular fluid (30). For the patient with ESRD, the underlying potential mild elevation of potassium that occurs during the intradialytic period may put the patient at greater risk for hyperkalemia at the time of induction of anesthesia and muscle relaxation.

Other drugs or clinical conditions that cause significant cell injury and lysis may contribute to hyperkalemia. These conditions include rhabdomyolysis from statins, seizures, compartment syndrome, or tumor lysis syndrome. Penicillin G is often administered as the potassium salt; penicillin VK contains significant amounts of potassium, so caution must be used with these medications (31). In patients with ESRD who still make urine or have early-stage CKD, medications that decrease the activity of the renin–angiotensin–aldosterone system (including ACE inhibitors, ARBs, and spironolactone) can reduce potassium excretion by the kidney and should be used with caution. These medications must be administered cautiously and require close monitoring in this group of patients; in general, the long-term benefits of these drugs outweigh this potential risk. For the patient with more advanced renal disease who is no longer making urine, renal excretion via the renin–angiotensin–aldosterone axis is not relevant; many of these patients will benefit, for example, from ACE inhibitors and ARBs for blood-pressure control without the same risk of hyperkalemia from the drugs themselves.

Prior to instituting treatment for hyperkalemia, the possibility of hemolysis during sample collection or pseudohyperkalemia should be considered (32). Any hemolysis that occurs during or after collection can result in spurious hyperkalemia; in contrast, hemolysis associated with sampling must be distinguished from intravascular hemolysis. Clinical laboratories will report whether hemolysis is present in a sample; if there is hemolysis present, the laboratory measurement should be repeated on a fresh sample. If hemolysis is persistent, the possibility of an ongoing hemolytic process must be considered. Other causes of pseudohyperkalemia include severe thrombocytosis, leukocytosis, or erythrocytosis. A confirmatory second sample can be helpful in differentiating real from artifactual hyperkalemia, but is also useful to determine if the potassium is rapidly increasing.

Given the life-threatening complications of hyperkalemia, confirmatory testing should never delay further patient evaluation and consideration of treatment. An electrocardiogram (ECG) should be obtained promptly, because different patients have different thresholds for cardiac conduction abnormalities. In general, patients with ESRD have mild hyperkalemia predialysis (serum potassium of 5–6 mmol/L), although this is not always the case. More importantly, some ESRD patients will have ECG changes with a minimal increase in serum potassium. Classically, the first manifestation of hyperkalemia is peaking of the T waves, followed by P-R interval prolongation, QRS widening, and ultimately a sinusoidal tracing (33). Although the changes evolve with increasing potassium, treatment should be initiated whenever there are changes from the baseline ECG; the urgency of treatment depends on the nature of the ECG changes, the potassium level (e.g., >6.0 mmol/L), and the rate at which the potassium level is increasing.

Although dialysis is the definitive treatment of hyperkalemia in the anuric ESRD patient, other treatments may be needed to temporarily lower the serum potassium. Acutely, if ECG changes are present, treatment with intravenous calcium should be provided to stabilize the membrane of cardiomyocytes and to decrease myocardial excitability. Either calcium gluconate or calcium chloride may be administered. Because of differences in the molecular weight of the gluconate and chloride moieties, calcium chloride is approximately 3 times as potent as calcium gluconate, although either calcium therapy is appropriate. When administering calcium, special care must be taken to avoid extravasation of the solutions into the tissue as they can cause a local thrombophlebitis and/or skin necrosis. Other therapies can be provided to drive potassium into cells and to reduce plasma concentrations. Such temporizing measures include insulin with glucose, β-2 receptor agonists, and, in the setting of acidosis, possibly bicarbonate.

Insulin is also an effective treatment to acutely reduce the serum potassium level. By activating several transport pathways, insulin stimulates the uptake of potassium into cells. Ten units of regular insulin given intravenously, along with 25 g of dextrose (50 mL of 50% dextrose), has been shown to effectively decrease serum potassium within 10–20 minutes. Although this option is a reliable method for acute management of hyperkalemia, it may frequently cause hypoglycemia within an hour after administration (34). Blood glucose levels should therefore be frequently measured after administration of insulin.

Like insulin, β-2 adrenergic agonists also stimulate cell membrane transporters to shift potassium into cells. Nebulized or inhaled albuterol can decrease serum potassium levels within 30–120 minutes (35, 36). Low doses (0.5 mg) of albuterol may be effective, if given intravenously (37), although this form is not readily available in the United States. In addition to its independent effect, albuterol seems to potentiate the therapeutic effect of insulin in correcting hyperkalemia (27). Patients who receive albuterol may experience tremor or tachycardia, but these effects usually do not limit its use.

Sodium bicarbonate was for many years considered a first-line agent in the management of acute hyperkalemia (38). In the last two decades, however, a number of studies have shown its lack of efficacy in acutely lowering serum potassium levels, particularly when used to treat hyper-kalemia in dialysis patients (39–41). Furthermore, sodium bicarbonate, especially if given as hypertonic solution, predisposes the dialysis-dependent renal failure patient to expansion of extracellular fluid, volume overload, and its sequelae including the possible need for ventilatory support or emergent dialysis for volume removal. Thus, bicarbonate is at best an adjunct treatment for hyperkalemia in the ESRD patient. Despite this limitation, when given in combination with insulin and glucose, bicarbonate may synergistically facilitate potassium shift into the intracellular compartment in the setting of metabolic acidosis (42).

After treating the acute hyperkalemia by providing stabilization of the myocardium and temporizing measures to shift potassium into cells, the focus of therapy should be removal of potassium from the body rather than redistribution. Dialysis is the definitive management of hyper-kalemia in the ESRD patient. When there are life-threatening ECG changes, dialysis should be performed emergently. If dialysis cannot be performed and additional treatment for hyperkalemia is needed, a cation-exchange resin, such as sodium polystyrene sulfonate (Kayexalate), may be given orally with a cathartic (e.g., lactulose or sorbitol) to promote excretion of the resin or alone as an enema. The dose of Kayexalate typically ranges from 15 to 30 g depending on the degree of hyperkalemia and the route of administration (orally versus rectally). Kayexalate has been associated with intestinal necrosis, in particular in premature infants (43) and critically ill adults (44), so in adults with ESRD, the threshold for treatment with dialysis (rather than treatment with Kayexalate) should be low. Whenever these agents are used, serum potassium should be serially monitored. Because resins will require >2 hours to decrease serum potassium, they are not necessarily helpful in acute management of significant hyperkalemia with cardiac conduction defects.

In patients with some residual renal function who continue to make urine, diuretics, particularly those acting on the thick ascending loop of Henle, such as furosemide and bumetanide, may promote potassium wasting. However, these medications are of no use in managing hyper-kalemia in anuric patients. Based on limited data, mineralocorticoid activity in the bowel epithelium may increase potassium secretion at that site (45). The degree to which medications such as fludrocortisone may have clinical value is questionable and still being investigated (46).

The most rapid and effective way to treat hyperkalemia is with IHD. IHD is most effective because it can be initiated with a low potassium dialysate fluid (a potassium concentration of 0–1 mmol/L) to facilitate rapid removal of potassium. CRRT and PD will also effectively lower serum potassium but more slowly, so they are of limited value in acute hyperkalemia. It should be noted that, following completion of a hemodialysis session, it takes 2–4 hours for serum potassium to reequilibrate; prior to that, serum potassium may be spuriously low and should not be repleted.

Acid Base

The normally functioning kidney reabsorbs bicarbonate and excretes acid, and therefore is crucial in maintaining acid–base homeostasis. The anephric patient will accumulate protons (H+) and anions such as phosphate, sulfate, and hippurate. As a result, the patient with ESRD will predictably develop an anion gap acidosis between IHD treatments. Hemodialysis, hemofiltration, or hemodiafiltration delivers base equivalents to the patient to neutralize the metabolic acidosis, most commonly by administration of bicarbonate, although other buffers such as lactate and acetate can be used, because the liver will metabolize these moieties to bicarbonate. After dialysis or hemofiltration, the bicarbonate level will normalize; between dialysis treatments, the bicarbonate will gradually decrease at a rate determined by the patient's diet (protein intake) and daily acid production. Continuous forms of therapy including PD will minimize the bicarbonate changes. As a result, for the critically ill patient with severe metabolic acidosis and ongoing acid production, CRRT may be a more effective way to control acidosis.

The endpoint for therapy of metabolic acidosis should be the pH, rather than the absolute bicarbonate level. Depending on the chronicity of the acidemia, some nephrologists have advocated that severe metabolic acidosis ($HCO_3 < 10$ mmol/L) be corrected slowly utilizing lower bicarbonate dialysate to minimize the "paradoxical" acidification of the cerebrospinal fluid (47) and its influence on intracranial compliance.

Under normal circumstances, although metabolic compensation for acute respiratory acidosis is limited, the kidney is able to generate bicarbonate over the course of several days. As a result, for the patient with ESRD who is not able to develop this compensatory response, any acute change in alveolar ventilation or worsening of respiratory acidosis will have a profound and sustained effect on the serum pH. Intravenous bicarbonate may be of temporary help in addressing the pH alone, but with significant sequelae. The bicarbonate can contribute to hypervolemia and the need for acute dialysis. In addition, the patient's $PaCO_2$ will increase because the patient already has respiratory failure and will not be able to increase the spontaneous minute ventilation. In many cases, mechanical ventilatory support with increased alveolar ventilation will be required to correct the pH toward normal. Tromethamine [tris(hydroxymethyl)aminomethane, (THAM)], a nonbicarbonate buffer, has been advocated to treat the severely acidotic patient, because it does not increase the $PaCO_2$. In the patient with ESRD THAM should be avoided, because it is associated with hyperkalemia and hypoglycemia and is renally excreted (48–50).

Alkalosis is also a risk in the patient with ESRD, from both a metabolic and respiratory cause, and has significant consequences. Metabolic alkalosis is common in the perioperative period for a number of reasons, including vomiting, nasogastric suctioning (depending on the pH of the gastric secretions), lactate- or acetate-based *total parenteral nutrition* solutions, and transfusion with citrate anticoagulation. Dialysis with a "standard" bicarbonate dialysate (~35 mmol/L) will also exacerbate alkalosis. The alkalemia has a number of effects. The elevated pH shifts the oxyhemoglobin dissociation curve to the left, with marked impairment of peripheral unloading of oxygen (51). Hypocalcemia will also occur as a result of acute binding of active (ionized) calcium by albumin. The resulting hypocalcemia can cause cardiac arrhythmias, decreased myocardial contractility, obtundation, paresthesias, muscle cramping, tetany, and seizures.

Other Electrolytes

Phosphate, calcium, and magnesium imbalances are commonly seen in ESRD. The ESRD patient is frequently hyperphosphatemic, because phosphate is poorly cleared by dialysis. Phosphate binders are of some value, at least to minimize the effects of dietary phosphate intake. They reduce serum phosphate by binding dietary phosphorus in the gastrointestinal tract and preventing systemic absorption and include calcium carbonate, calcium acetate, aluminum hydroxide, sevelemer, and lanthanum. They must be taken with meals to be effective. Patients must be instructed to avoid foods and medications with high concentrations of phosphorus (e.g., Fleet phospho-soda, commonly administered to constipated patients) (52).

Other disease processes that result in tissue breakdown and therefore intracellular phosphate release (e.g., rhabdomyolysis, tumor lysis syndrome, seizure) will further predispose the patient to hyperphosphatemia. Whereas hyperphosphatemia alone is generally asymptomatic, the consequent metabolic abnormalities (including hypocalcemia) have serious consequences, including cardiac conduction abnormalities and neuromuscular symptoms. In general, patients are at higher risk of hypocalcemia with sudden, acute hyperphosphatemia (e.g., tumor lysis) than with chronic hyperphosphatemia associated with ESRD.

Severe hyperphosphatemia should generally be treated with hemodialysis. Unless the patient is symptomatic, intravenous calcium repletion should be avoided in these cases, because it can cause precipitation and calciphylaxis (skin and soft tissue necrosis from small vessel calcification) (53). When treating with calcium, the generally accepted guideline is to closely monitor both calcium and phosphate and target a calcium–phosphate product of < 55 (54).

In contrast to many cardiac patients who waste magnesium in the urine with diuretic use, the anuric ESRD patient is unable to excrete magnesium and is more commonly hypermagnesemic. The primary cause for exogenous hypermagnesemia is the intravenous administration of magnesium, although other sources include cathartic bowel preparations (55). As a result, magnesium must be administered cautiously in the patient with ESRD. Although rarely symptomatic, severe hypermagnesemia can cause bradycardia, hypotension, and respiratory muscle weakness and failure (56). The definitive management of symptomatic hypermagnesemia is hemodialysis.

Hematologic Complications

Patients with ESRD usually have chronic anemia. A deficiency of endogenous erythropoietin, 90% of which is produced by the kidneys, is a primary cause of chronic anemia in ESRD (57). Other causes for anemia include iron deficiency, shortened red-cell survival, bone-marrow suppression from uremic toxins, and bleeding as a result of uremic platelet dysfunction. Since the introduction of recombinant human erythropoietin in the mid-1980s, erythropoiesis-stimulating agents (ESAs) have become a mainstay in management of chronic anemia in ESRD (58, 59). For patients with ESRD, ESAs are usually administered in the outpatient setting. The target hemoglobin is 10–12 g/dL (60, 61); dosing is adjusted to achieve this target. When chronic erythropoietin has not been administered, some investigators have advocated acute administration prior to surgery to minimize transfusion requirements (62). This acute therapy is rarely effective in the perioperative period because the effects of erythropoietin are not usually seen until about 2 weeks after administration.

Bleeding is one of the most worrisome complications of uremia, particularly in patients undergoing cardiac surgery. Uremia increases bleeding time as a result of dysfunction of clotting factors, most notably von Willebrand factor (vWF), and impaired platelet aggregation. Compared to patients with normal renal function, those with severe renal dysfunction (GFR < 40 mL/min) are 6 times more likely to have postoperative bleeding after coronary artery bypass graft (63). Although dialysis results in improved clearance of uremic toxins and decreases the risk of bleeding, ESRD patients are still at higher risk of bleeding than is the general population.

Multiple therapeutic strategies are recommended for managing the bleeding diatheses in patients with ESRD, particularly those undergoing surgery. DDAVP (1-deamino-8-D-arginine-vasopressin) is a first-line treatment (64). DDAVP stimulates endothelial release of vWF and factor VIII and may be used acutely to shorten bleeding time in uremic patients. It can be administered at a dose of 0.3 µg/kg every 12 hours for up to 48 hours. After several doses, it is less effective; some patients develop tachyphylaxis. For surgical patients, the initial dose should be administered 30–60 minutes prior to the procedure. Conjugated estrogens have also been used to treat bleeding in surgical patients with uremia. Estrogens have been demonstrated to improve hemostasis within 6 hours of intravenous administration (65). Postoperative bleeding is reduced with estrogens that are administered for as long as 5 days after surgery. Cryoprecipitate has also been used. It provides replacement of decreased or dysfunctional vWF, fibrinogen, factor VIII, and factor XIII. Although it may be given for uremic bleeding, it is expensive and carries the risk of blood-borne infection (65). Dialysis should also be considered in uremic patients both preoperatively and postoperatively, because it will correct dysfunctional hemostasis through clearance of uremic toxins.

Transfusion is also advocated for the patient with ESRD scheduled for surgery, although transfusions must be provided with caution. Treatment of anemia will foster intravascular distribution of platelets toward endothelium and decrease bleeding time (66). Historically, at least in the acute setting, some nephrologists have advocated red-blood-cell transfusion to achieve a hematocrit >30% in any patient with renal failure (67). This approach is no longer routinely advocated, although since erythropoietin therapy has become available, anemia is rarely an acute clinical problem in this group of patients. Another factor that must be taken into account in deciding whether to transfuse the patient with ESRD is the impact of transfusion on tissue matching. For patients who are or may become candidates for heart, kidney, or other organ transplantation, blood transfusion carries the risk of human leukocyte antigen presensitization, subsequent tissue mismatch or rejection, and possibly worse transplant outcomes (68, 69). In such patients, blood transfusions should be used judiciously.

Another source of concern for the anesthesiologist caring for the patient with ESRD is the use of heparin both during dialysis and as part of the routine maintenance of venous access. In the chronic hemodialysis setting, patients routinely receive heparin during their treatments to prevent circuit clotting and blood loss. The chronic administration of heparin during dialysis should not pose any problem in the perioperative management of the dialysis-dependent patient. In the acute setting, particularly if dialysis is required immediately before surgery, it can be performed without anticoagulation. It is critical for the anesthesiologist and nephrologist to coordinate management during this period of time. For long-term management of dialysis catheters, both tunneled and non-tunneled heparin is usually inserted into the catheter to prevent clotting. The heparin is aspirated from the catheter prior to dialysis and should not reach the systemic circulation. In an increasing number of cases, heparin is no longer being used as part of catheter management. Catheters can be managed with alternative anticoagulants (typically sodium citrate or *tissue plasminogen activator*), particularly for patients with a history of heparin-induced thrombocytopenia and during periop-erative care. Recent studies have demonstrated the value of instillation of an antibiotic solution rather than heparin for catheter maintenance. The antibiotic lock solution decreases the risk of catheter-related infec-tions 7.72-fold without an increased risk of thrombosis (70).

Cardiovascular System

Cardiovascular disease continues to be the leading cause of mortality in patients with ESRD with or without diabetes mellitus. It accounts for >50% of deaths in ESRD (71). These patients are 10–20 times more likely to die from cardiovascular causes compared with patients in the general population of similar age, gender, and race (72). Among dialysis patients, 40% have coronary artery disease, 75% have left ventricular hypertro-phy, and 40% have heart failure (73, 74). As a result, a large percentage of these patients will require cardiac surgery. An important characteris-tic of cardiovascular disease is the presentation of acute complications. Recent data suggest that acute myocardial infarction may present with atypical symptoms more frequently in patients with ESRD than in the general population (75); these data emphasize the importance of a high index of suspicion for myocardial ischemia in this at-risk population at any time, but particularly during the perioperative period.

The significant overlap and interaction of renal and cardiovascular diseases have long been recognized. Common risk factors, including hypertension and diabetes mellitus, contribute to development and pro-gression of both disease processes. In addition, a number of issues related to renal dysfunction contribute to increased cardiovascular risk. For example, anemia associated with ESRD may worsen left ventricular hypertrophy (76, 77). Abnormal calcium–phosphorous metabolism in ESRD is associated with accelerated coronary artery calcification (78) and increased risk of cardiovascular disease and poor outcome (25, 79). Cardiac arrhythmias and conduction defects associated with metabolic derangements are likely to contribute to the risk of sudden cardiac death in ESRD patients (80).

COMPLICATIONS OF DIALYSIS THERAPY

Hypotension

The most common complication during dialysis therapy is hypotension, generally attributed to acute fluid shifts and volume removal (ultrafiltration). The speed with which intracellular and interstitial fluid shifts into the vascular compartment during dialysis varies among patients. Depending on comorbidities, such as arteriosclerosis or autonomic dysfunction, some patients also lack the physiologic capacity to compensate for rapid changes intravascular volume. Intradialytic hypotension will often limit the rate and/or amount of volume removal that can be achieved during dialysis treatment.

Concurrent use of antihypertensive medications may contribute to hypotension related to dialysis. These medications may need to be given in smaller doses or held altogether on days of dialysis treatment. Rarely, hypotension may result from various types of hypersensitivity reactions to the dialysis membrane or any aspect of the extracorporeal dialysis circuit, the solvents used in dialysate, or other medications administered during dialysis, such as heparin (81, 82).

The rate and degree of fluid removal in PD patients is dictated by the formulation and frequency of the peritoneal dialysate exchange prescribed by the nephrologist. Hypotension in PD patients may be managed by changing the PD regimen or, more acutely, by enteral or parenteral salt and volume repletion. In general, because fluid removal is continuous, PD is better tolerated from a hemodynamic standpoint than is hemodialysis, and may be preferable in patients with severe heart failure. Although the degree of hypotension associated with dialysis is variable, if the therapy is effective at removing intravascular volume, the recently dialyzed patient is usually clinically intravascularly volume depleted; if the acute volume shifts associated with dialysis are not recognized by the anesthesiologist, the patient is at risk for severe hypotension during and after anesthesia induction and with initiation of positive pressure ventilation. A careful assessment of volume status immediately prior to induction of anesthesia and judicious fluid administration will minimize this risk.

Infection

Patients with ESRD are at increased risk of infections—and probably infectious complications after surgery. Infection is the second leading cause of death among ESRD patients after cardiovascular disease (83). The risk is multifactorial, and contributed to by the renal dysfunction and (for some patients) the risk of infection related to the dialysis access site. A variety of access sites are used for dialysis with varying incidence of infectious complications. Permanent AVFs carry the lowest risk of infection. AVGs are also used, but carry a higher infection risk. Hemodialysis catheters, whether tunneled or not, carry a high risk for septicemia, with the risk increasing with increasing access of the catheter (84). These catheters should be restricted to use for dialytic therapy and not used for routine medication administration.

Although the anesthesiologist will rarely have any reason to either access or manage a PD catheter, it is important to consider the peritoneal catheter as a source for unexplained sepsis in the surgical patient with ESRD. Peritonitis can occur as a complication of chronic PD. Signs of peritonitis may include nausea, vomiting, abdominal pain, and cloudy peritoneal fluid (85). Because the dialysate fluid contains dextrose, the white blood cell count cutoff for the diagnosis of PD-associated peritonitis is only 100 white blood cells/mm^3. If PD-associated peritonitis is suspected, the dialysate should be sent for Gram stain and culture, and empiric antibiotic therapy should cover gram-negative rod gastrointestinal flora and skin pathogens.

Most importantly, the anesthesiologist must be attentive to the proper sterile management of both hemodialysis access and PD catheters. Exit sites of all catheters should be inspected regularly (including prior to cardiac surgery) for erythema, tenderness, fluctuance, or other signs of infection. The potential complications including bacteremia and peritonitis can be devastating with exceptionally high morbidity and mortality (85).

Vascular Complications

Anesthesiologists are well aware of the complications associated with vascular access catheters. A review of the complications is beyond the scope of this chapter. However, the anesthesiologist caring for the dialysis-dependent patient should be aware of some issues that are relatively specific to this patient population. In addition to the usual infectious risks associated with venous access, the patients are at risk for intravascular clotting and stenosis after repeated catheterization or manipulation of the access sites. If the patient has an AVF or AVG, venipuncture and blood-pressure monitoring should be avoided on that limb. For those patients with central venous catheters, there is a risk of venous thrombosis, which limits access site options and may be associated with superior vena cava syndrome or other complications. Patients with AVFs, for example, have high regional flow through the extremity. If the patient also has any evidence of central stenosis associated with previous venous cannulation, there is a risk of ipsilateral fistula thrombosis

(86). In addition, even small-bore peripherally inserted central catheters (PICCs) can result in subclavian stenosis and are relatively contraindicated in ESRD patients (87).

During surgery for the patient with dialysis-dependent renal failure, extra attention must be paid to padding and positioning of the extremity with the vascular access to prevent thrombosis or other injury to the graft or fistula. A well-functioning fistula or graft should have a palpable thrill and audible bruit on auscultation. Ideally, the anesthesiologist should be able to assess the fistula intraoperatively to assure that it is functioning, although it can be difficult to position the patient for the procedure and still have access to the extremity. The fistula should be carefully evaluated both before and after the procedure to ensure patency. In addition, although the fistulas and grafts should generally not be accessed for routine care, they can provide an emergency access site. When used, the smallest needle possible should be inserted, and special care should be taken when applying pressure to ensure hemostasis to minimize the risk of compromise to the fistula or graft.

OTHER CONSIDERATIONS

Pharmacokinetics

Because the kidneys play such an important role in the metabolism and clearance of many medications, the patient with renal insufficiency may have markedly altered pharmacokinetics. The effects of ESRD also include changes in plasma protein binding and volume of distribution of medications, as well as changes in their hepatic metabolism (88, 89). Many medications, including antimicrobial and cardiovascular agents, require dose adjustment in ESRD patients; additional modifications may have to be made based on the dialysis treatment methodology (hemodialysis, PD, or CRRT) and schedule. Consultation with a pharmacist, nephrologist, or reliable reference is advised to determine the appropriate loading and maintenance doses of drugs and to guide management (90).

The drug dispositions of some anesthetic agents warrant emphasis. For medications that are highly protein bound, the acidosis (and possible hypoalbuminemia) of ESRD increases their unbound, active fraction. For this reason, the dose of barbiturates (such as thiopental) and benzodiazepines (such as diazepam) are often reduced by as much as 50% (91, 92).

Other anesthetics, particularly some opioid analgesics, are metabolized by hepatic biotransformation. Although they themselves are not affected by renal failure, their water-soluble metabolites cannot be cleared by renal excretion. Accumulation of these active metabolites may result in prolonged sedation or intoxication. Repeated doses of morphine, for example, to an ESRD patient increases plasma levels of morphine-6-glucuronide (among other metabolites), which may cause severe respiratory depression (93). Similarly, prolonged use of meperidine leads to accumulation of normeperidine, a neuroexcitatory substance associated with seizures (94, 95). Other opioids such as fentanyl or hydromorphone are therefore preferred over morphine or meperidine in ESRD patients.

Nonsteroidal antiinflammatory drugs should be avoided in the patient with residual renal function, including the PD patient who continues to make urine. The anuric ESRD patient, however, may be given these medications if other risks associated with their use (including gastrointestinal bleeding and hypertension) are acceptable.

The effects of neuromuscular blocking agents may be substantially influenced by metabolic and pharmacokinetic disturbances in ESRD. The risk of hyperkalemia from succinylcholine is discussed earlier in this chapter. Nondepolarizing neuromuscular blocking drugs such as pancuronium are themselves or their metabolites excreted by the kidneys and should be avoided in ESRD (96).

Although vecuronium and rocuronium have been used safely in ESRD (96, 97), their durations of action may be longer in renal failure because of slower clearance of the medications or active metabolites (98–101). Atracurium, cisatracurium, and mivacurium are cleared by Hofmann degradation or plasma cholinesterase, so the half-lives of these drugs are not thought to be substantially affected by end-stage renal failure (102, 103). As is always the case with use of these agents, the degree of neuromuscular blockade should be monitored with train-of-four stimulation.

CONCLUSION

The dialysis-dependent ESRD patient poses unique challenges in perioperative management. The anesthesiologist must be aware of the pathophysiology of ESRD and its consequences for perioperative management. It is critical to consider the patient's comorbidities and, for these patients, to pay close attention to the preoperative volume and metabolic status and recent dialysis history. The anesthesiologist must take into account the pharmacokinetic changes that occur as a result of the renal failure and select agents and adjust drug dosage accordingly. Ongoing communication among all providers is essential to ensure a smooth transition to and from the operating room and to coordinate dialysis, anesthesia, surgery, and postoperative management to minimize the likelihood of complications in this vulnerable population.

Acknowledgment

K.D.L. is supported by National Institutes of Health/National Center for Research Resources/OD, University of California San Francisco-Clinical and Translational Science Institute Grant KL2 RR024130. We thank Daniel Burkhardt and Kristina Kudelko for their helpful comments.

References

1. Kogan A, Medalion B, Kornowski R, et al.: Cardiac surgery in patients on chronic hemodialysis: short and long-term survival. Thorac Cardiovasc Surg 2008; 56(3):123–7
2. Rahmanian PB, Adams DH, Castillo JG, Vassalotti J, Filsoufi F: Early and late outcome of cardiac surgery in dialysis-dependent patients: single-center experience with 245 consecutive patients. J Thorac Cardiovasc Surg 2008; 135(4):915–22
3. Coresh J, Selvin E, Stevens LA, et al.: Prevalence of chronic kidney disease in the United States. JAMA 2007; 298(17):2038–47
4. Lewis EJ, Hunsicker LG, Bain RP, Rohde RD: The effect of angio-tensin-converting-enzyme inhibition on diabetic nephropathy. The Collaborative Study Group. N Engl J Med 1993; 329(20):1456–62
5. Ravid M, Savin H, Jutrin I, Bental T, Katz B, Lishner M: Long-term stabilizing effect of angiotensin-converting enzyme inhibition on plasma creatinine and on proteinuria in normotensive type II diabetic patients. Ann Intern Med 1993; 118(8):577–81
6. Maschio G, Alberti D, Janin G, et al.: Effect of the angiotensin-con-verting-enzyme inhibitor benazepril on the progression of chronic renal insufficiency. The Angiotensin-Converting-Enzyme Inhibition in Progressive Renal Insufficiency Study Group. N Engl J Med 1996; 334(15):939–45
7. Randomised placebo-controlled trial of effect of ramipril on decline in glomerular filtration rate and risk of terminal renal failure in pro-teinuric, non-diabetic nephropathy. The GISEN Group (Gruppo Italiano di Studi Epidemiologici in Nefrologia). Lancet 1997; 349 (9069):1857–63
8. Hsu CY, Vittinghoff E, Lin F, Shlipak MG: The incidence of end-stage renal disease is increasing faster than the prevalence of chronic renal insufficiency. Ann Intern Med 2004; 141(2):95–101
9. System URD. USRDS 2008 annual data report: atlas of chronic kid-ney disease and end-state renal disease in the United States. Bethesda, MD, 2008.
10. K/DOQI clinical practice guidelines for chronic kidney disease: evaluation, classification, and stratification. Am J Kidney Dis 2002; 39(2 Suppl 1):S1–266

11. Cockcroft DW, Gault MH: Prediction of creatinine clearance from serum creatinine. Nephron 1976; 16(1):31–41

12. Levey AS, Bosch JP, Lewis JB, Greene T, Rogers N, Roth D: A more accurate method to estimate glomerular filtration rate from serum creatinine: a new prediction equation. Modification of Diet in Renal Disease Study Group. Ann Intern Med 199916; 130(6):461–70

13. Levey AS, Coresh J, Greene T, et al.: Expressing the Modification of Diet in Renal Disease Study equation for estimating glomerular filtration rate with standardized serum creatinine values. Clin Chem 2007; 53(4):766–72

14. Johnson WJ, Hagge WW, Wagoner RD, Dinapoli RP, Rosevear JW: Effects of urea loading in patients with far-advanced renal failure. Mayo Clin Proc 1972; 47(1):21–9

15. Meyer TW, Hostetter TH: Uremia. N Engl J Med 2007; 357(13): 1316–25

16. Liu K, Chertow G: Dialysis in the treatment of renal failure. In: Fauci AS, Braunwald E, Kasper DL, Hauser SL, Longo DL, Jameson JL, Loscalzo J, eds. Harrison's principles of internal medicine, 17th Edition. New York, NY, McGraw Hill Medicine, 2008

17. Daugirdas J, Blake P, Ing T: Handbook of dialysis. Philadelphia, PA, Lippincott Williams and Wilkins, 2007

18. Cheung A: Hemodialysis and hemofiltration. In: Greenberg A, ed. Primer on kidney diseases, 4th Edition. Philadelphia, PA, Saunders, 2005:464–76

19. Forni LG, Hilton PJ: Continuous hemofiltration in the treatment of acute renal failure. N Engl J Med 1997; 336(18):1303–9

20. Vinsonneau C, Camus C, Combes A, et al.: Continuous venovenous haemodiafiltration versus intermittent haemodialysis for acute renal failure in patients with multiple-organ dysfunction syndrome: a multicentre randomised trial. Lancet 2006; 368(9533):379–85

21. Augustine JJ, Sandy D, Seifert TH, Paganini EP: A randomized controlled trial comparing intermittent with continuous dialysis in patients with ARF. Am J Kidney Dis 2004; 44(6):1000–7

22. Mehta RL, McDonald B, Gabbai FB, et al. A randomized clinical trial of continuous versus intermittent dialysis for acute renal failure. Kidney Int 2001; 60(3):1154–63

23. Stevens LA, Levey AS: Chronic kidney disease: staging and principles of management. In: Greenberg A, editor. Primer on kidney diseases, 4th Edition. Saunders Book Company, Philadelphia, PA, 2005:455–63

24. Foley RN, Parfrey PS, Harnett JD, Kent GM, Murray DC, Barre PE: Impact of hypertension on cardiomyopathy, morbidity and mortality in end-stage renal disease. Kidney Int 1996; 49(5):1379–85

25. Blacher J, Guerin AP, Pannier B, Marchais SJ, London GM: Arterial calcifications, arterial stiffness, and cardiovascular risk in end-stage renal disease. Hypertension 2001; 38(4):938–42
26. Thier SO: Potassium physiology. Am J Med 1986; 80(4A):3–7
27. Putcha N, Allon M: Management of hyperkalemia in dialysis patients. Semin Dial 2007; 20(5):431–9
28. Hamad A, Salameh M, Zihlif M, Feinfeld DA, Carvounis CP: Life-threatening hyperkalemia after intravenous labetolol injection for hypertensive emergency in a hemodialysis patient. Am J Nephrol 2001; 21(3):241–4
29. Arthur S, Greenberg A: Hyperkalemia associated with intravenous labetalol therapy for acute hypertension in renal transplant recipients. Clin Nephrol 1990; 33(6):269–71
30. Martyn JA, Richtsfeld M: Succinylcholine-induced hyperkalemia in acquired pathologic states: etiologic factors and molecular mechanisms. Anesthesiology 2006; 104(1):158–69
31. Thiele A, Rehman HU: Hyperkalemia caused by penicillin. Am J Med 2008; 121(8):e1–2
32. Sevastos N, Theodossiades G, Archimandritis AJ. Pseudohyperkalemia in serum: a new insight into an old phenomenon. Clin Med Res 2008; 6(1):30–2
33. Parham WA, Mehdirad AA, Biermann KM, Fredman CS: Hyperkalemia revisited. Tex Heart Inst J 2006; 33(1):40–7
34. Allon M, Copkney C: Albuterol and insulin for treatment of hyperkalemia in hemodialysis patients. Kidney Int 1990; 38(5):869–72
35. Allon M, Dunlay R, Copkney C: Nebulized albuterol for acute hyperkalemia in patients on hemodialysis. Ann Intern Med 1989; 110(6):426–9
36. Montoliu J, Almirall J, Ponz E, Campistol JM, Revert L: Treatment of hyperkalaemia in renal failure with salbutamol inhalation. J Intern Med 1990; 228(1):35–7
37. Montoliu J, Lens XM, Revert L: Potassium-lowering effect of albuterol for hyperkalemia in renal failure. Arch Intern Med 1987; 147(4):713–7
38. Iqbal Z, Friedman EA: Preferred therapy of hyperkalemia in renal insufficiency: survey of nephrology training-program directors. N Engl J Med 1989; 320(1):60–1
39. Blumberg A, Weidmann P, Shaw S, Gnadinger M: Effect of various therapeutic approaches on plasma potassium and major regulating factors in terminal renal failure. Am J Med 1988; 85(4):507–12
40. Gutierrez R, Schlessinger F, Oster JR, Rietberg B, Perez GO: Effect of hypertonic versus isotonic sodium bicarbonate on plasma potas-

sium concentration in patients with end-stage renal disease. Miner Electrolyte Metab 1991; 17(5):297–302

41. Allon M, Shanklin N: Effect of bicarbonate administration on plasma potassium in dialysis patients: interactions with insulin and albuterol. Am J Kidney Dis 1996; 28(4):508–14

42. Kim HJ: Combined effect of bicarbonate and insulin with glucose in acute therapy of hyperkalemia in end-stage renal disease patients. Nephron 1996; 72(3):476–82

43. Rugolotto S, Gruber M, Solano PD, Chini L, Gobbo S, Pecori S: Necrotizing enterocolitis in a 850 gram infant receiving sorbitol-free sodium polystyrene sulfonate (Kayexalate): clinical and histopathologic findings. J Perinatol 2007; 27(4):247–9

44. Rogers FB, Li SC: Acute colonic necrosis associated with sodium polystyrene sulfonate (Kayexalate) enemas in a critically ill patient: case report and review of the literature. J Trauma 2001; 51(2):395–7

45. Imbriano LJ, Durham JH, Maesaka JK: Treating interdialytic hyperkalemia with fludrocortisone. Semin Dial 2003; 16(1):5–7

46. Kim DM, Chung JH, Yoon SH, Kim HL: Effect of fludrocortisone acetate on reducing serum potassium levels in patients with end-stage renal disease undergoing haemodialysis. Nephrol Dial Transplant 2007; 22(11):3273–6

47. Daugirdas J, Ross E, Nissenson A: Acute hemodialysis prescription. In: Daugirdas J, Blake P, Ing T, editors. Handbook of dialysis. Philadelphia, PA, Lippincott Williams and Wilkins, 2007

48. Hoste EA, Colpaert K, Vanholder RC, et al.: Sodium bicarbonate versus THAM in ICU patients with mild metabolic acidosis. J Nephrol 2005; 18(3):303–7

49. Nahas GG, Sutin KM, Fermon C, et al.: Guidelines for the treatment of acidaemia with THAM. Drugs 1998; 55(2):191–224

50. Kallet RH, Jasmer RM, Luce JM, Lin LH, Marks JD: The treatment of acidosis in acute lung injury with tris-hydroxymethyl aminomethane (THAM). Am J Respir Crit Care Med 2000; 161(4 Pt 1):1149–53

51. Adrogue HJ, Madias NE: Management of life-threatening acid-base disorders. Second of two parts. N Engl J Med 1998; 338(2):107–11

52. Hsu HJ, Wu MS: Extreme hyperphosphatemia and hypocalcemic coma associated with phosphate enema. Intern Med 2008; 47(7):643–6

53. Fine A, Zacharias J: Calciphylaxis is usually non-ulcerating: risk factors, outcome and therapy. Kidney Int 2002; 61(6):2210–7

54. K/DOQI clinical practice guidelines for bone metabolism and disease in chronic kidney disease. Am J Kidney Dis 2003; 42(4 Suppl 3):S1–201

55. Smilkstein MJ, Smolinske SC, Kulig KW, Rumack BH: Severe hyper-magnesemia due to multiple-dose cathartic therapy. West J Med 1988; 148(2):208–11
56. Schelling JR: Fatal hypermagnesemia. Clin Nephrol 2000; 53(1):61–5
57. Eschbach JW: The anemia of chronic renal failure: pathophysiology and the effects of recombinant erythropoietin. Kidney Int 1989; 35(1):134–48
58. Winearls CG: Historical review on the use of recombinant human erythropoietin in chronic renal failure. Nephrol Dial Transplant 1995; 10 Suppl 2:3–9
59. Stubbs JR: Alternatives to blood product transfusion in the critically ill: erythropoietin. Crit Care Med 2006; 34(5 Suppl):S160–9
60. Locatelli F, Nissenson AR, Barrett BJ, et al.: Clinical practice guidelines for anemia in chronic kidney disease: problems and solutions. A position statement from Kidney Disease: Improving Global Outcomes (KDIGO). Kidney Int 2008; 74(10):1237–40
61. KDOQI Clinical Practice Guideline and Clinical Practice Recommendations for anemia in chronic kidney disease: 2007 update of hemoglobin target. Am J Kidney Dis 2007; 50(3):471–530
62. Corwin HL, Gettinger A, Fabian TC, et al.: Efficacy and safety of epoetin alfa in critically ill patients. N Engl J Med 2007; 357(10): 965–76
63. Winkelmayer WC, Levin R, Avorn J: Chronic kidney disease as a risk factor for bleeding complications after coronary artery bypass surgery. Am J Kidney Dis 2003; 41(1):84–9
64. Mannucci PM, Remuzzi G, Pusineri F, et al.: Deamino-8-D-arginine vasopressin shortens the bleeding time in uremia. N Engl J Med 1983; 308(1):8–12
65. Hedges SJ, Dehoney SB, Hooper JS, Amanzadeh J, Busti AJ: Evidence-based treatment recommendations for uremic bleeding. Nat Clin Pract Nephrol 2007; 3(3):138–53
66. Turitto VT, Weiss HJ: Red blood cells: their dual role in thrombus formation. Science 1980; 207(4430):541–3
67. Remuzzi G: Bleeding in renal failure. Lancet 1988; 1(8596):1205–8
68. Bishay ES, Cook DJ, El Fettouh H, et al.: The impact of HLA sensitization and donor cause of death in heart transplantation. Transplantation 2000; 70(1):220–2
69. Susal C, Opelz G: Kidney graft failure and presensitization against HLA class I and class II antigens. Transplantation 2002; 73(8): 1269–73
70. Jaffer Y, Selby NM, Taal MW, Fluck RJ, McIntyre CW: A meta-analysis of hemodialysis catheter locking solutions in the prevention of catheter-related infection. Am J Kidney Dis 2008; 51(2):233–41

71. Collins AJ: Cardiovascular mortality in end-stage renal disease. Am J Med Sci 2003; 325(4):163-7

72. Levey AS, Beto JA, Coronado BE, et al. Controlling the epidemic of cardiovascular disease in chronic renal disease: what do we know? What do we need to learn? Where do we go from here? National Kidney Foundation Task Force on Cardiovascular Disease. Am J Kidney Dis 1998; 32(5):853-906

73. Foley RN, Parfrey PS, Sarnak MJ: Epidemiology of cardiovascular disease in chronic renal disease. J Am Soc Nephrol 1998; 9(12 Suppl):S16-23

74. Foley RN, Parfrey PS, Harnett JD, et al.: Clinical and echocardiographic disease in patients starting end-stage renal disease therapy. Kidney Int 1995; 47(1):186-92

75. Herzog CA, Littrell K, Arko C, Frederick PD, Blaney M: Clinical characteristics of dialysis patients with acute myocardial infarction in the United States: a collaborative project of the United States Renal Data System and the National Registry of Myocardial Infarction. Circulation 2007; 116(13):1465-72

76. Parfrey PS: Cardiac disease in dialysis patients: diagnosis, burden of disease, prognosis, risk factors and management. Nephrol Dial Transplant 2000; 15 Suppl 5:58-68

77. Frank H, Heusser K, Hoffken B, Huber P, Schmieder RE, Schobel HP. Effect of erythropoietin on cardiovascular prognosis parameters in hemodialysis patients. Kidney Int 2004; 66(2):832-40

78. Goodman WG, Goldin J, Kuizon BD, et al.: Coronary-artery calcification in young adults with end-stage renal disease who are undergoing dialysis. N Engl J Med 2000; 342(20):1478-83

79. Raggi P, Boulay A, Chasan-Taber S, et al.: Cardiac calcification in adult hemodialysis patients. A link between end-stage renal disease and cardiovascular disease? J Am Coll Cardiol 2002; 39(4):695-701

80. Meier P, Vogt P, Blanc E: Ventricular arrhythmias and sudden cardiac death in end-stage renal disease patients on chronic hemodialysis. Nephron 2001; 87(3):199-214

81. Kraske GK, Shinaberger JH, Klaustermeyer WB: Severe hypersensitivity reaction during hemodialysis. Ann Allergy Asthma Immunol 1997; 78(2):217-20

82. Acute allergic-type reactions among patients undergoing hemodialysis—multiple states, 2007–2008. MMWR Morb Mortal Wkly Rep 2008; 57(5):124-5

83. Sarnak MJ, Jaber BL: Mortality caused by sepsis in patients with end-stage renal disease compared with the general population. Kidney Int 2000; 58(4):1758-64

84. Hoen B, Paul-Dauphin A, Hestin D, Kessler M: EPIBACDIAL: a multicenter prospective study of risk factors for bacteremia in chronic hemodialysis patients. J Am Soc Nephrol 1998; 9(5):869–76
85. Piraino B, Bailie GR, Bernardini J, et al.: Peritoneal dialysis-related infections recommendations: 2005 update. Perit Dial Int 2005; 25(2):107–31
86. Agarwal AK, Patel BM, Haddad NJ: Central vein stenosis: a nephrologist's perspective. Semin Dial 2007; 20(1):53–62
87. Gonsalves CF, Eschelman DJ, Sullivan KL, DuBois N, Bonn J: Incidence of central vein stenosis and occlusion following upper extremity PICC and port placement. Cardiovasc Intervent Radiol 2003; 26(2):123–7
88. Dreisbach AW, Lertora JJ: The effect of chronic renal failure on drug metabolism and transport. Expert Opin Drug Metab Toxicol 2008; 4(8):1065–74
89. Nolin TD, Frye RF, Matzke GR: Hepatic drug metabolism and transport in patients with kidney disease. Am J Kidney Dis 2003; 42(5):906–25
90. Brier M, Aronoff G: Drug prescribing in renal failure, 5th Edition. Philadelphia, PA, American College of Physicians, 2007
91. Burch PG, Stanski DR: Decreased protein binding and thiopental kinetics. Clin Pharmacol Ther 1982; 32(2):212–7
92. Schmith VD, Piraino B, Smith RB, Kroboth PD: Alprazolam in end-stage renal disease. II. Pharmacodynamics. Clin Pharmacol Ther 1992; 51(5):533–40
93. D'Honneur G, Gilton A, Sandouk P, Scherrmann JM, Duvaldestin P: Plasma and cerebrospinal fluid concentrations of morphine and morphine glucuronides after oral morphine. The influence of renal failure. Anesthesiology 1994; 81(1):87–93
94. Hassan H, Bastani B, Gellens M: Successful treatment of normeperidine neurotoxicity by hemodialysis. Am J Kidney Dis 2000; 35(1):146–9
95. Szeto HH, Inturrisi CE, Houde R, Saal S, Cheigh J, Reidenberg MM: Accumulation of normeperidine, an active metabolite of meperidine, in patients with renal failure of cancer. Ann Intern Med 1977; 86(6):738–41
96. Sirotzky L, Lewis EJ: Anesthesia related muscle paralysis in renal failure. Clin Nephrol 1978; 10(1):38–42
97. Dhonneur G, Rebaine C, Slavov V, Ruggier R, De Chaubry V, Duvaldestin P: Neostigmine reversal of vecuronium neuromuscular block and the influence of renal failure. Anesth Analg 1996; 82(1):134–8

98. Khuenl-Brady KS, Pomaroli A, Puhringer F, Mitterschiffthaler G, Koller J: The use of rocuronium (ORG 9426) in patients with chronic renal failure. Anaesthesia 1993; 48(10):873–5

99. Lynam DP, Cronnelly R, Castagnoli KP, et al.: The pharmacodynamics and pharmacokinetics of vecuronium in patients anesthetized with isoflurane with normal renal function or with renal failure. Anesthesiology 1988; 69(2):227–31

100. Beauvoir C, Peray P, Daures JP, Peschaud JL, D'Athis F: Pharmacodynamics of vecuronium in patients with and without renal failure: a meta-analysis. Can J Anaesth 1993; 40(8):696–702

101. Robertson EN, Driessen JJ, Booij LH: Pharmacokinetics and pharmacodynamics of rocuronium in patients with and without renal failure. Eur J Anaesthesiol 2005; 22(1):4–10

102. Frampton JE, McTavish D: Mivacurium. A review of its pharmacology and therapeutic potential in general anaesthesia. Drugs 1993; 45(6):1066–89

103. Della Rocca G, Pompei L, Coccia C, et al.: Atracurium, cisatracurium, vecuronium and rocuronium in patients with renal failure. Minerva Anestesiol 2003; 69(7–8):605–11, 12, 5

Thomas F. Slaughter, MD
David C. Sane, MD

Heparin-Induced Thrombocytopenia in Patients Requiring

6 Cardiovascular Surgery

INTRODUCTION

Heparin-induced thrombocytopenia (HIT) characterizes an immune system–mediated adverse reaction to heparin. It represents a prothrombotic state characterized by thrombocytopenia and thrombosis. As many as 5% of patients exposed to unfractionated heparin therapy for extended periods develop HIT; if unrecognized, HIT can contribute to increased mortality (1, 2). In contrast to other drug-induced thrombocytopenias, HIT is characterized by platelet activation and elevated risk for both venous and arterial thromboses (odds ratio, 20–40; absolute risk, 35%–75%) (2–4). In a recent case–control study assessing financial impact of HIT on inpatient costs, each additional case of HIT was associated with a financial loss of $14,387 and an increased length of hospital stay of 14.5 days. Based on a conservative estimate of a 0.2% incidence of HIT within a tertiary academic medical center (50 episodes of HIT per year), overall institutional financial impact was projected to be between $700,000 and $1,000,000 in losses annually (5). As a result, it is critical for the anesthesiologist to be aware of the factors associated with HIT, its clinical presentation, and methods to address it.

CLINICAL PRESENTATION

HIT is defined as an adverse clinical event (most often thrombocytopenia and/or thrombosis) in a patient with recent heparin exposure who tests

Medically Challenging Patients Undergoing Cardiothoracic Surgery, edited by Neal H. Cohen, MD, MPH, MS, Lippincott Williams & Wilkins, Baltimore © 2009.

positive for platelet factor 4 (PF4) and/or heparin-dependent antibodies. Thrombocytopenia is the most common clinical sequela of HIT occurring in 90% or more of patients; however, despite the low platelet count, in most patients there appears to be no increased propensity for bleeding (6, 7). In most cases, thrombocytopenia is moderate in severity, with a nadir platelet count between $20 \times 10^9/L$ and $150 \times 10^9/L$ (8). Rather than relying on absolute platelet count, a 50% reduction in platelet count from baseline values has proved a more sensitive indicator of HIT. One of the interesting features of HIT is the high incidence of thrombosis, despite the low platelet count. If untreated, a majority of patients with HIT will experience a thrombotic complication; in some cases, thrombosis precedes or occurs concurrently with reductions in platelet count (2, 9).

Four patient variables have impact on the frequency with which HIT occurs: 1) type of heparin administered (bovine unfractionated heparin > porcine unfractionated heparin > low-molecular-weight heparin (LMWH) > fondaparinux); 2) duration of heparin therapy; 3) patient population (postoperative >> medical > obstetric); and 4) gender (female > male) (6, 10). Estimates for incidence of HIT vary widely; however, consensus estimates suggest that overall incidence of HIT may vary from 3% to 5% in perioperative patient populations exposed to unfractionated heparin therapy to 0.1% after exposure to LMWH (4, 11–13).

Characteristically, clinical presentation of HIT conforms to 1 of 4 patterns in relation to timing of heparin exposure: 1) typical-onset HIT; 2) rapid-onset HIT; 3) delayed-onset HIT; or 4) acute spontaneous systemic reactions. Typical-onset HIT is the most common variant occurring after 5–10 days of heparin exposure. Rapid-onset HIT may occur within 1 day of heparin administration in individuals with recent prior heparin exposure (6). Delayed-onset HIT, a less common presentation, may occur days after heparin discontinuation (14–16). Most recently, HIT has been implicated in acute systemic (i.e., anaphylactoid) reactions occurring within 30 minutes of heparin administration (9, 13).

In most cases, HIT will be identified after development of thrombocytopenia; however, an important consideration necessitating vigilance is that thrombosis may precede or occur concurrent with thrombocytopenia in as many as 40%–50% of patients (2, 17). Contrary to popular belief, venous thromboses (i.e., deep venous thromboses, pulmonary embolism) prove more common in HIT than do arterial thrombotic complications (venous/arterial: 4–10:1) (2, 18). Limb ischemia and/or necrosis are more commonly associated with acute HIT after administration of vitamin K antagonists (i.e., warfarin) (19, 20). Less common presentations of HIT include necrotizing skin lesions at heparin injection sites, bilateral adrenal infarction, or cerebral sinus thrombosis (21–23).

PATHOGENESIS

An immune-mediated response to heparin underlies the seemingly paradoxical association between heparin therapy, thrombocytopenia, and thrombosis. Heparin, a highly anionic molecule, readily binds cationic PF4 molecules in circulating plasma (24). PF4, a 70-amino-acid positively charged protein of the CXC chemokine family, is synthesized in megakaryocytes and stored within platelet α-granules. A subset of patients exposed to heparin generates immunoglobulin G (IgG) directed against an immune complex composed of heparin and PF4. During platelet activation, PF4 is released to bind heparin and cell surface anionic glycosaminoglycans (i.e., heparan sulfate) (25, 26). After heparin (or heparan sulfate) binds PF4, conformational changes within the complex expose novel antigenic sites capable of binding IgG antibodies directed against the PF4/heparin complex. PF4/heparin immune complexes then bind FcγRIIa (CD32) receptors on platelet surfaces resulting in platelet activation (18). Despite low copy numbers (1000–2000/platelet surface), FcγRIIa receptors have proved potent platelet activators. After being activated, platelets rapidly are cleared from the circulation, accounting for the thrombocytopenia observed with HIT. HIT-associated thrombocytopenia differs from that of other drug-induced thrombocytopenias in that platelets are activated before clearance (27, 28). Although immunoglobulin M (IgM) and immunoglobulin A (IgA) antibodies directed against PF4/heparin complexes are generated with IgG, their role in pathogenesis of HIT remains unclear (29, 30). Similarly, both neutrophil-activating peptide 2 and interleukin 8 (IL-8) may substitute for PF4 in HIT-related immune complexes but appear to contribute minimally to HIT pathogenesis (31, 32).

Platelet activation leads to release of potent mediators of coagulation, including platelet-derived microparticles, promoting thrombin generation with resultant hypercoagulable or prothrombotic state (33). Platelet activation alone may enhance potential for thrombotic complications through increased platelet binding to vascular endothelium and platelet–leukocyte aggregate formation (34, 35). In addition, HIT immune complexes bound to heparan sulfate and other glycosaminoglycans on vascular endothelial surfaces have been implicated in vascular injury via monocyte activation and enhanced vascular endothelial tissue factor expression (36–38). Plasma concentrations of von Willebrand factor and soluble thrombomodulin, surrogate markers for vascular endothelial injury, are elevated in patients with HIT (38, 39). Further evidence for vascular endothelial damage is reflected in elevated concentrations of intercellular adhesion molecule-1 (ICAM-1) and vascular cell adhesion molecule-1 (VCAM-1) in patients with PF4/heparin antibodies (40). Vascular injury sites, with an overabundance of tissue factor expression, may enhance thrombotic potential—partially explaining the higher prevalence of thrombotic events among surgical patients with HIT. Needless to say, platelet activation releases additional PF4 from α granules providing a positive feedback mechanism to facilitate PF4/heparin immune complex formation (11).

LABORATORY ASSESSMENT

Given the variability in clinical presentation of HIT and potential for other clinical conditions to masquerade as HIT ("pseudo-HIT"), laboratory assessment is essential to make a definitive diagnosis. Laboratory tests for HIT may be categorized as either 1) functional (platelet activation) assays; or 2) immunologic (PF4/heparin antibody–dependent) assays (9). The basis for functional assays relates to the propensity for serum from patients with HIT to activate healthy donor platelets in the presence of therapeutic heparin concentrations. Donor platelets, washed in apyrase (degrades platelet agonist adenosine diphosphate) and resuspended in a physiologic buffer with calcium and magnesium, are incubated with the test patient's serum and heparin (41, 42). PF4/heparin antibodies in the serum test sample activate platelets and may be detected by monitoring platelet aggregation or release of radioactively tagged serotonin ("gold standard") (9). Functional assays for detection of HIT display high specificity for detecting clinically relevant pathogenic HIT antibodies. However, functional assays prove technically demanding and have slow turnaround times (42, 43). For this reason, performance of these assays typically has been restricted to a limited number of centers, and immunologic assays have proved the more commonly employed method for initial laboratory screening for HIT.

Immunologic assays for HIT most often employ enzyme-linked immunosorbent assay (ELISA) technology with PF4/heparin or PF4/polyvinyl sulfonate as the target complex coated onto polystyrene microtiter plates. HIT antibodies in test serum incubated within the microtiter wells bind PF4/heparin targets and, after washing, may be quantitated using colorimetric detectors directed against human immunoglobulins (9). ELISA-based immunoassays have proved highly sensitive for detection of PF4/heparin antibodies. In fact, a negative test result using an ELISA for HIT essentially rules out the diagnosis (i.e., high negative predictive value). However, immunologic assays do not provide the specificity associated with functional assays (41, 44). In other words, PF4/heparin antibodies may be detected in some asymptomatic nonthrombocytopenic patients. Therefore, when using immunologic assays alone, HIT may be overdiagnosed. In some cases, this overdiagnosis may relate to potential for immunoassays to detect nonpathogenic

TABLE 6–1. Pretest probability of HIT–4 Ts scoring system

Points for Each Parameter

	2	1	0
Thrombocytopenia	>50% decline (or nadir 20–100 × 10⁹/L)	30%–50% decline (or nadir 10–19 × 10⁹/L)	<30% decline (or nadir <10 × 10⁹/L)
Timing (of platelet count decrease)	Onset after 5–10 d heparin therapy (or ≤1 d with prior heparin exposure)	Consistent with heparin exposure but unclear (or onset after day 10)	Onset ≤4 d after heparin therapy (or without recent heparin exposure)
Thrombosis (or other sequelae)	New thrombosis; skin necrosis; acute anaphylactoid reaction	Progressive or recurrent thrombosis; suspicious thrombosis or skin lesion	None
Thrombocytopenia (Other possible etiologies)	No evidence	Possible	Definite

Pretest probability for HIT (Maximum possible score = 8): High: 6–8; Intermediate: 4–5; Low: 0–3. Modified from (6, 52).

IgM and IgA antibodies (45, 46). In contrast, functional assays for HIT lack the sensitivity of the immunoassays and may misclassify some suspected cases of HIT as negative when, in fact, HIT is present. Clearly, the optimal approach would be to employ both immunologic and functional assays during diagnostic evaluation for HIT. High antibody titers as measured by ELISA appear to be associated with greater probability for HIT and thromboembolic complications; however, in cases with only moderate or low titers of PF4/heparin antibodies as measured by immunoassay, functional testing might better clarify the diagnosis and provide an improved assessment for thromboembolic risk (46, 47).

Given the sensitivity of immunoassays for HIT and knowledge that preexisting variables may influence development of clinical manifestations of HIT, PF4/heparin antibodies are detected in significant numbers of patients who do not develop thrombocytopenia, thrombosis, or other obvious sequelae of HIT; therefore, incorporation of pretesting probabilities for HIT based on clinical signs and symptoms offers potential to refine risk estimates based on laboratory testing alone (9, 48).

One of the more popular clinical scoring systems for defining pretest probability for HIT has been described as the "4 Ts" (Table 6–1). By incorporating scores for 1) severity of *T*hrombocytopenia; 2) *T*iming of thrombocytopenia onset; 3) occurrence of *T*hrombosis or other sequelae; and

TABLE 6–2. Management of the patient with high clinical suspicion for HIT

- Discontinue all heparin exposure (including LMWH)
- Administer an alternative nonheparin anticoagulant
- Avoid vitamin K antagonists (i.e., warfarin) in the acute phase
- Perform laboratory screening tests for HIT
- Obtain duplex ultrasonography of lower extremities to assess for DVTs
- Avoid platelet transfusions in the absence of significant bleeding

Adapted from (6).

4) whether o*T*her explanations for thrombocytopenia exist, a composite score is developed (49, 50). Higher scores are associated with greater likelihood for HIT. The use of this scoring system in combination with the testing options can provide a rational approach to the diagnosis of HIT. From a practical standpoint, a low clinical probability for HIT (as determined by the 4 Ts clinical scoring system) accompanied by negative immunologic testing eliminates a diagnosis of HIT. In contrast, a moderate or high score by the 4 Ts clinical scoring system accompanied by a highly positive immunologic assay (or a positive functional assay) would prove diagnostic for HIT. Cases for which 4 Ts scoring suggests HIT, but immunoassay results prove inconclusive, may necessitate the addition of functional testing to clarify the diagnosis. In addition, functional testing offers an advantage in that it may detect HIT in rare cases where the heparin immune complex incorporates an alternative protein to PF4 such as neutrophil-activating peptide 2 or IL-8 (31, 32, 51).

GENERAL PRINCIPLES OF TREATMENT

The mainstays of treatment (Table 6–2) for HIT include 1) immediate discontinuation of all heparin (including LMWH); 2) avoidance of vitamin K antagonists in the acute setting; 3) administration of an alternative nonheparin anticoagulant; 4) assessment for "subclinical" deep venous thrombosis (i.e., duplex ultrasonography of lower extremities); 5) laboratory assessment via immunologic and/or functional assay; and 6) avoidance of platelet transfusions (6, 52). In the presence of HIT, continued exposure to heparin or heparin-related compounds poses high risk for catastrophic thrombotic complications and death (2). LMWHs pose a risk for cross-reactivity with PF4/heparin antibodies and should be avoided (13, 53, 54). Even heparin-bonded catheters and heparin-containing catheter flush solutions must be avoided (55, 56).

Despite heparin discontinuation, patients with HIT remain hypercoagulable for days to weeks after exposure to heparin. In fact, failure to provide appropriate anticoagulation during this period has been associated with a 50% incidence of thrombosis in the 30 days immediately after diagnosis of HIT (2). For this reason, an appropriate nonheparin anticoagulant must be substituted for heparin immediately in settings where HIT is suspected. Vitamin K antagonists (i.e., warfarins) are contraindicated in the acute phase of HIT because of the potential for inducing limb ischemia and/or necrosis (13). Thrombosis in this setting appears related to deficiencies of protein C (a potent intrinsic anticoagulant protein) superimposed on the hypercoagulable state induced by HIT (20, 57). Protein C concentrations decline precipitously after administration of vitamin K antagonists. To minimize potential for thrombotic complications, warfarin therapy is initiated in HIT only after resolution and stabilization of the platelet count after administration of a direct thrombin inhibitor or other alternative nonheparin anticoagulant. Furthermore, loading doses of warfarin should not be administered, and the direct thrombin inhibitor should be continued until stable therapeutic warfarin concentrations are achieved over a period of days (13). In patients who inadvertently receive a vitamin K antagonist before diagnosis of HIT, vitamin K should be administered for reversal concomitant with initiation of a direct thrombin inhibitor (13). Long-term anticoagulation for patients with HIT appears prudent—particularly for those patients experiencing a thrombotic complication, although the specific duration of anticoagulation must be based on the clinical situation and careful monitoring of the patient (13).

In nonoperative settings, alternative anticoagulants most often employed in HIT include the following: 1) lepirudin; 2) bivalirudin; 3) argatroban; and 4) danaparoid. Within the United States, lepirudin and argatroban have been approved by the U.S. Food and Drug Administration (FDA) for treatment of HIT, whereas bivalirudin has received approval for prevention of HIT during percutaneous coronary interventions. Danaparoid is no longer commercially available in the United States (13).

Lepirudin, a 65-amino-acid recombinant derivative of hirudin (leech anticoagulant) and direct thrombin inhibitor, poses no risk for cross-reactivity with PF4/heparin antibodies. The half-life of lepirudin is approximately 80 minutes, and it is administered by continuous infusion (58, 59). The terminal elimination half-life is substantially prolonged in patients with severe renal insufficiency. No reversal agent is available for lepirudin; therefore, reduced dosing in settings of renal impairment must be administered (60–62). In nonoperative settings, lepirudin infusions have been adjusted to target activated partial thromboplastin time (aPTT) values 1.5–2 times baseline; however, at higher concentrations (such as those employed during cardiopulmonary bypass [CPB] for cardiac surgery), the dose-response curve of the aPTT flattens such that the ecarin clotting time (ECT) proves a more accurate measure (58, 63, 64).

Unfortunately, at present the ECT remains unavailable commercially in the United States. Given that the molecular origin for lepirudin is a "foreign" leech-derived protein, the potential for anaphylactoid reactions exists. In fact, fatal anaphylaxis has been reported after lepirudin administration (65, 66). Antibodies directed against lepirudin may reduce clearance and contribute to prolongation of the aPTT (67). In addition, lepirudin-associated antibodies may cross-react with bivalirudin (68).

Much like lepirudin, bivalirudin is a direct thrombin inhibitor with no potential for cross-reactivity with PF4/heparin antibodies. A synthetic peptide analog of hirudin 20 amino acids in length, bivalirudin is eliminated with a half-life of 25 minutes necessitating administration by continuous infusion (69, 70). Elimination occurs via plasma-mediated enzymatic degradation and, to a lesser degree, by renal excretion (≈20%). Dosing must be reduced in patients with renal insufficiency or failure (58). As with lepirudin, no reversal agent exists for bivalirudin; however, the more favorable pharmacokinetic profile may reduce potential for bleeding complications. Monitoring of bivalirudin in nonoperative settings has relied on the aPTT and/or ECT (70). At high dose ranges, such as those used during CPB, the activated clotting time (ACT) has demonstrated utility for monitoring anticoagulant effects of bivalirudin (71). In contrast to lepirudin, the small molecular size of bivalirudin appears to pose no risk for anaphylactoid reactions.

Argatroban, a small (527 Da) synthetic peptide, is a direct thrombin inhibitor derived from L-arginine. It has no cross-reactivity with PF4/heparin antibodies. Argatroban reversibly binds the thrombin active site with a terminal elimination half-life of approximately 45 minutes (72–74). Dependent almost entirely on hepatobiliary clearance, argatroban dosing must be modified in settings of hepatic dysfunction (75). Administered by continuous infusion, in nonoperative settings argatroban is monitored using the aPTT targeted to a value of 1.5–3 times baseline values (58, 76). Given its small size and synthetic preparation, argatroban does not appear to pose a risk for adverse immune responses (13). Prolongation of the international normalized ratio (INR) by argatroban may complicate transition to vitamin K antagonists during the recovery phase of HIT.

Although unavailable in the United States, danaparoid proved a popular alternative anticoagulant for management of HIT before emergence of direct thrombin inhibitors (77). Danaparoid, derived from porcine mucosal extracts, is composed primarily of heparin, dermatan, and chondroitin sulfates. With a half-life of 24 hours, after a therapeutic concentration has been achieved danaparoid may be administered either intravenously or subcutaneously (78, 79). Because its clearance is dependent on renal elimination, doses must be adjusted in patients with renal insufficiency. Danaparoid has a risk for cross-reactivity with PF4/heparin antibodies; therefore, before administration, laboratory testing should be completed to ensure absence of cross-reactivity (58). Despite its shortcomings, danaparoid offers potential advantages in HIT including dual inhibition of thrombin as well as factor Xa, lack of effects on the INR, ease of monitoring with antifactor Xa measurements, and a prolonged half-life, which simplifies administration (33).

More recently, fondaparinux, another factor Xa inhibitor—composed of a synthetic pentasaccharide with a half-life of 17–21 hours—has been advanced by some authors as a potential bridging anticoagulant for transition from direct thrombin inhibitors to longer term therapy with vitamin K antagonists (80). Administered by once-daily subcutaneous injection, fondaparinux is eliminated renally (81). Fondaparinux may be monitored by the antifactor Xa assay; however, given its favorable pharmacokinetics and bioavailability, routine monitoring has not been recommended. Considering its limited chain length and lack of additional sulfated chains, fondaparinux has been thought to pose little risk for interaction with PF4/heparin immune complexes; however, a small potential for cross-reactivity has been demonstrated in laboratory settings (53, 82). Although potential for fondaparinux to induce HIT appears low, questions about its safety in patients with preexisting HIT limit its use at this time. Fondaparinux is not FDA approved for administration in patients with HIT (13).

INTRAOPERATIVE ANTICOAGULATION STRATEGIES FOR THE PATIENT WITH HIT

For those patients with HIT (or suspected HIT) requiring anticoagulation for cardiac and/or vascular surgery, there are no FDA "approved" alternatives to unfractionated heparin. Several recent reviews provide guidelines for clinical management strategies for intraoperative anticoagulation of the patient with HIT (13, 71, 83–86). Generally, these patients may be categorized in one of three broad categories: 1) patients with a remote history of HIT now testing negative for PF4/heparin antibodies; 2) patients with acute HIT; and 3) patients with subacute HIT for whom thrombocytopenia has resolved, but laboratory testing for HIT remains positive. In patients testing negative for PF4/heparin antibodies by immunoassay, and requiring only intraoperative anticoagulation, consensus guidelines recommend administration of unfractionated heparin (13). Anecdotal evidence supports safety of this strategy with the caveat that additional heparin exposure both pre- and postoperatively must be avoided. In patients testing negative for PF4/heparin antibodies by ELISA, a single intraoperative exposure to unfractionated heparin is thought to pose less risk than the possibility of excessive bleeding associated with alternative anticoagulants such as a direct thrombin inhibitors. In this situation it is important to document that the patient did not receive any heparin as part of the preoperative evaluation.

In patients with acute HIT (or suspected HIT) requiring intraoperative anticoagulation, consensus guidelines recommend strict avoidance of heparin (i.e., unfractionated or LMWH). If possible, surgery should be delayed to allow for clearance of PF4/heparin antibodies such that unfractionated heparin might be administered (13). In most cases, PF4/heparin antibodies prove undetectable within 4 months of an acute episode of HIT. In one study, the median time to seroconversion to a negative assay for HIT approximated 50 days using functional assays and 85 days by immunoassay (87). When surgery cannot be delayed, substitution of a direct thrombin inhibitor is recommended (Table 6–3) (13). Although case reports and clinical series have demonstrated successful administration of lepirudin (88–90), argatroban (91), and various platelet inhibitors (92, 93) in these settings, the limited half-life of bivalirudin and accumulation of published data to date suggest that, at present, bivalirudin offers the most favorable profile for intraoperative anticoagulation of patients with PF4/heparin antibodies and/or HIT (71).

Bivalirudin elimination is largely dependent on plasma-mediated enzymatic degradation; however, dosing should be reduced in patients with severe renal dysfunction (creatinine clearance <30 ml/min) (70, 71). Although recommended for use, the specific dosing and monitoring recommendations for bivalirudin for surgical patients is not well defined; however, case series and two small open-label trials of bivalirudin administration for CPB and off-pump coronary artery bypass graft (CABG) surgery provide guidance (94–97). These series recommend bivalirudin administration for CPB at a bolus dose of 1 mg/kg followed by a 2.5 mg/kg/h continuous infusion. In addition, 50 mg of bivalirudin can be added to the extracorporeal circuit preceding CPB and additional boluses of 0.1–0.5 mg/kg can be administered if needed to maintain the ACT >2.5 times baseline values. In settings of off-pump CABG surgery, bivalirudin has been administered successfully in a bolus dose of 0.75 mg/kg followed by a 1.75 mg/kg/h infusion (13). Target plasma concentrations for bivalirudin of 10–15 mcg/ml (ECT values: 400–500 seconds) have been recommended for CPB; however, institution-specific calibration curves should be prepared to validate ECT accuracy before clinical application (89). Although the ECT provides a validated method for determining bivalirudin plasma concentrations, this testing currently remains unavailable commercially in the United States. Anecdotal evidence suggests that the ACT may provide a useful guide to intraoperative bivalirudin administration by adjusting ACT values to exceed 2.5 times the institutional

TABLE 6–3. Alternative intraoperative anticoagulants to heparin

Drug	Pharma-cology	Plasma T$_{1/2}$	Elimination	Monitoring	Concerns
Direct Thrombin Inhibitors					
Bivalirudin	Synthetic peptide	0.5 h	Plasma enzymatic degradation	(80%); renal (20%)	aPTT; ECT
Lepirudin	Recombinant hirudin	1–2 h	Renal (90%)	aPTT; ECT	Potential for anaphylactoid reactions; prolonged T$_{1/2}$
Argatroban	Synthetic peptide	0.8 h	Hepato-biliary	aPTT	Minimal experience
Factor Xa Inhibitors					
Danaparoid	Heparinoid	24 h	Renal	Anti-Xa	10% cross-reactivity with PF4/heparin antibodies; unavailable in U.S.
Fonda-parinux	Synthetic penta-saccharide	18 h	Renal	Anti-Xa	Potential cross-reactivity with PF4/heparin antibodies; prolonged T$_{1/2}$
Platelet Inhibitors					
Heparin + Epoprostenol	Prostacyclin analogue	3–6 min	Plasma enzymatic degradation	None	Potential for severe hypotension; minimal experience
Heparin + Tirofiban	GPIIb/IIIa inhibitor	2 h	Renal	None	Minimal experience; bleeding; manufacturer opposes indication

GP: glycoprotein.
Modified from (13)

baseline ACT for procedures performed using CPB and 300 seconds for off-pump CABG surgery (13). In vascular surgery settings, bivalirudin administration and monitoring using strategies similar to those for off-pump CABG surgery are probably reasonable; however, consensus recommendations pertaining to these indications are lacking.

One unique consideration for intraoperative bivalirudin administration is the fact that plasma esterases in stagnant blood consume bivalirudin resulting in clot formation. Clot formation within pericardial collections of blood may falsely suggest the need for additional anticoagulant. Similarly, failure to provide for continued anticoagulation of blood within the CPB circuit after completion of CPB—or blood within the cell saver reservoir—may result in clot formation with loss of retained blood volume. Continuous internal recirculation of the extracorporeal circuit after CPB has been recommended by incorporating bivalirudin (50 mg bolus and 50 mg/h continuous infusion) to the CPB reservoir immediately after completion of CPB (70, 83). Alternatively, the entire extracorporeal circuit blood volume may be transferred to a cell saver for immediate processing at completion of CPB. Cell saver processing removes the majority of bivalirudin from plasma (83). To maintain patency of the extracorporeal circuit in this setting, crystalloid and sodium citrate are added to the circuit, allowing for continuous recirculation after transfer of blood to the cell saver.

HEPARIN ANTIBODIES AS INDEPENDENT RISK PREDICTORS

Although HIT characteristically is defined by thrombocytopenia and/or thrombosis in association with PF4/heparin antibodies, there has been growing appreciation that heparin-dependent antibodies alone, in the absence of other overt signs of HIT, may increase risk for adverse outcomes (98). Several investigations have examined the correlation between clinical events and PF4/heparin antibodies in nonthrombocytopenic patients with cardiovascular disease (99–103). In a comparison of patients with unstable angina, patients with PF4/heparin antibodies experienced elevated rates of death, myocardial infarction (MI), recurrent angina, stroke, and urgent revascularization at 1 year as compared to antibody-negative patients. Williams and colleagues (100) analyzed sera in a subset of patients enrolled in the GUSTO IV-ACS (Global Utilization of Streptokinase and Tissue Plasminogen Activator for Occluded Coronary Arteries IV-Acute Coronary Syndrome trial. Patients testing positive for PF4/heparin antibodies were significantly more likely to experience MI and/or death within 30 days. Similarly, in a Japanese population with acute coronary syndrome, Matsuo and colleagues (104) reported a 28% incidence of a thromboembolic event in subjects testing positive for PF4/heparin antibodies as compared to 3% in those without antibodies.

Two studies examined the effect of PF4/heparin antibodies on cardiac surgical outcomes. Bennett-Guerrero and colleagues (103) prospectively assessed patients undergoing CABG surgery, valve surgery, or combined CABG and valve surgery. The primary endpoint included a postoperative hospital length of stay exceeding 10 days and/or in-hospital death. The primary endpoint occurred in 34% of subjects testing positive for PF4/heparin antibodies by ELISA as compared to 22% of those who were antibody negative. Although Bennett-Guerrero and colleagues did not evaluate patients for a clinical diagnosis of HIT, the authors identified a statistically significant association between PF4/heparin antibodies as measured by ELISA preoperatively and adverse perioperative outcomes. Kress and colleagues (105) reported an observational study of patients undergoing cardiac surgery including CABG, valve surgery, or both. Of their 1114 patients, 5.4% tested positive for PF4/heparin antibodies preoperatively. Preoperative presence of antibodies proved to be an independent predictor for adverse postoperative outcomes. Serologically positive patients experienced a prolonged postoperative length of stay as well as a higher incidence of mechanical ventilatory assistance exceeding 96 hours, acute limb ischemia, and renal complications (including requirement for dialysis). The authors concluded that PF4/heparin antibody status should be determined preoperatively as a component of cardiac surgical risk assessment and mitigation.

A number of plausible hypotheses may explain the increased morbidity and mortality associated with PF4/heparin antibodies—despite absence of thrombocytopenia and/or thrombosis. Certain antibodies may activate platelets without concomitant reductions in platelet concentration (98). It is possible that the culprit antibodies do not bind platelets, but instead bind endothelial cells or monocytes—inducing tissue factor expression (35, 37, 106, 107). Alternatively, in some subjects heparin-dependent antibodies may serve as surrogate markers for a heightened inflammatory or autoimmune state and associated risk for thrombosis and other adverse outcomes (98, 107).

Evidence that PF4/heparin antibodies impact outcomes in the absence of thrombocytopenia should be considered in the context of the challenges associated with estimating the platelet concentration trends during and after surgery. Hemodilution, platelet consumption, drug-mediated effects, infection, and platelet transfusion can obfuscate identification of thrombocytopenia and its etiology (13). However, these data support the necessity for vigilance to identify HIT in perioperative settings. Further prospective investigations assessing the relationship between PF4/heparin antibodies and long-term outcomes in nonthrombocytopenic patients will clarify the role of heparin immune complexes as a clinical risk predictor; however, broader perioperative testing for PF4/heparin antibodies appears to be a reasonable consideration for risk reduction in perioperative settings.

CONCLUSION

HIT is a serious complication of heparin administration. For the patient scheduled for cardiac surgery, the anesthesiologist must be aware of the potential for HIT, the characteristics of the complication, and management strategies to address them. As importantly, when a patient is known to have HIT, it is important to understand when it occurred and the circumstances associated with its onset to define an appropriate perioperative anticoagulation plan.

References

1. Hirsh J, Heddle N, Kelton JG: Treatment of heparin-induced thrombocytopenia: a critical review. Arch Intern Med 2004; 164:361–9
2. Warkentin TE, Kelton JG: A 14-year study of heparin-induced thrombocytopenia. Am J Med 1996; 101:502–7
3. Warkentin TE: Heparin-induced thrombocytopenia: pathogenesis and management. Br J Haematol 2003; 121:535–55
4. Girolami B, Prandoni P, Stefani PM, et al.: The incidence of heparin-induced thrombocytopenia in hospitalized medical patients treated with subcutaneous unfractionated heparin: a prospective cohort study. Blood 2003; 101:2955–9
5. Smythe MA, Koerber JM, Fitzgerald M, Mattson JC: The financial impact of heparin-induced thrombocytopenia. Chest 2008; 134:568–73
6. Warkentin TE: Heparin-induced thrombocytopenia. Hematol Oncol Clin North Am 2007; 21:589–607, v
7. Warkentin TE, Roberts RS, Hirsh J, Kelton JG: An improved definition of immune heparin-induced thrombocytopenia in postoperative orthopedic patients. Arch Intern Med 2003; 163:2518–24
8. Greinacher A, Warkentin TE: Recognition, treatment, and prevention of heparin-induced thrombocytopenia: review and update. Thromb Res 2006; 118:165–76
9. Warkentin TE: New approaches to the diagnosis of heparin-induced thrombocytopenia. Chest 2005; 127:35S–45S

10. Warkentin TE, Sheppard JA, Sigouin CS, Kohlmann T, Eichler P, Greinacher A: Gender imbalance and risk factor interactions in heparin-induced thrombocytopenia. Blood 2006; 108:2937–41

11. Greinacher A: Heparin-induced thrombocytopenia: frequency and pathogenesis. Pathophysiol Haemost Thromb 2006; 35:37–45

12. Prandoni P, Siragusa S, Girolami B, Fabris F: The incidence of heparin-induced thrombocytopenia in medical patients treated with low-molecular-weight heparin: a prospective cohort study. Blood 2005; 106:3049–54

13. Warkentin TE, Greinacher A, Koster A, Lincoff AM: Treatment and prevention of heparin-induced thrombocytopenia: American College of Chest Physicians Evidence-Based Clinical Practice Guidelines, 8th Edition. Chest 2008; 133:340S–80S

14. Rice L, Attisha WK, Drexler A, Francis JL: Delayed-onset heparin-induced thrombocytopenia. Ann Intern Med 2002; 136:210–5

15. Warkentin TE, Kelton JG: Delayed-onset heparin-induced thrombocytopenia and thrombosis. Ann Intern Med 2001; 135:502–6

16. Warkentin TE, Bernstein RA: Delayed-onset heparin-induced thrombocytopenia and cerebral thrombosis after a single administration of unfractionated heparin. N Engl J Med 2003; 348:1067–9

17. Greinacher A, Farner B, Kroll H, Kohlmann T, Warkentin TE, Eichler P: Clinical features of heparin-induced thrombocytopenia including risk factors for thrombosis. A retrospective analysis of 408 patients. Thromb Haemost 2005; 94:132–5

18. Kelton JG: The pathophysiology of heparin-induced thrombocytopenia: biological basis for treatment. Chest 2005; 127:9S–20S

19. Warkentin TE, Elavathil LJ, Hayward CP, Johnston MA, Russett JI, Kelton JG: The pathogenesis of venous limb gangrene associated with heparin-induced thrombocytopenia. Ann Intern Med 1997; 127:804–12

20. Smythe MA, Warkentin TE, Stephens JL, Zakalik D, Mattson JC: Venous limb gangrene during overlapping therapy with warfarin and a direct thrombin inhibitor for immune heparin-induced thrombocytopenia. Am J Hematol 2002; 71:50–2

21. Warkentin TE, Greinacher A: Thrombosis of the cerebral veins and sinuses. N Engl J Med 2005; 353:314–5

22. Warkentin TE, Sikov WM, Lillicrap DP: Multicentric warfarin-induced skin necrosis complicating heparin-induced thrombocytopenia. Am J Hematol 1999; 62:44–8

23. Warkentin TE, Roberts RS, Hirsh J, Kelton JG: Heparin-induced skin lesions and other unusual sequelae of the heparin-induced thrombocytopenia syndrome: a nested cohort study. Chest 2005; 127:1857–61

24. Rauova L, Poncz M, McKenzie SE, et al.: Ultralarge complexes of PF4 and heparin are central to the pathogenesis of heparin-induced thrombocytopenia. Blood 2005; 105:131–8

25. Poncz M, Rauova L, Cines DB: The role of surface PF4: glycosaminoglycan complexes in the pathogenesis of heparin-induced thrombocytopenia (HIT). Pathophysiol Haemost Thromb 2006; 35:46–9

26. Rauova L, Zhai L, Kowalska MA, Arepally GM, Cines DB, Poncz M: Role of platelet surface PF4 antigenic complexes in heparin-induced thrombocytopenia pathogenesis: diagnostic and therapeutic implications. Blood 2006; 107:2346–53

27. Greinacher A, Eichler P, Lubenow N, Kiefel V: Drug-induced and drug-dependent immune thrombocytopenias. Rev Clin Exp Hematol 2001; 5:166–200; discussion 311–2

28. McKenzie SE, Reilly MP: Heparin-induced thrombocytopenia and other immune thrombocytopenias: lessons from mouse models. Semin Thromb Hemost 2004; 30:559–68

29. Juhl D, Eichler P, Lubenow N, Strobel U, Wessel A, Greinacher A: Incidence and clinical significance of anti-PF4/heparin antibodies of the IgG, IgM, and IgA class in 755 consecutive patient samples referred for diagnostic testing for heparin-induced thrombocytopenia. Eur J Haematol 2006; 76:420–6

30. Warkentin TE, Sheppard JA, Moore JC, Moore KM, Sigouin CS, Kelton JG: Laboratory testing for the antibodies that cause heparin-induced thrombocytopenia: how much class do we need? J Lab Clin Med 2005; 146:341–6

31. Regnault V, de Maistre E, Carteaux JP, et al.: Platelet activation induced by human antibodies to interleukin-8. Blood 2003; 101:1419–21

32. Amiral J: Antigens involved in heparin-induced thrombocytopenia. Semin Hematol 1999; 36:7–11

33. Kelton JG, Warkentin TE: Heparin-induced thrombocytopenia: a historical perspective. Blood 2008; 112:2607–16

34. Khairy M, Lasne D, Brohard-Bohn B, Aiach M, Rendu F, Bachelot-Loza C: A new approach in the study of the molecular and cellular events implicated in heparin-induced thrombocytopenia. Formation of leukocyte-platelet aggregates. Thromb Haemost 2001; 85:1090–6

35. Khairy M, Lasne D, Amelot A, et al.: Polymorphonuclear leukocyte and monocyte activation induced by plasma from patients with heparin-induced thrombocytopenia in whole blood. Thromb Haemost 2004; 92:1411–9

36. Pouplard C, May MA, Iochmann S, et al.: Antibodies to platelet factor 4-heparin after cardiopulmonary bypass in patients anticoagulated with unfractionated heparin or a low-molecular-weight heparin: clinical implications for heparin-induced thrombocytopenia. Circulation 1999; 99:2530–6
37. Arepally GM, Mayer IM: Antibodies from patients with heparin-induced thrombocytopenia stimulate monocytic cells to express tissue factor and secrete interleukin-8. Blood 2001; 98:1252–4
38. Davidson SJ, Wadham P, Rogers L, Burman JF: Endothelial cell damage in heparin-induced thrombocytopenia. Blood Coagul Fibrinolysis 2007; 18:317–20
39. Blank M, Shoenfeld Y, Tavor S, et al.: Anti-platelet factor 4/heparin antibodies from patients with heparin-induced thrombocytopenia provoke direct activation of microvascular endothelial cells. Int Immunol 2002; 14:121–9
40. Mascelli MA, Deliargyris EN, Damaraju LV, et al.: Antibodies to platelet factor 4/heparin are associated with elevated endothelial cell activation markers in patients with acute coronary ischemic syndromes. J Thromb Thrombolysis 2004; 18:171–5
41. Warkentin TE, Heddle NM: Laboratory diagnosis of immune heparin-induced thrombocytopenia. Curr Hematol Rep 2003; 2:148–57
42. Prechel M, Jeske WP, Walenga JM: Laboratory methods for heparin-induced thrombocytopenia. Methods Mol Med 2004; 93:83–93
43. Warkentin TE: Laboratory testing for heparin-induced thrombocytopenia. J Thromb Thrombolysis 2000; 10 Suppl 1:35–45
44. Francis JL: A critical evaluation of assays for detecting antibodies to the heparin-PF4 complex. Semin Thromb Hemost 2004; 30:359–68
45. Warkentin TE, Crowther MA: When is HIT really HIT? Ann Thorac Surg 2007; 83:21–3
46. Warkentin TE: Confirmatory procedure and other maneuvers to assess pathogenicity of platelet factor 4 (PF4)-dependent antibodies—distinguishing "signal" from "noise." Thromb Haemost 2008; 100:523–4
47. Warkentin TE, Sheppard JI, Moore JC, Sigouin CS, Kelton JG: Quantitative interpretation of optical density measurements using PF4-dependent enzyme-immunoassays. J Thromb Haemost 2008; 6:1304–12
48. Lo GK, Sigouin CS, Warkentin TE: What is the potential for overdiagnosis of heparin-induced thrombocytopenia? Am J Hematol 2007; 82:1037–43

49. Gruel Y, Regina S, Pouplard C: Usefulness of pretest clinical score (4Ts) combined with immunoassay for the diagnosis of heparin-induced thrombocytopenia. Curr Opin Pulm Med 2008; 14:397–402

50. Lo GK, Juhl D, Warkentin TE, Sigouin CS, Eichler P, Greinacher A: Evaluation of pretest clinical score (4 T's) for the diagnosis of heparin-induced thrombocytopenia in two clinical settings. J Thromb Haemost 2006; 4:759–65

51. Bounameaux C, Boehlen F, Membre A, et al.: Heparin-induced thrombocytopenia associated with interleukin-8-dependent platelet activation in a patient with antiphospholipid syndrome. Eur J Haematol 2007; 79:550–3

52. Girolami B, Girolami A: Heparin-induced thrombocytopenia: a review. Semin Thromb Hemost 2006; 32:803–9

53. Warkentin TE, Maurer BT, Aster RH: Heparin-induced thrombocytopenia associated with fondaparinux. N Engl J Med 2007; 356:2653–5

54. Warkentin TE, Cook RJ, Marder VJ, et al.: Anti-platelet factor 4/heparin antibodies in orthopedic surgery patients receiving antithrombotic prophylaxis with fondaparinux or enoxaparin. Blood 2005; 106:3791–6

55. Mayo DJ, Cullinane AM, Merryman PK, Horne MK, 3rd: Serologic evidence of heparin sensitization in cancer patients receiving heparin flushes of venous access devices. Support Care Cancer 1999; 7:425–7

56. Kadidal VV, Mayo DJ, Horne MK: Heparin-induced thrombocytopenia (HIT) due to heparin flushes: a report of three cases. J Intern Med 1999; 246:325–9

57. Srinivasan AF, Rice L, Bartholomew JR, et al.: Warfarin-induced skin necrosis and venous limb gangrene in the setting of heparin-induced thrombocytopenia. Arch Intern Med 2004; 164:66–70

58. Dager WE, Dougherty JA, Nguyen PH, Militello MA, Smythe MA: Heparin-induced thrombocytopenia: treatment options and special considerations. Pharmacotherapy 2007; 27:564–87

59. Greinacher A, Warkentin TE: The direct thrombin inhibitor hirudin. Thromb Haemost 2008; 99:819–29

60. Wittkowsky AK, Kondo LM: Lepirudin dosing in dialysis-dependent renal failure. Pharmacotherapy 2000; 20:1123–8

61. Dager WE, White RH: Use of lepirudin in patients with heparin-induced thrombocytopenia and renal failure requiring hemodialysis. Ann Pharmacother 2001; 35:885–90

62. Saxer SB, Smith BS, Gandhi PJ, Tataronis GR, Krikorian SA: Recommended and actual lepirudin doses in patients with renal insufficiency. Am J Health Syst Pharm 2003; 60:2588–93

63. Koster A, Hansen R, Grauhan O, et al.: Hirudin monitoring using the TAS ecarin clotting time in patients with heparin-induced thrombocytopenia type II. J Cardiothorac Vasc Anesth 2000; 14:249–52

64. Fabrizio MC: Use of ecarin clotting time (ECT) with lepirudin therapy in heparin-induced thrombocytopenia and cardiopulmonary bypass. J Extra Corpor Technol 2001; 33:117–25

65. Greinacher A, Lubenow N, Eichler P: Anaphylactic and anaphylactoid reactions associated with lepirudin in patients with heparin-induced thrombocytopenia. Circulation 2003; 108:2062–5

66. Badger NO, Butler K, Hallman LC: Excessive anticoagulation and anaphylactic reaction after rechallenge with lepirudin in a patient with heparin-induced thrombocytopenia. Pharmacotherapy 2004; 24:1800–3

67. Eichler P, Friesen HJ, Lubenow N, Jaeger B, Greinacher A: Antihirudin antibodies in patients with heparin-induced thrombocytopenia treated with lepirudin: incidence, effects on aPTT, and clinical relevance. Blood 2000; 96:2373–8

68. Eichler P, Lubenow N, Strobel U, Greinacher A: Antibodies against lepirudin are polyspecific and recognize epitopes on bivalirudin. Blood 2004; 103:613–6

69. Warkentin TE, Koster A: Bivalirudin: a review. Expert Opin Pharmacother 2005; 6:1349–71

70. Warkentin TE, Greinacher A, Koster A: Bivalirudin. Thromb Haemost 2008; 99:830–9

71. Czosnowski QA, Finks SW, Rogers KC: Bivalirudin for patients with heparin-induced thrombocytopenia undergoing cardiovascular surgery. Ann Pharmacother 2008; 42:1304–9

72. Yeh RW, Jang IK: Argatroban: update. Am Heart J 2006; 151:1131–8

73. Serebruany MV, Malinin AI, Serebruany VL: Argatroban, a direct thrombin inhibitor for heparin-induced thrombocytopaenia: present and future perspectives. Expert Opin Pharmacother 2006; 7:81–9

74. Boggio LN, Oza VM: Argatroban use in heparin-induced thrombocytopenia. Expert Opin Pharmacother 2008; 9:1963–7

75. Levine RL, Hursting MJ, McCollum D: Argatroban therapy in heparin-induced thrombocytopenia with hepatic dysfunction. Chest 2006; 129:1167–75

76. Francis JL, Hursting MJ: Effect of argatroban on the activated partial thromboplastin time: a comparison of 21 commercial reagents. Blood Coagul Fibrinolysis 2005; 16:251–7

77. Magnani HN, Gallus A: Heparin-induced thrombocytopenia (HIT). A report of 1,478 clinical outcomes of patients treated with dana-

paroid (Orgaran) from 1982 to mid-2004. Thromb Haemost 2006; 95:967–81

78. Acostamadiedo JM, Iyer UG, Owen J: Danaparoid sodium. Expert Opin Pharmacother 2000; 1:803–14

79. Ibbotson T, Perry CM: Danaparoid: a review of its use in thromboembolic and coagulation disorders. Drugs 2002; 62:2283–314

80. Warkentin TE: Fondaparinux versus direct thrombin inhibitor therapy for the management of heparin-induced thrombocytopenia (HIT)—bridging the River Coumarin. Thromb Haemost 2008; 99:2–3

81. Bauer KA: New anticoagulants. Hematology Am Soc Hematol Educ Program 2006; 450–6

82. Greinacher A, Alban S, Omer-Adam MA, Weitschies W, Warkentin TE: Heparin-induced thrombocytopenia: a stoichiometry-based model to explain the differing immunogenicities of unfractionated heparin, low-molecular-weight heparin, and fondaparinux in different clinical settings. Thromb Res 2008; 122:211–20

83. Riess FC: Anticoagulation management and cardiac surgery in patients with heparin-induced thrombocytopenia. Semin Thorac Cardiovasc Surg 2005; 17:85–96

84. Murphy GS, Marymont JH: Alternative anticoagulation management strategies for the patient with heparin-induced thrombocytopenia undergoing cardiac surgery. J Cardiothorac Vasc Anesth 2007; 21:113–26

85. Levy JH, Tanaka KA, Hursting MJ: Reducing thrombotic complications in the perioperative setting: an update on heparin-induced thrombocytopenia. Anesth Analg 2007; 105:570–82

86. Slaughter TF, Greenberg CS: Heparin-associated thrombocytopenia and thrombosis: implications for perioperative management. Anesthesiology 1997; 87:667–75

87. Warkentin TE, Kelton JG: Temporal aspects of heparin-induced thrombocytopenia. N Engl J Med 2001; 344:1286–92

88. Sun Y, Greilich PE, Wilson SI, Jackson MR, Whitten CW: The use of lepirudin for anticoagulation in patients with heparin-induced thrombocytopenia during major vascular surgery. Anesth Analg 2001; 92:344–6

89. Warkentin TE, Greinacher A: Heparin-induced thrombocytopenia and cardiac surgery. Ann Thorac Surg 2003; 76:2121–31

90. Greinacher A: Lepirudin: a bivalent direct thrombin inhibitor for anticoagulation therapy. Expert Rev Cardiovasc Ther 2004; 2:339–57

91. Edwards JT, Hamby JK, Worrall NK: Successful use of argatroban as a heparin substitute during cardiopulmonary bypass: heparin-

induced thrombocytopenia in a high-risk cardiac surgical patient. Ann Thorac Surg 2003; 75:1622–4

92. Mertzlufft F, Kuppe H, Koster A: Management of urgent high-risk cardiopulmonary bypass in patients with heparin-induced thrombocytopenia type II and coexisting disorders of renal function: use of heparin and epoprostenol combined with on-line monitoring of platelet function. J Cardiothorac Vasc Anesth 2000; 14:304–8

93. Aouifi A, Blanc P, Piriou V, et al.: Cardiac surgery with cardiopulmonary bypass in patients with type II heparin-induced thrombocytopenia. Ann Thorac Surg 2001; 71:678–83

94. Dyke CM, Smedira NG, Koster A, et al.: A comparison of bivalirudin to heparin with protamine reversal in patients undergoing cardiac surgery with cardiopulmonary bypass: the EVOLUTION-ON study. J Thorac Cardiovasc Surg 2006; 131:533–9

95. Dyke CM, Aldea G, Koster A, et al.: Off-pump coronary artery bypass with bivalirudin for patients with heparin-induced thrombocytopenia or antiplatelet factor four/heparin antibodies. Ann Thorac Surg 2007; 84:836–9

96. Koster A, Dyke CM, Aldea G, et al.: Bivalirudin during cardiopulmonary bypass in patients with previous or acute heparin-induced thrombocytopenia and heparin antibodies: results of the CHOOSE-ON trial. Ann Thorac Surg 2007; 83:572–7

97. Merry AF: Bivalirudin, blood loss, and graft patency in coronary artery bypass surgery. Semin Thromb Hemost 2004; 30:337–46

98. Stribling WK, Slaughter TF, Houle TT, Sane DC: Beyond the platelet count: heparin antibodies as independent risk predictors. Am Heart J 2007; 153:900–6

99. Mattioli AV, Bonetti L, Sternieri S, Mattioli G: Heparin-induced thrombocytopenia in patients treated with unfractionated heparin: prevalence of thrombosis in a 1 year follow-up. Ital Heart J 2000; 1:39–42

100. Williams RT, Damaraju LV, Mascelli MA, et al.: Anti-platelet factor 4/heparin antibodies: an independent predictor of 30-day myocardial infarction after acute coronary ischemic syndromes. Circulation 2003; 107:2307–12

101. Matsuo T, Tomaru T, Kario K, Hirokawa T, HIT Research Group of Japan: Incidence of heparin-PF4 complex antibody formation and heparin-induced thrombocytopenia in acute coronary syndrome. Thromb Res 2005; 115:475–81

102. Gluckman TJ, Segal JB, Fredde NL, et al.: Incidence of antiplatelet factor 4/heparin antibody induction in patients undergoing percutaneous coronary revascularization. Am J Cardiol 2005; 95:744–7

103. Bennett-Guerrero E, Slaughter TF, White WD, et al.: Preoperative anti-PF4/heparin antibody level predicts adverse outcome after cardiac surgery. J Thorac Cardiovasc Surg 2005; 130:1567–72

104. Matsuo T, Tomaru T, Kario K, Hirokawa T: Incidence of heparin-PF4 complex antibody formation and heparin-induced thrombocytopenia in acute coronary syndrome. Thromb Res 2005; 115:475–81

105. Kress DC, Aronson S, McDonald ML, et al.: Positive heparin-platelet factor 4 antibody complex and cardiac surgical outcomes. Ann Thorac Surg 2007; 83:1737–43

106. Pouplard C, Iochmann S, Renard B, et al.: Induction of monocyte tissue factor expression by antibodies to heparin-platelet factor 4 complexes developed in heparin-induced thrombocytopenia. Blood 2001; 97:3300–2

107. Walenga JM, Jeske WP, Prechel MM, Bakhos M: Newer insights on the mechanism of heparin-induced thrombocytopenia. Semin Thromb Hemost 2004; 30 Suppl 1:57–67

Julie L. Huffmyer, MD
George F. Rich, MD, PhD

Managing the Patient with Pulmonary Hypertension Who Requires Cardiac
7 Surgery

INTRODUCTION

Pulmonary hypertension (PH) is a risk factor for increased morbidity and mortality in patients requiring either noncardiac and cardiac surgery (1, 2). Furthermore, PH may induce right ventricular (RV) failure, which is also a predictor of poor outcome (3). Managing the patient with PH during cardiac surgery requires an understanding of pulmonary physiology and how certain factors alter pulmonary blood flow and pulmonary vascular resistance (PVR). As part of the management strategy, the clinician must be able to define the presence of PH and assess its implications. A variety of methods are available to assess the degree of PH, its manifestations, and RV function. They include such modalities as transthoracic echocardiography, transesophageal echocardiography (TEE), and cardiac magnetic resonance imaging (MRI). Therapeutic options, although limited, include intravenous and/or inhaled vasodilators to decrease PVR and inotropic agents to support underlying RV failure resulting from PH. This discussion will review PH and its implications and describe some of the challenges associated with its management for the patient who is scheduled to undergo cardiac surgery.

PULMONARY PHYSIOLOGY

The pulmonary circulation is normally a low pressure and low resistance circuit. The normal systolic, diastolic, and mean pulmonary artery pres-

Medically Challenging Patients Undergoing Cardiothoracic Surgery, edited by Neal H. Cohen, MD, MPH, MS, Lippincott Williams & Wilkins, Baltimore © 2009.

sure (PAP) are 22 mmHg, 10 mmHg, and 15 mmHg, respectively. The PVR is normally between 90 and 120 dynes.s.cm^{-5}. PH is defined as a mean PAP of >25 mmHg at rest or >30 mmHg with exercise, or a PVR >300 dynes.s.cm^{-5} (4). A mean PAP >50 mmHg or a PVR >600 dynes.s.cm^{-5} is considered severe PH. The PVR is the important parameter because it represents the afterload of the RV, and therefore influences RV function and cardiac output (CO). PVR may also influence blood flow within the heart, particularly is there is either real or potential intracardiac shunting through septal defects. In the clinical situation in which there is intracardiac shunting, PVR will have a direct influence on oxygenation.

In contrast to the systemic circulation, the pulmonary vessels have relatively thin walls and the vascular smooth muscle is sparsely distributed in the smaller arterioles. As such, increases in CO distend open pulmonary vessels and recruit previously closed vessels. Clinically, increasing CO through the administration of inotropic agents or increasing blood volume will passively decrease PVR. This relationship becomes less pronounced in those disease states of the pulmonary circulation in which vessels become less distensible. The vascular endothelium plays an important role in maintaining low resting pulmonary vascular tone. Normally, endogenous endothelial vasodilators such as nitric oxide (NO) and prostacyclin (PGI$_2$) predominate, although endothelial vasoconstrictors (endothelin, thromboxane) may also modulate PVR (5). Shear stress and stimulation of endothelial receptors modulate the NO/3'5'cyclic guanosine monophosphate (cGMP) and PGI$_2$/3'5'cyclic adenosine monophosphate (cAMP) pathways to promote vasodilation (6). Exogenous sources of these vasodilating agents are an important line of therapy in treating PH. Endothelial dysfunction and alterations of endogenous vasodilators are associated with the development of PH. PH is associated with increases in endothelial vasoconstrictors, primarily endothelin-1 (5). As a result, in the presence of PH, exogenous sources of these or other vasodilators become increasingly important (7).

Airway pressure and gravity affect the pulmonary circulation as well and are more significant in the pulmonary circulation than in the systemic circulation because of the lower intravascular pressure. Intraalveolar vessels are compressed when the transpulmonary pressure is increased during inspiration. In contrast, the extraalveolar vessels' resistance decreases during inspiration. The contribution of the two vessel beds accounts for the U-shaped relationship between lung volume and PVR, which is minimal at functional residual capacity (FRC) and increased at high and low lung volumes (8). Clinically, this may be important in some situations because extremes in ventilation that result in hyperinflation or underinflation of the lungs increase PVR. The distribution of blood flow in the pulmonary circulation is influenced by the relationship among alveolar, pulmonary arterial, and pulmonary venous pressures. Blood flow and to a lesser extent ventilation increase significantly in the dependent areas of the lung. Ventilation and perfusion are normally well matched; however, in certain disease states lung units are relatively under- or overventilated and result in ventilation/perfusion mismatching. In patients with lung disease primarily in the dependent zones, the blood flow to well-ventilated areas in the upper zones may be reduced if the PAP or CO is decreased as the result of treatment of PH. As a result, patients with PH are at risk for significant changes in gas exchange, particularly oxygenation with institution of positive pressure ventilation as often occurs after induction of anesthesia.

FACTORS AFFECTING PVR

The most important aspect of treating PH is understanding how certain factors or interventions alter PVR. Oxygenation has a large influence on PVR; alveolar hypoxia is a potent vasoconstrictor (9). Small areas of alveolar hypoxia cause diversion of blood flow to other areas of the lung and have minimal effect on PVR. In this situation, hypoxic pulmonary vasoconstriction (HPV) is a protective mechanism that improves ventilation/perfusion matching. An understanding of the effects of HPV on gas exchange is important, because the treatment of PH with intravenous vasodilators may inhibit HPV and decrease PaO_2 (10). Larger areas of hypoxia within the lung have greater impact on PVR. PVR will increase as the proportion of the lung affected increases. Atelectasis can increase PVR via stimulation of HPV and mechanical compression; therefore, the lungs should be adequately expanded in patients with PH. Acidosis is also a potent vasoconstrictor of the pulmonary circulation, whereas alkalosis vasodilates it (11). Hypercapnia and hypocapnia alter PVR primarily through their effects on pH, although hypercapnia itself may increase PVR (12). Adequate oxygenation and treatment of acidosis (respiratory or metabolic) represent the most important and first line treatments for PH. Sympathetic stimulation, cold, and catecholamines are also important factors that increase PVR (13, 14).

Alpha-1 adrenoreceptors and beta-2 adrenoreceptors are the most clinically relevant receptors in the pulmonary vasculature (15). Beta-2 agonists decrease PVR, whereas alpha-1 agonists increase PVR. These receptors are less densely distributed in the pulmonary circulation than in the systemic circulation, so one would expect the effects of agonists to be decreased (16). The tone of the pulmonary circulation is normally low; therefore, beta-2 stimulation normally has little effect. In the presence of PH, however, beta-2 agonists decrease PVR. Beta-2 receptors responsible for vasodilation are on the endothelial surface of the lung;

therefore, their effect may be decreased in the presence of endothelial dysfunction. Alpha-1 agonists increase PVR, but not to the same degree as they increase systemic vascular resistance (SVR), because there is relatively less vascular smooth muscle in the pulmonary circulation.

PULMONARY HYPERTENSION (PH)

PH is classified by etiology and pathophysiology (5). For those patients undergoing cardiac surgery, underlying cardiac and/or pulmonary disease are the most common causes for PH. Left ventricular (LV) failure, mitral valve disease, and decreased LV compliance result in elevations in left atrial (LA) pressure. The increase in LA pressure passively increases the pulmonary venous pressure, PAP, and PVR. Congenital cardiac diseases that cause left-to-right shunting result in chronic increases in pulmonary blood flow that eventually lead to pulmonary vasoconstriction, vascular remodeling, and an elevated PVR. Respiratory disorders such as chronic obstructive airway disease may lead to PH, at least in part, via hypoxia-induced vasoconstriction. PH may present as arterial hypertension in which the Pulmonary Artery Occlusion Pressure (PAOP) may be normal (i.e., respiratory diseases) or venous hypertension in which both the PAP and PAOP are elevated (i.e., mitral valve disease).

PH is a progressive disease. The efficacy of therapeutic interventions is dependent on the extent of the pathology. PH may initially be caused by vasoconstriction, which is easily reversible with vasodilator therapy. However, as PH continues, vasoconstriction results in smooth muscle hypertrophy and narrowing of the vascular lumen (17). Reversal of smooth muscle hypertrophy is possible over weeks to months with vasodilator therapy, but has limited effect acutely (18). Further progression of the disease leads to inflammation, fibrosis, and more fixed disease (17). Therapy at this point becomes difficult, and attempts to decrease PVR with vasodilators after the disease has progressed may be ineffective and, in fact, only dilate the systemic circulation and reduce peripheral perfusion. Endothelial dysfunction also may lead to the loss of receptors and important vasodilating factors. The main focus of acute treatment of PH during cardiac surgery is reversal of vasoconstriction and/or replacement of endothelial vasodilators although, as the PH progresses, even these approaches may be ineffective.

THE RIGHT VENTRICLE (RV)

The RV is a thin walled, crescent-shaped structure that is anatomically and histologically suited for volume work, in contrast to the thick-walled LV that is suited for pressure work (19, 20). Thus, the RV is less preload-dependent than the LV and, for any given increase in preload, a smaller increase in stroke work would be expected. Whereas the LV maintains a constant output over a relatively wide range of afterloads, RV function is more sensitive to changes in PAP. An acute increase in mean PAP above 40 mmHg results in a decrease in RV ejection fraction, even in the presence of normal RV contractility (21). In the presence of decreased RV contractility, the RV is even more sensitive to acute increases in afterload. In contrast, more gradual changes in PAP may allow time for the RV to hypertrophy and sustain a relatively normal output.

Coronary blood flow to the RV occurs throughout systole and diastole because of the continuous pressure gradient (coronary perfusion pressure) between the aorta and the RV. The RV blood/oxygen supply is proportional to the systemic pressure and inversely proportional to the RV pressure. Systemic hypotension (or attempts to treat PH or systemic hypertension) or increased RV pressure may result in decreased RV coronary perfusion pressure. RV oxygen demand is proportional to the RV pressure, RV volume, and heart rate. Hence, increased RV pressure not only decreases RV oxygen supply but also increases oxygen demand. Therefore, decreasing PAP with the use of vasodilators to decrease RV pressure is critically important in treating PH and RV ischemia. At the same time it is important to avoid decreasing systemic pressure and coronary perfusion pressure.

RV FAILURE

RV failure is most commonly caused by acute or chronic pressure overload. Whereas acute increases in RV afterload are poorly tolerated, more gradual increases in pressure or volume overload of the RV are sometimes remarkably well tolerated for years before symptoms and signs of RV failure, including an elevated central venous pressure (CVP), become evident. In the presence of chronic increase in PVR, the RV may hypertrophy and be able to generate systemic pressures. Despite this apparent compensatory change in the RV, PH eventually leads to RV dilation, decreased RV ejection fraction, decreased stroke volume, and decreased global cardiac function. Ischemia and infarction may also contribute to RV failure as a result of reduced coronary flow to the RV. Although angina generally occurs because of LV ischemia, ischemia may also arise from this decrease in RV coronary blood flow or increased RV oxygen demand. RV ischemia may also result from inadequate myocardial protection during cardiopulmonary bypass (CPB) (22). Volume overload caused by tricuspid regurgitation (TR) or the presence of atrial communications through an atrial septal defect or patent foramen ovale may also contribute to RV failure.

The most common preoperative symptoms that occur as a result of PH and RV failure are dyspnea, fatigue, reduced exercise tolerance, syncope, chest pain, and peripheral edema. Electrocardiogram (ECG) changes such as right-axis deviation, right bundle branch block, and inferior wall ST segment changes may be consistent with RV enlargement or RV ischemia. Signs of PH and RV failure may include tachypnea and tachycardia with neck vein distension. RV lifts are usually palpable, and the murmur associated with TR can be heard on cardiac auscultation. RV failure may be diagnosed on echocardiography by RV dilation, decreased movement of the RV free wall and/or septum, and TR (see next section). As the RV failure progresses, neck veins will become distended. The CVP, which is normally <5 mmHg, may increase to 20 mmHg or higher in the presence of RV failure.

PH may not only decrease RV function, but can also affect LV function (23). Interdependence between the ventricles occurs in the presence of increased PVR and RV end-diastolic volume and pressure, such that the intraventricular septum shifts toward the LV cavity. Consequently, RV failure may decrease LV filling, increase PAOP, and decrease LV output. RV dilation also may cause an increase in intrapericardial pressure that decreases LV distensibility. Hence, RV failure may significantly impair global cardiac performance and CO from either RV failure itself or by impacting LV function.

EVALUATION OF PH AND RV FAILURE BY TEE

The TEE assessment of the RV is not as straightforward as is echocardiographic evaluation of the LV. The nongeometric and asymmetric crescent RV shape make its evaluation by TEE more challenging not only in obtaining adequate views but also in both qualitative and quantitative assessment of function.

Using TEE, the following views are used to focus on the right side of the heart.

- Midesophageal four-chamber view: With rotation of the probe from the midesophageal four-chamber view to focus on the right side, the apical, mid, and basal segments of the RV can be investigated. The normal length of the RV is 2/3 that of the LV (24) (Figure 7–1).
- Midesophageal RV inflow–outflow: The right atrium (RA), RV, and PA are seen to wrap around the aortic valve and left atrium (LA). This view assists in evaluation of the tricuspid valve and RV free wall and RV outflow tract (RVOT) (Figure 7–2).
- Transgastric midpapillary short-axis view: Similar to looking at the LV in cross-section, the RV free wall and interventricular septum can be visualized and qualitative function may be assessed.

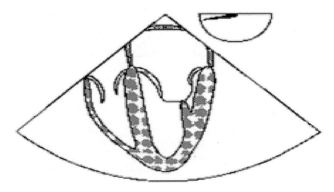

FIGURE 7–1. Transesophageal echocardiograph depiction of midesophageal four-chamber view with focus on the right side of the heart. Note that the normal length of the right ventricle is 2/3 that of the left ventricle.

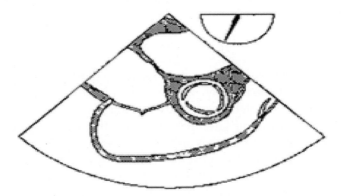

FIGURE 7–2. Transesophageal echocardiograph depiction of the midesophageal right ventricle (RV) inflow–outflow view. The right atrium, RV, and pulmonary artery wrap around the aortic valve and left atrium. Note ability to evaluate the tricuspid valve, RV free wall, and RV outflow tract.

- Transgastric RV inflow view: This long-axis view of the RV can be obtained either by getting the transgastric short-axis view and then advancing the multiplane angle to 90 degrees or by visualizing first the transgastric two-chamber LA and LV and then rotating the probe clockwise until the RV and RA are brought into view (Figure 7–3).

GLOBAL ASSESSMENT OF RV FUNCTION

The normal thickness of the RV free wall is less than half that of the LV and should be <5 mm at end-diastole. RV hypertrophy (RVH) is charac-

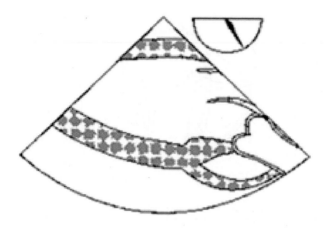

FIGURE 7–3. Transesophageal echocardiograph depiction of the transgastric right ventricle (RV) inflow view, which may assist in evaluation of the tricuspid valve and the long axis of the RV.

terized by RV free wall thickness >5 mm at end-diastole (25). Although there is some overlap between pressure and volume overload of the RV, it is commonly accepted that RVH is a compensation for RV pressure overload and that it indicates that a patient either has some degree of PH or pulmonic valve stenosis and RVOT obstruction (26). In patients who develop RVH and RV dysfunction caused by PH, RV wall thickness may exceed 10 mm (26). In addition, with TEE assessment of the RV, it is common to see more prominent intraventricular trabeculation in patients with RVH.

Whereas RV pressure overload leads to RVH, RV volume overload most frequently leads to RV dilation. The normal RV end-diastolic cross-sectional area (CSA) is 60% of the LV CSA. Severity of RV dilation progresses from mild (RV CSA 60%–100% of LV CSA) to moderate (RV CSA = LV CSA) to severe (RV CSA > LV CSA) (27). As the RV dilates, its shape changes from triangular to more rounded and often forms part of the cardiac apex (Figure 7–4).

Signs of RV dysfunction that are evident on TEE examination include severe hypokinesis or akinesis of the RV free wall, RV enlargement, and change in normal crescent RV shape to round, as well as flattening or bulging of the interventricular septum from right to left (25). Normally, the interventricular septum functions as part of the LV and has a convex curvature toward the RV throughout the cardiac cycle. In contrast, as the RV dilates or becomes thickened and of greater mass than

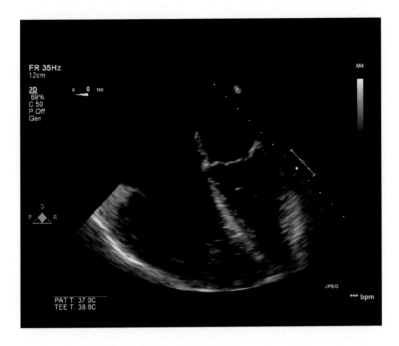

FR 35Hz
12cm

2D
69%
C 50
P Off
Gen

PAT T: 37.0C
TEE T: 38.6C

FIGURE 7–4.   Transesophageal echocardiograph, midesophageal four-chamber view demonstrating dilated, rounded right ventricle forming part of the cardiac apex.

the LV, the interventricular septum flattens and paradoxical motion of the septum can occur (Figure 7–5).

QUANTITATIVE EVALUATION OF THE RV FUNCTION AND PAP

In the absence of RVOT obstruction and pulmonic valve disease, the (TR) jet can be used to estimate PA systolic pressure. The continuous-wave Doppler beam is placed across the TR jet and, using the simplified Bernoulli equation, the transvalvular pressure gradient is calculated as $\Delta P = 4v2$, where v = peak velocity of the TR jet (26). To estimate the PA systolic pressure, this estimate of RV systolic pressure is added to the RA pressure or CVP.

There are quantitative echocardiographic approaches to evaluation of RV function as well. Tricuspid annular plane systolic excursion (TAPSE) is visualized in the four-chamber view by measuring the degree of systolic excursion of the lateral aspect of the tricuspid annulus toward the cardiac apex, reflecting the longitudinal motion of the descent of the

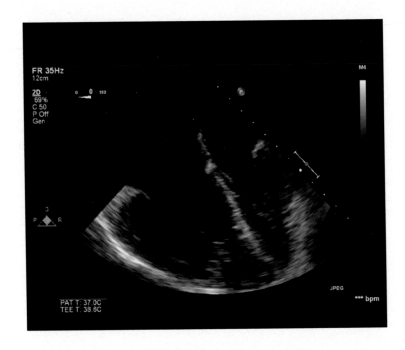

FIGURE 7–5. Transesophageal echocardiograph, midesophageal four-chamber view noting right ventricle (RV) dilation and flattened interventricular septum instead of normal convex curvature toward the RV.

RV base. For patients with normal RV function, the normal TAPSE is 20–25 mm. With each decrement of 5 mm in excursion of the tricuspid annulus during systole, the RV ejection fraction is estimated to decrease by 10% (28).

A second method for quantitatively evaluating the RV function is the myocardial performance index (RVMPI), which involves the following ratio:

[isovolumic contraction time + isovolumic relaxation time]
÷ RV ejection time

RVMPI can also be calculated by Doppler imaging of the tricuspid valve:

TR duration − RV ejection time ÷ RV ejection time

Normal RVMPI is >0.40 (29) (Figure 7–6). The myocardial performance index has the advantage of being relatively unaffected by heart rate, loading conditions, or presence and degree of TR (30).

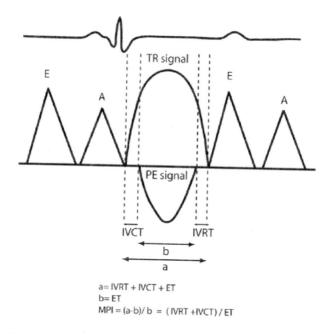

a= IVRT + IVCT + ET
b= ET
MPI = (a-b)/ b = (IVRT +IVCT) / ET

FIGURE 7–6. RVMPI = [isovolumic contraction time + isovolumic relaxation time] ÷ RV ejection time; IVCT = isovolumic contraction time; IVRT = isovolumic relaxation time; ET = ejection time; E = tricuspid rapid filling velocity; A = atrial rapid filling velocity; PE = pulmonary ejection; TR = tricuspid regurgitation.

RV fractional area change (RVFAC) is another quantitative method to assess RV function. It is measured in the midesophageal four-chamber view by tracing the RV endocardium at end-diastole and then performing a simple calculation as below. It can also be measured by transthoracic echocardiography using the apical four-chamber view.

RV end-diastolic area − RV end-systolic area ÷ end diastolic area

Normal reference value for RVFAC is >45%. Anavekar et al. (31) demonstrated that with each 5% decrease in RVFAC, there was a significantly increased risk for both fatal and nonfatal cardiovascular outcomes.

Haddad et al. (32) hypothesized that preoperative RVMPI and RVFAC could be used to predict in-hospital mortality and circulatory failure after valvular surgery. They measured the RVMPI and RVFAC using TEE in 50 patients undergoing mitral or aortic valve surgery; their results indicated that RVMPI and RVFAC were significantly related to the duration of intensive care unit (ICU) and hospital stay and suggested that this information might be used to risk stratify cardiac surgical patients.

MRI is also increasingly utilized to assess both RV and LV volumes and function. Several aspects of the RV can be evaluated including anatomy, function, shape, stress and strain, and viability of the myocardium including coronary artery anatomy (33). A number of studies have documented both the accuracy of the MRI technique and its reproducibility (34, 35). Contrast-enhanced MRI allows a heavily T1 weighted image to be captured which maximizes the difference in contrast between scarred and normal myocardium in that the scar appears bright white and normal myocardium appears dark (24). Despite the increasing use of MRI to assess RV function, it has several disadvantages. It can be time-consuming to acquire and analyze the images, and MRI requires a cooperative patient who can his or her breath to eliminate thoracic motion. Patients with pacemakers who would potentially benefit from MRI cardiac analysis cannot undergo the study because of the magnet interference.

THERAPEUTIC OPTIONS FOR PH AND/OR RV FAILURE

Treatment of PH and/or RV failure is based on the understanding of the impact of each on global hemodynamic function. As was noted previously, PH increases RV afterload, which may increase RV pressure and volume, while decreasing RV ejection fraction and stroke volume. These changes may cause a shift of the intraventricular septum, increase pericardial pressure and PAOP, and decrease CO. Increased RV volume and pressure may also decrease coronary blood flow and worsen RV ischemia and RV failure, which will have a further impact on CO. A decrease in CO may cause metabolic acidosis and worsen PH. Treatment of PH may include vasodilators to decrease PVR, inotropic agents to improve RV function (optimizing ventricular volume), and correction of acid base and/or oxygenation status.

To treat the patient with PH and RV failure, continuous assessment of hemodynamics is required. Patients presenting for cardiac surgery are best monitored with an arterial line and a PA catheter for continuous monitoring of these pressures, because small changes in ventilation, oxygenation, or cardiac function can have a major impact on PVR. An ECG for ST analysis of the RV and TEE are necessary to optimize global hemodynamics and guide therapy for improvements. A PA catheter and thermodilution CO measurements are helpful, if the tricuspid valve is not insufficient as a result of the RV failure.

A careful assessment of the management strategies used to control the PH prior to surgery must be performed. Patients with chronic PH presenting for cardiac surgery are often receiving therapy that includes alpha-adrenergic antagonist, calcium channel blockers, endothelin recep-

TABLE 7–1.   Treatments for right ventricular (RV) failure, pulmonary hypertension (PH) alone, or the presence of both

−RV, +PH	Vasodilator (intravenous/inhaled) ± vol
++RV, −PH	Inotrope, ± vol/diuretic, ± vasoconstrictor
++RV, +PH	Inotrope, vasodilator (intravenous/inhaled)

−RV = no RV failure; +RV = RV failure present; −PH = no PH; +PH = PH.

tor blockers, phosphodiesterase (PDE) III or V inhibitors, and prostacyclin (36). In general, these medications should be continued, but it must be realized that these therapies modify the effects of inotropic agents and vasodilators that may be added during cardiac surgery.

It is important to understand whether the patient has RV failure, PH, or both. Treatment of patients with PH without RV failure consists primarily of the use of vasodilators. In contrast, patients with RV failure without PH may be treated primarily with inotropic agents and possibly diuretics or vasoconstrictors. Patients with PH and RV failure may require both vasodilators and inotropic agents (Table 7–1).

ANESTHETIC MANAGEMENT OF THE PATIENT WITH PH

Anesthetic induction in patients with PH may be particularly challenging. Patients with PH often have high baseline sympathetic tone and may be catecholamine deficient. As such, these patients are prone to severe hemodynamic compromise upon anesthetic induction. Although there are no studies evaluating the effects of specific anesthetic agents during induction of anesthesia in cardiac surgical patients with PH, it may be reasonable to consider using titrated doses of synthetic narcotics, etomidate, or ketamine, to minimize changes in systemic blood pressure or heart rate. Maintenance of baseline systemic pressures is critical to the management of these tenuous patients.

Most patients with PH and RV failure presenting for cardiac surgery will require a narcotic/relaxant technique, supplemented with an amnestic. NO and ketamine are generally avoided in patients with PH. Each may increase PVR in adult patients with PH, although neither increases PVR in pediatric patients (37, 38). Clinically, it is probably prudent to avoid these agents in patients with PH, although ketamine may allow for a stable induction. Volatile anesthetics have minimal effect on PVR, but they may depress myocardial contractility and should be used sparingly in patients with severe RV failure.

GAS EXCHANGE STRATEGIES

It is well recognized that hypoxia, acidosis, and hypercarbia may greatly increase PVR. Although these factors must be avoided, hyperventilation may passively increase PVR and alter preload of the RV if there is gas trapping within the lung. Mechanical positive pressure ventilation may have significant negative hemodynamic effects. As lung volumes increase and FRC decreases with positive pressure ventilation, PVR increases and thus RV afterload increases (39). In patients with normal RV function, this may have negligible effects, but for patients with PH, lung hyperinflation and either inadequate or excessive positive end expiratory pressure (PEEP) can result in catastrophically reduced CO. Thus, optimal ventilation management for patients with PH may be a low tidal volume and low PEEP (3–8 cm H_2O) (39). This strategy is similar to that used to ventilate patients with acute respiratory distress syndrome (ARDS), but extreme care must be taken to avoid hypercapnia as PVR has been shown to increase by 54% and mean PAP by 30% with hypercapnia (40). The positive pressure ventilation may also reduce RV filling as a result of decreased venous return, further compromising pulmonary blood flow.

FLUID MANAGEMENT

Volume loading will increase RV output in the absence of PH, if RV contractility is normal. Particularly when the CVP is <12–15 mmHg, increasing preload may increase RV ejection fraction and stroke volume (41). However, if decreased contractility and PH accompany RV failure, then volume loading may be detrimental. In this situation, volume loading may cause RV dilation and result in a decrease in LV volume and systemic CO through the mechanisms of increasing wall tension, decreased contractility, increased ventricular interdependence, and impaired LV filling (41). This is particularly true after the CVP reaches approximately 20 mmHg and in the presence of RV infarction. The most appropriate way of managing fluids in these patients is to cautiously assess the effects of fluid administration by measuring the CO and/or following RV and LV function by TEE. In the presence of RV volume overload, venous vasodilation with nitroglycerin or diuretic therapy may be beneficial in improving RV function.

INTRAVENOUS VASODILATORS TO TREAT PH

Virtually all vasodilators have been shown to decrease PVR in patients undergoing cardiac surgery. Specific choices may be related to the potency of the pulmonary vasodilator and effects of the vasodilator on the systemic circulation as opposed to the pulmonary vasculature. Drugs that act via the NO/cGMP pathway will cause vasodilation in the presence of pulmonary vasoconstriction. As such, nitroglycerin or sodium nitroprusside may be useful in patients with isolated PH and in patients with combined PH and RV failure (42). Nitroglycerin not only decreases PVR but also has the added advantage over sodium nitroprusside of improving coronary blood flow to ischemic myocardium. Alternatively, sodium nitroprusside may be particularly useful in the presence of pulmonary *and* systemic hypertension, because it has effects on both vascular beds. Drugs that increase cAMP will also cause pulmonary vasodilation. Prostacyclin stimulates adenylate cyclase, thus increasing cAMP, which causes vasodilation and may promote increased CO and heart rate and decreased mean PAP and RA pressure (5). Prostaglandin E_1 (PGE$_1$) and PGI$_2$ are potent vasodilators, and the ability of these agents to vasodilate the pulmonary vasculature and improve RV function has been demonstrated in cardiac surgical patients (43). Although helpful for many patients, these drugs must be used with caution because they have known side effects that may undermine their value, particular in some clinical circumstances. Side effects of prostaglandins and prostacyclins for cardiac surgical patients include high-output cardiac failure, flushing, diarrhea, and thrombocytopenia (36).

Intravenous vasodilators used to treat PH are not selective for the pulmonary circulation and, therefore, may decrease systemic pressure. Decreasing systemic pressure results in decreased coronary perfusion pressure, which may worsen RV ischemia. The degree to which intravenous vasodilators may preferentially vasodilate the pulmonary circulation depends on the PVR/SVR ratio (i.e., if the PVR is elevated more than the SVR, all intravenous agents may produce relatively more pulmonary vasodilation than systemic vasodilation). These effects have been demonstrated with vasodilators such as nitroglycerin and milrinone used during cardiac surgery (42, 44). The decrease in systemic pressure secondary to intravenous vasodilators may also be minimized if RV afterload reduction results in an increase in RV stroke volume. The resulting increase in RV output may increase CO and limit the decrease of (or actually increase) systemic pressure (Figure 7–7). In contrast, if pulmonary vasodilation does not improve RV stroke volume, a decrease in systemic pressure may not be avoided. Therefore, in determining the potential benefits of intravenous vasodilators, it is important to evaluate the effects of the vasodilator on RV function and CO. It is important to recognize that RV afterload reduction nearly always results in a decrease in RV end-systolic and -diastolic volume. This translates to an increase in RV ejection fraction but not necessarily an increase in RV stroke volume.

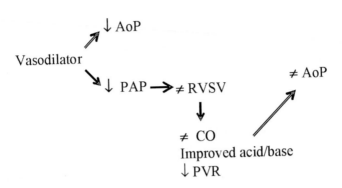

FIGURE 7–7. Potential effects of an intravenous vasodilator on right ventricular (RV) function and CO. AoP = aortic pressure; PAP = pulmonary artery pressure; RVSV = RV stroke volume; CO = cardiac output; PVR = pulmonary vascular resistance.

PDE III INHIBITORS

The PDE III inhibitors decrease the breakdown of cAMP and hence are vasodilators and positive inotropic agents. The PDE III inhibitors have been shown to be effective in the presence of PH and RV failure in the perioperative period. Known as an inodilator, milrinone has been shown to cause pulmonary vasodilation in addition to increasing CO, and hence may be useful for RV failure and PH. In weaning patients successfully from CPB, milrinone has been shown in multiple studies to be efficacious (45–48).

Milrinone, like other vasodilators, is not specific to the pulmonary circulation and may cause systemic hypotension; however, the PVR may be preferentially decreased in the presence of high PVR/SVR ratios (44, 49). Yamada et al. (50) showed, that although milrinone leads to higher cardiac index in patients with both low and normal pre-CPB cardiac index, it caused a significant decrease in SVR, especially in the low pre-CPB cardiac index group, requiring therapy with norepinephrine to maintain adequate systemic perfusion pressure. Milrinone also decreases PAOP and CVP. Amrinone is another PDE III inhibitor, and in studies comparing milrinone and amrinone, there was no significant difference found in hemodynamic variables (45). The half-life of amrinone is significantly longer than that of milrinone (3.5 hours vs. 30–60 minutes), which has limited its usefulness in the cardiac surgical population (51). Amrinone has also been reported to cause impairments in coagulation caused by reduced platelet count and function, thus its use has been limited, particularly in the patient who is undergoing cardiac surgery (52).

PDE III inhibitors are also beneficial in patients with severely decreased myocardial contractility because the effects of these drugs potentiate the effects of beta-adrenergic agonists. Beta agonists used for inotropic support stimulate adenylate cyclase to increase cAMP; hence prevention of breakdown of cAMP by PDE III inhibitors enhances the effects of inotropic agents such as epinephrine and norepinephrine.

OTHER VASODILATORS

PDE V inhibitors decrease the breakdown of cGMP, and hence are vasodilators. Sustained pulmonary vasodilation has been demonstrated with the PDE V inhibitor sildenafil alone and in combination with other pulmonary vasodilators (53). Sildenafil has been used as an oral premedication prior to cardiac surgery to decrease perioperative PH. Two patients with severe PH as a result of mitral valve disease undergoing cardiac surgery were successfully treated with nasogastric sildenafil (54). Sildenafil may also enhance the effects of drugs that work by stimulating the cGMP pathway. For example, sildenafil enhances and prolongs the effects of inhaled NO (55, 56).

Endothelin-1 acts on endothelin-A receptors to cause vasoconstriction, and on endothelin-B receptors to cause vasodilation. There is evidence that endothelin A is upregulated in PH and hence contributes to vasoconstriction (57, 58). The nonselective endothelin antagonist bosentan has been demonstrated to decrease PVR in several studies, although it is only relatively selective to the pulmonary circulation (59, 60). Channick et al. (59) demonstrated an increase in cardiac index and 6-minute walk distance as well as a decrease in PVR in patients with PH treated with bosentan as compared to placebo. Currently, there are trials in cardiac surgical patients using the selective endothelin-A antagonist sitaxsentan. Given its selectivity for blocking the endothelin-A receptor, sitaxsentan decreases the pulmonary vasoconstriction associated with PH but does not affect the vasodilation associated with endothelin B (36, 61, 62).

Adenosine has been demonstrated to cause selective pulmonary vasodilation if administered in the PA in the correct dose, and its short half-life allows for pulmonary vasodilation but no systemic vasodilation. Fullerton et al. (63) showed that central venous infusion of adenosine produced significant pulmonary vasodilation measured by decreased PAP and PVR, and also increased the CO in a group of 10 cardiac surgical patients.

INOTROPIC AGENTS

If the primary etiology for the RV failure is decreased contractility, all beta-1 adrenergic agonists will be effective in improving RV function.

Many studies have demonstrated that epinephrine, norepinephrine, dobutamine, isoproterenol, and dopamine may be beneficial in managing RV failure secondary to decreased contractility during cardiac surgery. The particular agent of choice depends in large part on the severity of myocardial dysfunction. In the presence of mildly decreased RV contractility, dopamine or dobutamine may be appropriate. Of the two, dobutamine may be better than dopamine in treating patients with PH and RV failure because it lacks alpha-1 adrenergic agonist effects and the subsequent increase in PVR. Although dobutamine has positive inotropic effects, an observational study by Romson et al. (64) concluded that, in post-CPB patients, the dominant method by which dobutamine raises CO is through increasing heart rate. The Milrinone Multicentre Trial Group studied the effects of dobutamine versus milrinone and found that dobutamine increased cardiac index by 55% versus 36% with milrinone but also found that dobutamine use was associated with more episodes of tachycardia and hypertension (65). Thus, it seems that although dobutamine may improve CO more than milrinone may, the tachycardia associated with dobutamine limits its usefulness in the cardiac surgical patient population and may make milrinone more appropriate in treating PH and mild RV failure. Isoproterenol may also be used because it has positive inotropic effects and it vasodilates the pulmonary circulation; however, its usefulness is limited by its effect on myocardial oxygen consumption and its profound tachycardic effects.

Patients with more severely decreased RV contractility may require treatment with more potent beta-adrenergic agonists such as epinephrine or norepinephrine. Epinephrine is a naturally occurring catecholamine that binds to both alpha and beta receptors, and at low doses its beta effects predominate but at higher doses alpha agonism becomes more prominent. A study comparing epinephrine to amrinone in patients with low CO showed that epinephrine produced a greater increase in cardiac index, heart rate, and mean arterial pressure than did amrinone, but epinephrine also caused a greater increase in myocardial workload and oxygen consumption (66). In the presence of systemic hypotension, norepinephrine may be an appropriate choice because it not only provides inotropic support but it may also increase RV coronary perfusion pressure via its relatively potent alpha-1 adrenergic effects in comparison to its beta-2 vasodilating effects.

The calcium sensitizer levosimendan is an investigational drug in a new class of inotropes that may augment myocardial contractility and cause vasodilation (67). Studies are currently being undertaken in cardiac surgical patients; the indications for the drug are still being defined. It may be beneficial for some patients because it has been shown to improve heart failure symptoms. Recent pilot studies found that levosimendan increased cardiac index and stroke volume while decreasing PAOP and PA pressures as well (68, 69).

Pure alpha-adrenergic agonists may also be useful in RV failure, because they increase coronary perfusion pressure. If decreased coronary perfusion is the etiology of ischemia, as may occur after CPB, increasing systemic pressure may reverse RV ischemia and improve contractility. However, it is important to realize that all alpha-1 agonists may increase PVR. Vasopressin may be useful to improve systemic and coronary perfusion pressure in states of low SVR with patients who have PH. A study in postcardiotomy patients by Tayama et al. (70) demonstrated increases in mean systemic arterial pressure and SVR, maintenance of CO, but no significant alteration of the PVR.

COMBINATION THERAPY FOR PH AND RV FAILURE

In the presence of PH and decreased RV contractility, a combination of inotropic agents and vasodilators usually will be required. In an attempt to decrease PVR and increase CO, various combinations of vasodilators and inotropic agents have been demonstrated to be effective. The precise combination of agents to select will depend on the degree of inotropic support and vasodilation required. PH with mild RV dysfunction may be treated with dobutamine, milrinone, or combinations of dopamine or dobutamine plus nitroglycerin.

When the RV dysfunction is severe, the more potent inotropic agents epinephrine and norepinephrine may be required. Milrinone may potentiate the inotropic effects of epinephrine or norepinephrine while adding pulmonary vasodilation. Carceles et al. (71) showed that milrinone potentiated the contractile responses to both norepinephrine and epinephrine in atrial myocardial tissue of patients undergoing cardiac surgery. Nitroglycerin or sodium nitroprusside can be added to the more potent inotropic agents to dilate the pulmonary vasculature. Inhaled pulmonary vasodilators should also be considered, because they will decrease PH with little effect on systemic pressures (see Inhaled Pulmonary Vasodilator Therapy).

An intraaortic balloon pump (IABP), which is normally inserted to help manage LV failure, may also be beneficial for patients with RV failure. The IABP may augment CO, decrease Left Atrial Pressure (LAP), and subsequently decrease PAP and PVR. In an animal study, Nordhaug et al. (72) found that the use of IABP decreased PVR while improving arterial blood pressure, CO, and RV efficiency. RV assist devices (RVAD) that use a mechanical pump to withdraw blood from the RA and return blood to the PA have been demonstrated to support the failing RV. In a group of patients who developed acute RV failure after coronary artery bypass graft and/or valvular surgery, Moazami et al. (73) found that RVAD support allows for recovery of RV function. These devices should be considered in the patient whose RV function is deteriorating in the perioperative period.

INHALED PULMONARY VASODILATOR THERAPY

Inhaled pulmonary vasodilators have significant advantages for many patients with PH. Inhaled vasodilators are selective to the pulmonary circulation, meaning that they cause pulmonary vasodilation but not systemic vasodilation. The primary inhaled pulmonary vasodilators used clinically for cardiac surgery are NO and PGI_2. Inhaled NO acts by diffusing from the alveoli into the pulmonary vascular smooth muscle to stimulate the production of cGMP and subsequently results in vasodilation (74). NO is prevented from producing downstream systemic vasodilation because it rapidly combines with hemoglobin so it has no effect on the SVR. Inhaled PGI_2 increases vascular smooth muscle cAMP, which results in pulmonary arterial vasodilation, but is hydrolyzed before producing systemic effects (75). Inhaled vasodilators also have the potential to increase PaO_2 in patients with ventilation/perfusion abnormalities. Because these drugs are inhaled, vasodilation is primarily limited to areas that are ventilated, and hence, ventilation/perfusion matching is improved and shunt is decreased (74). The effect of inhaled vasodilators on oxygenation is in sharp contrast to that of intravenous vasodilators, which vasodilate all lung areas and potentially worsen oxygenation by inhibiting HPV in poorly ventilated areas.

Inhaled NO and PGI_2 have been demonstrated to selectively vasodilate the pulmonary circulation and improve RV function in pediatric and adult cardiac surgical patients in addition to patients with ARDS and newborn patients with persistent PH (74, 76). Furthermore, numerous case reports have demonstrated that inhaled NO and PGI_2 may facilitate weaning from CPB of patients with severe PH and RV failure (77, 78). RV afterload reduction translates to decreased RV pressure in addition to decreased RV end-systolic and -diastolic volumes (79). This results in a decrease in stroke work and an increase in RV ejection fraction. Although inhaled NO and PGI_2 almost always increase RV ejection fraction, the results of studies evaluating their benefit are mixed as to whether RV stroke volume and CO are increased. Some studies have demonstrated in patients with RV failure, PH, and cardiogenic shock that inhaled NO decreases PAP and PVR while increasing RV stroke volume and CO (80). Others have indicated that RV ejection fraction is increased but RV stroke volume is unchanged (79).

The primary advantage of inhaled vasodilators over intravenous vasodilators is that pulmonary vasodilation is not accompanied by systemic vasodilation and the resulting decrease in coronary perfusion pressure. Therefore, perhaps the greatest value of inhaled vasodilators is in patients with PH and systemic hypotension or in patients in whom a decrease in systemic pressure would critically decrease coronary perfusion pressure. Additionally, in patients with systemic hypotension, inhaled vasodilators may reverse the pulmonary effects of alpha agonists used to treat systemic hypotension.

Inhaled NO and PGI_2 also may be useful in treating cardiac surgical patients with PH who are hypoxemic secondary to having ventilation/perfusion abnormalities associated with respiratory diseases. Although many studies have demonstrated positive acute effects on RV function and oxygenation in patients with respiratory disease, long-term trials with inhaled NO in ARDS patients have shown that the positive effects on oxygenation are temporary. Inhaled NO is not associated with improved outcome in these patients (74, 81, 82).

A number of other inhaled agents in addition to NO and PGI_2 have been shown to be selective vasodilators (83). These include PGE_1, NO donors, sodium nitroprusside, nitroglycerin, PDE inhibitors specific to cAMP or cGMP, adenosine, and adrenomedullin. All have been shown to be effective and comparable to NO and PGI_2, and all of these inhaled agents work synergistically with other classes of drugs. For example, intravenous or inhaled milrinone may potentiate the effects of inhaled PGI_2 the same way that intravenous milrinone potentiates the effects of beta-adrenergic agonists (84). Sildenafil, an oral PDE V inhibitor, alone produces pulmonary vasodilation, but more importantly it potentiates and prolongs the effects of inhaled NO (85). Whereas inhaled NO is delivered as a gas via a specialized delivery system, PGI_2 and all other agents are delivered as nebulized drugs.

Either NO or PGI_2 is an appropriate agent to consider in the management of the patient with PH who is undergoing cardiac surgery. Most studies indicate that NO and PGI_2 are equally effective in decreasing PAP and PVR (76, 86). Both agents cause rapid onset of pulmonary vasodilation, proportional to the baseline PVR and the degree of vasoconstriction. Both have dose-dependent effects that may change over the course of the therapy. Both also may cause rebound PH because their prolonged use may downregulate endogenous vasodilator pathways (74, 87). Each drug has a different profile of potential side effects or complications. NO can cause methemoglobinemia, although this effect is minimal with low-dose NO (74). Nitrogen dioxide formation in the airway is also a potential for toxicity but unlikely at low clinical inhaled NO concentrations. Inhaled PGI_2 may have toxic effects in the airway,

TABLE 7–2. Effects of inhaled and intravenous vasodilators on hemodynamics

PAP	↓	↓
PAOP	±	↓
AoP	↔	↓
CVP	±	↓

PAP = pulmonary artery pressure; PAOP = pulmonary artery occlusion pressure; AoP = aortic pressure; CVP = central venous pressure.

but it has not been studied to the extent of NO. Both NO and PGI$_2$ can increase bleeding because of platelet inhibition, although this is usually not clinically significant (74, 81).

A number of studies have compared the effectiveness of inhaled and intravenous vasodilators. Most of these studies have indicated that the effect on PAP and PVR are similar (88). However, there are important differences between the effects of intravenous and inhaled vasodilators that dictate their clinical utility. Intravenous vasodilators decrease PAOP, CVP, and systemic pressure in addition to decreasing PAP. In contrast, inhaled vasodilators decrease PAP but have minimal effect on LV preload and systemic pressure. In fact, inhaled vasodilators may increase LV end-diastolic pressure in patients with LV dysfunction (89). This increase is thought to be secondary to increased pulmonary blood flow in the absence of vasodilation of the pulmonary venous system. If the desired effect is to decrease preload or systemic pressure, then intravenous agents may be a more appropriate choice. If a decrease in PAP without a decrease in systemic pressure is critically important in the treatment of PH and RV failure, then inhaled agents may be a more appropriate choice (Table 7–2).

CONCLUSION

Patients presenting for cardiac surgery with PH are challenging to manage. The precise therapeutic approach to the management of the patient with PH undergoing cardiac surgery should be based on the understanding of pulmonary physiology and the rational use of pharmacologic agents. Although many studies have demonstrated that a wide variety of therapies are effective, there are limited data comparing the benefits of one agent over another.

Despite the limited comparative data, all patients with PH will benefit from both passive and active approaches to decreasing PVR. The most important initial approach should be to maintain normal acid–base status and to prevent hypoxemia. Volume status must also be optimized. Thereafter, the choice of vasodilators and inotropic agents should be based on a rational approach and guided by immediate feedback from invasive and noninvasive monitors.

Treatment of mild PH with or without RVH may be achieved with an intravenous vasodilator plus a less potent inotropic agent or with a PDE III inhibitor alone. More severe PH and or RV failure will require the use of an intravenous and/or inhaled vasodilator and a more potent inotropic agent. Administration of a PDE III inhibitor may be beneficial because of its ability to potentiate the effects of the inotropic agent while also promoting pulmonary vasodilation. Patients who have PH, systemic hypotension, and RV failure are the most challenging to manage. These patients will most often require a potent inotropic agent with alpha-1 properties to increase systemic pressure, in combination with a PDE III inhibitor to potentiate the effects of the inotropic agent and add pulmonary vasodilation, and an inhaled pulmonary vasodilator to maximize pulmonary vasodilation without altering SVR.

References

1. Ramakrishna G, Sprung J, Ravi BS, Chandrasekaran K, McGoon MD.: Impact of pulmonary hypertension on the outcomes of noncardiac surgery: predictors of perioperative morbidity and mortality. J Am Coll Cardiol 2005; 45:1691–9
2. Wencker D, Borer JS, Hochreiter C, et al: Preoperative predictors of late postoperative outcome among patients with nonischemic mitral regurgitation with 'high risk' descriptors and comparison with unoperated patients. Cardiology 2000; 93:37–42
3. Reichert CL, Visser CA, van den Brink RB, et al.: Prognostic value of biventricular function in hypotensive patients after cardiac surgery as assessed by transesophageal echocardiography. J Cardiothorac Vasc Anesth 1992; 6:429–32
4. Rubin LJ: Primary pulmonary hypertension. N Engl J Med 1997; 336:111–7
5. Blaise G, Langleben D, Hubert B: Pulmonary arterial hypertension: pathophysiology and anesthetic approach. Anesthesiology 2003; 99:1415–32
6. Jeffery TK, Morrell NW: Molecular and cellular basis of pulmonary vascular remodeling in pulmonary hypertension. Prog Cardiovasc Dis 2002; 45:173–202
7. Hoeper MM, Rubin LJ: Update in pulmonary hypertension 2005. Am J Respir Crit Care Med 2006; 173:499–505
8. Miro AM, Pinsky MR: Heart-lung interactions. In: Tobin MJ, ed. Principles and Practice of Mechanical Ventilation. New York, NY, McGraw-Hill, 1994:647–72

9. Medical Research Council Working Party: Long term domiciliary oxygen therapy in chronic hypoxic cor pulmonale complicating chronic bronchitis and emphysema: report of the Medical Research Council Working Party. Lancet 1981; 1:681–6

10. McFarlane PA, Mortimer AJ, Ryder WA, et al.: Effects of dopamine and dobutamine on the distribution of pulmonary blood flow during lobar ventilation hypoxia and lobar collapse in dogs. Eur J Clin Invest 1985; 15:53–9

11. Brimioulle S, Lejeune P, Vachiery JL, Leeman M, Melot C, Naeije R: Effects of acidosis and alkalosis on hypoxic pulmonary vasoconstriction in dogs. Am J Physiol 1990; 258:H347–53

12. Viitanen A, Salmenpera M, Heinonen J: Right ventricular response to hypercarbia after cardiac surgery. Anesthesiology 1990; 73:393–400

13. Marin JL, Orchard C, Chakrabarti MK, Sykes MK: Depression of hypoxic pulmonary vasoconstriction in the dog by dopamine and isoprenaline. Br J Anaesth 1979; 51:303–12

14. Benumof JL, Wahrenbrock EA: Dependency of hypoxic pulmonary vasoconstriction on temperature. J Appl Physiol 1977; 42:56–8

15. Bevan RD: Influence of adrenergic innervation on vascular growth and mature characteristics. Am Rev Respir Dis 1989; 140:1478–82

16. Nakaki T, Nakayama M, Yamamoto S, Kato R: Alpha 1-adrenergic stimulation and beta 2-adrenergic inhibition of DNA synthesis in vascular smooth muscle cells. Mol Pharmacol 1990; 37:30–6

17. Heath D, Smith P, Gosney J, et al.: The pathology of the early and late stages of primary pulmonary hypertension. Br Heart J 1987; 58:204–13

18. Ricciardi MJ, Knight BP, Martinez FJ, Rubenfire M: Inhaled nitric oxide in primary pulmonary hypertension: a safe and effective agent for predicting response to nifedipine. J Am Coll Cardiol 1998; 32:1068–73

19. Fischer LG, Van Aken H, Burkle H: Management of pulmonary hypertension: physiological and pharmacological considerations for anesthesiologists. Anesth Analg 2003; 96:1603–16

20. Brieke A, DeNofrio D: Right ventricular dysfunction in chronic dilated cardiomyopathy and heart failure. Coron Artery Dis 2005; 16(1):5–11

21. Woods J, Monteiro P, Rhodes A: Right ventricular dysfunction. Curr Opin Crit Care 2007; 13:532–40

22. Kaul TK, Fields BL: Postoperative acute refractory right ventricular failure: incidence, pathogenesis, management and prognosis. Cardiovasc Surg 2000; 8:1–9

23. Bristow MR, Zisman LS, Lowes BD, et al.: The pressure-overloaded right ventricle in pulmonary hypertension. Chest 1998; 114(1 Suppl):101S–106S

24. Bleeker GB, Steendijk P, Holman ER, et al.: Assessing right ventricular function: the role of echocardiography and complementary technologies. Heart 2006; 92:i19–26

25. Shanewise JS, Cheung AT, Aronson S, et al.: ASE/SCA guidelines for performing a comprehensive intraoperative multiplane transesophageal echocardiography examination: recommendations of the American Society of Echocardiography Council for Intraoperative Echocardiography and the Society of Cardiovascular Anesthesiologists Task Force for Certification in Perioperative Transesophageal Echocardiography. Anesth Analg 1999; 89:870–84

26. Schroeder RA, Sreeram GM, Mark JB: Right ventricle, right atrium, tricuspid valve and pulmonic valve. In: Perrino AC, Jr., and Reeves ST, eds. Transesophageal Echocardiography. 2nd Edition. Philadelphia, PA, Lippincott Williams & Wilkins, 2008:281–93

27. Otto CM: Textbook of Clinical Echocardiography. Philadelphia, PA, WB Saunders, 2000:120–2

28. Kaul S, Tei C, Hopkins JM, Shah PM: Assessment of right ventricular function using two-dimensional echocardiography. Am Heart J 1984; 107:526–31

29. Miller D, Farah MG, Liner A, Fox K, Schluchter M, Hoit BD: The relation between quantitative right ventricular ejection fraction and indices of tricuspid annular motion and myocardial performance. J Am Soc Echocardiogr 2004; 17:443–7

30. Tei C, Dujardin KS, Hodge DO, et al.: Doppler echocardiographic index for assessment of global right ventricular function. J Am Soc Echocardiogr 1996; 9:838–47

31. Anavekar NS, Skali H, Bourgoun M, et al.: Usefulness of right ventricular fractional area change to predict death, heart failure, and stroke following myocardial infarction (from the VALIANT ECHO Study). Am J Cardiol 2008; 101:607–12

32. Haddad F, Denault AY, Couture P, et al.: Right ventricular myocardial performance index predicts perioperative mortality or circulatory failure in high-risk valvular surgery. J Am Soc Echocardiogr 2007; 20:1065–72

33. Greil GF, Beerbaum P, Razavi R, Miller O: Imaging the right ventricle: non-invasive imaging. Heart 2008; 94:803–8

34. Mogelvang J, Stubgaard M, Thomsen C, Henriksen O: Evaluation of right ventricular volumes measured by magnetic resonance imaging. Eur Heart J 1988; 9:529–33

35. Grothues F, Moon JC, Bellenger NG, Smith GS, Klein HU, Pennell DJ: Interstudy reproducibility of right ventricular volumes, function, and mass with cardiovascular magnetic resonance. Am Heart J 2004; 147:218–23
36. Sastry BK: Pharmacologic treatment for pulmonary arterial hypertension. Curr Opin Cardiol 2006; 21:561–8
37. Schulte-Sasse U, Hess W, Tarnow J: Pulmonary vascular responses to nitrous oxide in patients with normal and high pulmonary vascular resistance. Anesthesiology 1982; 57:9–13
38. Gooding JM: A physiologic analysis of cardiopulmonary responses to ketamine anesthesia in noncardiac patients. Anesth Analg 1977; 56:813–6
39. Zamanian RT, Haddad F, Doyle RL, Weinacker AB: Management strategies for patients with pulmonary hypertension in the intensive care unit. Crit Care Med 2007; 35:2037–50
40. Viitanen A, Salmenpera M, Heinonen J: Right ventricular response to hypercarbia after cardiac surgery. Anesthesiology 1990; 73:393–400
41. Piazza G, Goldhaber SZ: The acutely decompensated right ventricle: pathways for diagnosis and management. Chest 2005; 128: 1836–52
42. Ziskind Z, Pohoryles L, Mohr R, et al.: The effect of low-dose intravenous nitroglycerin on pulmonary hypertension immediately after replacement of a stenotic mitral valve. Circulation 1985; 72:II164–9
43. D'Ambra MN, LaRaia PJ, Philbin DM, Watkins WD, Hilgenberg AD, Buckley MJ: Prostaglandin E1. A new therapy for refractory right heart failure and pulmonary hypertension after mitral valve replacement. J Thorac Cardiovasc Surg 1985; 89:567–72
44. Feneck RO: Intravenous milrinone following cardiac surgery: II. Influence of baseline hemodynamics and patient factors on therapeutic response. The European Milrinone Multicentre Trial Group. J Cardiothorac Vasc Anesth 1992; 6:563–7
45. Kikura M, Sato S: The efficacy of preemptive milrinone or amrinone therapy in patients undergoing coronary artery bypass grafting. Anesth Analg 2002; 94:22–30
46. De Hert SG, ten Broecke PW, Mertens E, Rodrigus IE, Stockman BA: Effects of phosphodiesterase III inhibition on length-dependent regulation of myocardial function in coronary surgery patients. Br J Anaesth 2002; 88:779–84
47. Lobato EB, Florete O, Jr., Bingham HL: A single dose of milrinone facilitates separation from cardiopulmonary bypass in patients with pre-existing left ventricular dysfunction. Br J Anaesth 1998; 81:782–4
48. Doolan LA, Jones EF, Kalman J, Buxton BF, Tonkin AM: A placebo-controlled trial verifying the efficacy of milrinone in weaning high-

risk patients from cardiopulmonary bypass. J Cardiothorac Vasc Anesth 1997; 11:37–41

49. Feneck RO. Intravenous milrinone following cardiac surgery: I. Effects of bolus infusion followed by variable dose maintenance infusion. The European Milrinone Multicentre Trial Group. J Cardiothorac Vasc Anesth 1992; 6:554–62

50. Yamada T, Takeda J, Katori N, Tsuzaki K, Ochiai R: Hemodynamic effects of milrinone during weaning from cardiopulmonary bypass: comparison of patients with a low and high prebypass cardiac index. J Cardiothorac Vasc Anesth 2000; 14:367–73

51. Bailey JM, Levy JH, Rogers HG, Szlam F, Hug CC, Jr.: Pharmacokinetics of amrinone during cardiac surgery. Anesthesiology 1991; 75:961–8

52. Ansell J, Tiarks C, McCue J, Parrilla N, Benotti JR: Amrinone-induced thrombocytopenia. Arch Intern Med 1984; 144:949–52

53. Haj RM, Cinco JE, Mazer CD: Treatment of pulmonary hypertension with selective pulmonary vasodilators. Curr Opin Anaesthesiol 2006; 19:88–95

54. Madden BP, Sheth A, Ho TB, Park JE, Kanagasabay RR: Potential role for sildenafil in the management of perioperative pulmonary hypertension and right ventricular dysfunction after cardiac surgery. Br J Anaesth 2004; 93:155–6

55. Bhatia S, Frantz RP, Severson CJ, Durst LA, McGoon MD: Immediate and long-term hemodynamic and clinical effects of sildenafil in patients with pulmonary arterial hypertension receiving vasodilator therapy. Mayo Clin Proc 2003; 78:1207–13

56. Michelakis E, Tymchak W, Lien D, Webster L, Hashimoto K, Archer S: Oral sildenafil is an effective and specific pulmonary vasodilator in patients with pulmonary arterial hypertension: comparison with inhaled nitric oxide. Circulation 2002; 105:2398–403

57. Cacoub P, Dorent R, Nataf P, et al.: Endothelin-1 in the lungs of patients with pulmonary hypertension. Cardiovasc Res 1997; 33:196–200

58. Stewart DJ, Levy RD, Cernacek P, Langleben D: Increased plasma endothelin-1 in pulmonary hypertension: marker or mediator of disease? Ann Intern Med 1991; 114:464–9

59. Channick RN, Simonneau G, Sitbon O, et al.: Effects of the dual endothelin-receptor antagonist bosentan in patients with pulmonary hypertension: a randomised placebo-controlled study. Lancet 2001; 358:1119–23

60. Newman JH: Treatment of primary pulmonary hypertension—the next generation. N Engl J Med 2002; 346:933–5

61. Langleben D, Brock T, Dixon R, Barst R: STRIDE-1 study group. STRIDE 1: effects of the selective ET(A) receptor antagonist, sitaxsen-

tan sodium, in a patient population with pulmonary arterial hypertension that meets traditional inclusion criteria of previous pulmonary arterial hypertension trials. J Cardiovasc Pharmacol 2004; 44:S80–4

62. Langleben D, Hirsch AM, Shalit E, Lesenko L, Barst RJ: Sustained symptomatic, functional, and hemodynamic benefit with the selective endothelin-A receptor antagonist, sitaxsentan, in patients with pulmonary arterial hypertension: a 1-year follow-up study. Chest 2004; 126:1377–81

63. Fullerton DA, Jaggers J, Jones SD, Brown JM, McIntyre RC, Jr.: Adenosine for refractory pulmonary hypertension. Ann Thorac Surg 1996; 62:874–7

64. Romson JL, Leung JM, Bellows WH, et al.: Effects of dobutamine on hemodynamics and left ventricular performance after cardiopulmonary bypass in cardiac surgical patients. Anesthesiology 1999; 91:1318–28

65. Feneck RO, Sherry KM, Withington PS, Oduro-Dominah A: European Milrinone Multicenter Trial Group. Comparison of the hemodynamic effects of milrinone with dobutamine in patients after cardiac surgery. J Cardiothorac Vasc Anesth 2001; 15:306–15

66. Gunnicker M, Brinkmann M, Donovan TJ, Freund U, Schieffer M, Reidemeister JC: The efficacy of amrinone or adrenaline on low cardiac output following cardiopulmonary bypass in patients with coronary artery disease undergoing preoperative beta-blockade. Thorac Cardiovasc Surg 1995; 43:153–60

67. Takaoka S, Faul JL, Doyle R: Current therapies for pulmonary arterial hypertension. Semin Cardiothorac Vasc Anesth 2007; 11:137–48

68. Labriola C, Siro-Brigiani M, Carrata F, Santangelo E, Amantea B: Hemodynamic effects of levosimendan in patients with low-output heart failure after cardiac surgery. Int J Clin Pharmacol Ther 2004; 42:204–11

69. Slawsky MT, Colucci WS, Gottlieb SS, et al.: Acute hemodynamic and clinical effects of levosimendan in patients with severe heart failure. Study Investigators. Circulation 2000; 102:2222–7

70. Tayama E, Ueda T, Shojima T, et al.: Arginine vasopressin is an ideal drug after cardiac surgery for the management of low systemic vascular resistant hypotension concomitant with pulmonary hypertension. Interact Cardiovasc Thorac Surg 2007; 6:715–9

71. Carceles MD, Fuentes T, Aroca V, Lopez J, Hernandez J: Effects of milrinone on contractility and cyclic adenosine monophosphate production induced by beta1- and beta2-adrenergic receptor activation in human myocardium. Clin Ther 2007; 29:1718–24

72. Nordhaug D, Steensrud T, Muller S, Husnes KV, Myrmel T: Intraaortic balloon pumping improves hemodynamics and right

ventricular efficiency in acute ischemic right ventricular failure. Ann Thorac Surg 2004; 78:1426–32

73. Moazami N, Pasque MK, Moon MR, et al.: Mechanical support for isolated right ventricular failure in patients after cardiotomy. J Heart Lung Transplant 2004; 23:1371–5

74. Steudel W, Hurford WE, Zapol WM: Inhaled nitric oxide: basic biology and clinical applications. Anesthesiology 1999; 91:1090–121

75. Rosenkranz B, Fischer C, Frolich J: Prostacyclin metabolites in human plasma. Clin Pharmacol Ther 1981; 29:420–4

76. Walmrath D, Schneider T, Schermuly R, Olschewski H, Grimminger F, Seeger W: Direct comparison of inhaled nitric oxide and aerosolized prostacyclin in acute respiratory distress syndrome. Am J Respir Crit Care Med 1996; 153:991–6

77. Rich GF, Lowson SM, Baum VC: Inhaled nitric oxide for cardiac disease. Respir Care 1999; 44(2):196–202

78. Morris GN, Rich GF, John RA: Exogenous inhaled nitric oxide as a selective pulmonary vasodilator. Semin Anesth 1996; 15:47–60

79. Fierobe L, Brunet F, Dhainaut J, et al.: Effect of inhaled nitric oxide on right ventricular function in adult respiratory distress syndrome. Am J Respir Crit Care Med 1998; 157:1483–8

80. Inglessis I, Shin JT, Lepore JJ, et al.: Hemodynamic effects of inhaled nitric oxide in right ventricular myocardial infarction and cardiogenic shock [see comment]. J Am Coll Cardiol 2004; 44:793–8

81. Griffiths MJ, Evans TW: Inhaled nitric oxide therapy in adults. N Engl J Med 2005; 353:2683–95

82. Dellinger RP, Zimmerman JL, Taylor RW, et al.: Inhaled Nitric Oxide in ARDS Study Group. Effects of inhaled nitric oxide in patients with acute respiratory distress syndrome: results of a randomized phase II trial. Crit Care Med 1998; 26:15–23

83. Lowson SM: Inhaled alternatives to nitric oxide. Anesthesiology 2002; 96:1504–13

84. Haraldsson A: The additive pulmonary vasodilatory effects of inhaled prostacyclin and inhaled milrinone in postcardiac surgical patients with pulmonary hypertension. Anesth Analg 2001; 93:439–45

85. Lepore JJ, Maroo A, Bigatello LM, et al.: Hemodynamic effects of sildenafil in patients with congestive heart failure and pulmonary hypertension: combined administration with inhaled nitric oxide. Chest 2005; 127:1647–53

86. Haraldsson A, Kieler-Jensen N, Nathorst-Westfelt U, Bergh CH, Ricksten SE: Comparison of inhaled nitric oxide and inhaled aerosolized prostacyclin in the evaluation of heart transplant candi-

dates with elevated pulmonary vascular resistance. Chest 1998; 114:780–6

87. Augoustides JG, Culp K, Smith S: Rebound pulmonary hypertension and cardiogenic shock after withdrawal of inhaled prostacyclin. Anesthesiology 2004 Apr; 100(4):1023–5

88. Schmid ER, Bürki C, Engel MHC, Schmidlin D, Tornic M, Seifer B: Inhaled nitric oxide versus intravenous vasodilators in severe pulmonary hypertension after cardiac surgery. Anesth Analg 1999; 89:1108

89. Semigran MJ, Cockrill BA, Kacmarek R, et al.: Hemodynamic effects of inhaled nitric oxide in heart failure. J Am Coll Cardiol 1994; 24:982–8

Katherine Arendt, MD
Martin Abel, MD

The Pregnant Patient and Cardiopulmonary

8 Bypass

INTRODUCTION

Improvements in the management of congenital heart disease (CHD) have led to increased survival and an increased number of women with CHD who now reach childbearing age. Furthermore, although the prevalence of rheumatic heart disease is decreasing in the United States, immigration of women with rheumatic heart disease and the trend in many developed countries toward increasing maternal age and obesity results in a sizable number of pregnant women with acquired heart disease (AHD). As a result, the number of women requiring cardiac interventions during pregnancy will likely increase in the coming decades. This chapter addresses some of the unique aspects of anesthetic management for the pregnant patient requiring cardiac surgery and cardiopulmonary bypass (CPB).

Historically, severe mitral stenosis in pregnancy was treated with closed mitral valvotomy, first described in 1952 (1, 2). This approach continued to be popular for decades (3–5). In 1958, CPB was first performed on a pregnant woman (6). In recent years, increasingly more complex cardiac procedures have been performed without CPB either employing percutaneous modalities or "off-pump." Although these less invasive approaches are useful in the nonpregnant patient, a number of concerns limit their use in the parturient. In the pregnant patient, for example, fetal radiation exposure during fluoroscopy limits the utility of some of the less invasive percutaneous techniques. Echocardiography

Medically Challenging Patients Undergoing Cardiothoracic Surgery, edited by Neal H. Cohen, MD, MPH, MS, Lippincott Williams & Wilkins, Baltimore © 2009.

imaging alone without fluoroscopy has been described in percutaneous balloon valvuloplasty (7, 8): however, experience with this technique is limited. For now, many cardiac procedures still necessitate that parturients undergo CPB for surgery involving the heart or aorta.

Multiple cases and series have been published describing CPB in pregnancy. Generally, maternal mortality with cardiac surgery does not appear to be affected by pregnancy, but the risk of fetal loss is significant. The overall goals for the anesthesiologist caring for the parturient undergoing CPB include maternal safety and fetal preservation through maintenance of uteroplacental sufficiency, detection of fetal distress, and prevention of preterm labor.

PHYSIOLOGIC CHANGES OF PREGNANCY

A number of physiologic changes occur during pregnancy that must be accounted for in the anesthetic management of the patient requiring CPB. Hemodynamic changes and alterations in pulmonary function and pulmonary reserve influence clinical decision making and management strategies for the parturient.

Cardiac Function and Hemodynamics

The hemodynamic changes of a normal pregnancy begin as early as the fourth week of gestation and continue into the postpartum period. A fall in systemic vascular tone induces a hyperdynamic cardiovascular state with a 30% increase in cardiac output by the end of the first trimester. Cardiac output plateaus at 40% above baseline around the 26th week of gestation and may decrease slightly by 10% toward term (30% above baseline). At term, the uterus and fetoplacental unit receive about 10% of the maternal cardiac output. During labor and delivery, the cardiac output can be greater than twice that of the nonpregnant state, with the most significant increase immediately after delivery of the fetus as the empty uterus contracts resulting in relief of aortocaval compression and an autotransfusion of uteroplacental blood.

Both systolic and diastolic blood pressure decrease by about 10 mm Hg and 5 mm Hg, respectively, until 30 weeks gestation because of a decreased peripheral vascular tone. Heart rate increases by about 15 bpm. Pulmonary vascular resistance decreases.

Oxygen Consumption

Oxygen consumption progressively increases throughout pregnancy. The metabolic needs of the fetus and placenta increase with growth. The maternal metabolic needs also increase as cardiac and respiratory work

TABLE 8–1. Physiologic changes of pregnancy

Parameter	Average change during pregnancy
Blood volume	↑35%
Cardiac output	↑40–43%
Stroke volume	↑30%
Heart Rate	↑15–17%
Systemic vascular resistance	↓15–21%
Mean arterial pressure	No significant change
Systolic blood pressure	↓3–5 mm Hg
Diastolic blood pressure	↓5–10 mm Hg
Central venous pressure	No significant change
Serum colloid osmotic pressure	↓14%
Hemoglobin	↓2.1 g/dl

From (10), p. 180.

increase. At term, maternal oxygen consumption can be up to 60% greater than baseline with carbon dioxide production similarly increased (9).

Blood Rheology

Colloid osmotic pressure decreases and a dilutional anemia occurs. The total red blood cell volume increases (1500 ml to 1800 ml) relatively less than the plasma volume (2500 ml to 3800 ml). The cardiovascular changes in a normal pregnancy are summarized in Table 8–1.

Pulmonary Function

Functional residual capacity (FRC) begins to decrease in the fifth month of pregnancy as the uterus increases in size. At term, FRC of the parturient is decreased by about 80% from the nonpregnant state. Decreased FRC, along with increased oxygen consumption, leads to a significant decrease in reserve and poorly tolerated apneic periods. Tidal volume increases by 45% throughout pregnancy with half of the increase occurring during the first trimester (11). Respiratory rate stays approximately the same as in the nonpregnant state. As a result, minute ventilation increases by 45%, primarily influenced by changes in tidal volume caused by progesterone stimulation and increased carbon dioxide production (12, 13). $PaCO_2$ decreases to 30 mm Hg by the 12th week of gestation and remains at that level for the duration of the pregnancy. Incomplete metabolic compensation for the respiratory alkalosis occurs with the bicarbonate concentration decreasing to about 20 meq/L, the

TABLE 8–2. **Blood gases during pregnancy**

	Nonpregnant	1st Trimester	2nd Trimester	3rd Trimester
PaCO2 (mmHg)	40	30	30	30
PaO2 (mm Hg)	100	107	105	103
pH	7.40	7.44	7.44	7.44
[HCO3]	24	21	20	20

Adapted from (14), p. 17.

base excess decreasing to –2 to –3 meq/L, and the blood pH increasing by 0.02–0.06 units, from 7.40 to between 7.42 and 7.46 (12). Blood gases during pregnancy are summarized in Table 8–2.

Airway

Pregnant women are known to have a higher incidence of difficulty with endotracheal intubation as a result of a number of factors (15, 16). Capillary engorgement results in pharyngolaryngeal edema beginning during the first trimester. This phenomenon coupled with the reduction in FRC and increased metabolic rate increase the risk of hypoxemia during a difficult or prolonged attempt to achieve endotracheal intubation. In addition, the change in body habitus makes optimal positioning of the patient more challenging, depending on the gestational age.

CARDIAC RISK ASSESSMENT DURING PREGNANCY

Valvular Stenosis and Left Ventricular Dysfunction

Siu and colleagues (17) prospectively followed 599 pregnancies of women with both AHD and CHD and developed a risk index for prediction of cardiac complications during pregnancy. The independent predictors of a "cardiac event" (defined as pulmonary edema, arrhythmia, stroke, cardiac arrest, or death) during pregnancy included those with left heart obstruction and those with preexisting left ventricular systolic dysfunction (17). These finding indicate that patients with obstruction of either the mitral and aortic valves or with left ventricular dysfunction adjust poorly to the physiologic changes of pregnancy and are more likely to decompensate to the point of requiring cardiac surgery during pregnancy.

In women younger than 40 years, half of all aortic dissections are associated with pregnancy (18). Surgical treatment carries a mortality rate of 22% for parturients equal only to that for pulmonary embolectomy in pregnancy (19). Therefore, women with preexisting abnormalities of the aorta are often encouraged not to become pregnant until after the abnormality is corrected; when they do become pregnant, they require close monitoring throughout the pregnancy.

Maternal and Fetal Risks of Cardiac Surgery Requiring CPB During Pregnancy

The risks associated with cardiac surgery for the pregnant patient are different than those for the nonpregnant patient, although the mortality rate is similar. Generally, pregnant women who require surgery under CPB do well, with a mortality rate similar to the rate for nonpregnant patients, ranging between 1.4% and 13.3%. Fetal loss, however, is a significant concern, with rates of fetal demise ranging from 16% to 38.5%. These quoted mortality rates are based on published results from a variety of clinical series. The first series of outcomes associated with CPB in pregnancy was published in 1969; it described 20 cases with 1 (5%) maternal death and 7 (33%) fetal deaths (20). A 1986 review of previously published outcomes found 1 (2.2%) maternal death and 9 (20%) fetal deaths in 45 cases of parturients undergoing cardiac surgery with CPB (21). A Mayo Clinic study described 10 cases of CPB in pregnancy from 1965 through 1989 with 2 maternal deaths and 2 fetal deaths (22). In a 1983 survey of the members of The Society of Thoracic Surgeons, only 1 maternal death (1.4%) and 11 (16%) fetal deaths were identified in 68 surgical procedures performed using CPB (23). A review of 69 cardiac procedures requiring CPB performed from 1958 through 1992 identified a maternal mortality of 2.9% and a fetal mortality of 20.2% (24). The highest fetal mortality was reported in a series of 15 parturients undergoing open heart surgery between 1972 and 1998 in Mexico, in which there were 2 (13.3%) maternal deaths and 5 (38.5%) fetal deaths.

One of the more recent series identified similar risks, despite advances in the perioperative management of the pregnant patient requiring cardiac surgery and CPB. Weiss and colleagues (19) describe 59 cases of cardiac surgery with CPB performed between 1984 and 1996 and reported 3 (5%) maternal deaths and a fetal/neonatal mortality rate of 29%. What is more notable from this series is the 25% rate of premature births, a rate that is significantly higher than that for healthy pregnancies.

Given the high fetal death rate with CPB, it is likely that fetal morbidity is similarly high in the neonates who initially survive, although there are limited published data to document the incidence of complications. At present, there are no long-term follow-up studies assessing the probable deleterious effects on those babies with fetal exposure to CPB. The confounding effects of fetal exposure to the mother's cardiac disease, pharmacologic management, and other cardiac interventions in addition to CPB would make such an assessment of the effects of CPB alone difficult.

Despite the many publications describing the risks associated with CPB during pregnancy, there is little clinical information correlating specific approaches to CPB techniques and the impact on maternal and fetal morbidity and mortality. A number of factors, including gestational age at the time of surgery, fetal heart rate (FHR) monitoring, high-flow CPB, normothermic CPB, and possibly pulsatile CPB have all been suggested to improve outcome. These factors are discussed later in the text.

Timing of Cardiac Surgery During Pregnancy

Cardiologists who care for women of child-bearing age with heart disease counsel these patients about the risks of pregnancy and the importance of optimizing their clinical status prior to conception. However, such optimization is not always possible, pregnancy is not always planned, and often the existence or extent of cardiac disease is unmasked for the first time because of the cardiovascular changes that occur during the pregnancy. Therefore, cardiologists and cardiovascular surgeons are often required to address the timing of surgery during pregnancy and, in some cases whether the surgical intervention is necessary prior to birth and, if so, the optimal gestational age to intervene.

Typically, in obstetric medicine, what is in the best interest of maternal health is in the best interest of the fetus. This may not be the case when deciding the timing of surgery in the parturient with a deteriorating cardiac status. In a systematic review from 1984 through 1996, Weiss and colleagues (19) compared maternal and fetal outcomes in cardiac surgeries performed during pregnancy, those performed immediately after delivery of the neonate, and those in which the surgery was delayed until after the postpartum period. *Fetal mortality* declined when cardiac surgery was delayed and the fetus was allowed to mature. Fetal mortality was highest in those surgeries performed during pregnancy (30%), better when the mother underwent surgery immediately after delivery (5%), and best when the mother delayed surgery until the postpartum period (0%). In contrast, however, the *maternal mortality* increased when the surgery was delayed until after birth. Therefore, it seems that the fetus benefits most from delaying maternal cardiac surgery until after birth, but the mother may benefit from an earlier intervention, while still pregnant. Clearly, these retrospective data may be confounded by the fact that the sickest parturients were unable to wait until after delivery; many of the procedures performed during the pregnancy were performed urgently because of clinical deterioration of the mother. Determining the optimal timing of cardiac surgical intervention is one of the most challenging and critical clinical decisions in the care of a deteriorating parturient: Early intervention will decrease maternal risk, but may result in fetal demise. Alternatively, delaying cardiac surgery until after delivery may result in maternal death.

In determining the optimal gestational timing for cardiac surgery, the effects of general anesthesia need to be considered separately from the effects of CPB. The most thorough evaluation of the risks of all types of anesthesia and surgery during pregnancy was a retrospective analysis of a population of 720,000 pregnant women who underwent 5405 surgical procedures (25). The incidence of congenital malformations or stillbirths was not increased in the offspring of women who underwent surgery, regardless of gestational age at the time of surgery. The incidence of prematurity was increased, the incidence of low-birth-weight neonates was increased, and the rate of infant death within one week of birth was also slightly increased. This increase, however, was not linked to gestational age at the time of surgery. Furthermore, patients who required surgery may have had underlying illnesses that affected the health of their pregnancy. This makes it difficult to determine the independent risk of anesthesia and surgery during pregnancy. Extrapolating the findings from this study to the pregnant patient requiring cardiac surgery and CPB is difficult. In this series, few patients had procedures performed using CPB. Therefore, although it appears that anesthesia at any time during pregnancy is quite safe, the risks of fetal exposure to CPB at various times during gestation are less clear.

There are a few case reports noting adverse fetal outcome after cardiac surgery with CPB when performed early in pregnancy (26–28). In one report, a parturient had mitral valve surgery during the sixth week of gestation, and fetal hydrocephalus was detected at 18 weeks gestation by ultrasound (27). A case report of fetal hydrocephalus and hydrops has also been described after CPB at 19 weeks gestational age, illustrating that the second trimester is not free from fetal risk, assuming that these complications are related to the surgical procedure and CPB (29). Also, in retrospective series of parturients undergoing CPB, fetal mortality has been described during every trimester of gestation (19, 20, 22, 23, 30).

Although anesthesia and CPB during organogenesis in the first trimester might theoretically increase fetal risk, there are few data to support this hypothesis. Nonetheless, many anesthesiologists, cardiologists, obstetricians, and cardiothoracic surgeons recommend that surgery, especially surgery requiring CPB, be delayed until after organogenesis is complete (i.e., by delaying any intervention until after the first trimester of pregnancy). In contrast, the physiologic changes that occur throughout the pregnancy may impact the timing of surgery. For example, late in the second trimester, the cardiac output of the parturient peaks. As a result, if the parturient is doing poorly at the beginning of second trimester, it is likely that she will deteriorate further as the pregnancy continues and may not survive into the third trimester. Under these circumstances, it may be ideal to perform cardiac surgery early in the second trimester. This approach minimizes further deterioration of the parturient and allows for completion of organogenesis of the fetus.

IMPACT OF CPB ON THE FETOPLACENTAL UNIT

Perfusion Flow and Pressure

Oxygen and nutrient transport to the fetus is supplied via the placenta. Deoxygenated blood from the fetus reaches the placenta via the two uterine arteries, branches of the internal iliac arteries. Oxygenated blood from the placenta then returns to the fetus in the umbilical vein and enters the inferior vena cava at the level of the liver via the ductus venosus. Sufficiency of the uterine blood flow (UBF), bathing the maternal side of the placenta, is directly linked to fetal oxygenation (31). As pregnancy progresses, the uterine arteries increase in diameter and become dilated from the effects of systemic hormones and endothelially released vasodilators. The uterine arteries become maximally dilated during pregnancy; UBF becomes pressure dependent and hence no autoregulation of UBF can occur. UBF is directly related to maternal arterial blood pressure and therefore inversely related to uterine vascular resistance.

Acute fetoplacental insufficiency results in fetal bradycardia. Long-term insufficiency produces chronic fetal hypoxia and acidosis, resulting in fetal tachycardia with minimal beat-to-beat variability in FHR as seen on an FHR tracing. During CPB, loss of pulsatile blood flow and decreases in mean arterial pressure in the parturient directly result in decreased uterine perfusion. The changes will be reflected on the FHR tracing. An example of FHR monitored throughout CPB is provided in Figure 8–1. The onset of CPB is typically characterized by fetal bradycardia, whereas at the conclusion of CPB, fetal tachycardia with minimal beat-to-beat variability is present (32, 33). The cause of this initial fetal bradycardia is thought to be placental hypoperfusion because it is reversible in most cases by increasing the perfusion flow rate and pressure. Other theories on the cause of this initial fetal bradycardia have included maternal hypothermia resulting in fetal bradycardia, fetal hypoxia from hemodilution acutely decreasing the maternal oxygen content, and uterine contractility at the onset of CPB increasing the uterine vascular resistance and decreasing placental sufficiency (34). Despite these other considerations, FHR directly correlates with perfusion during CPB such that when flow rate is increased, the FHR is restored (35). Thus, when the fetus has

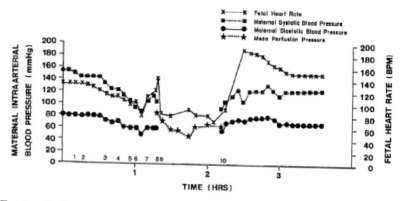

FIGURE 8–1. Example of fetal heart rate tracing as it relates to perfusion pressure during CPB. From (33; p. 113)

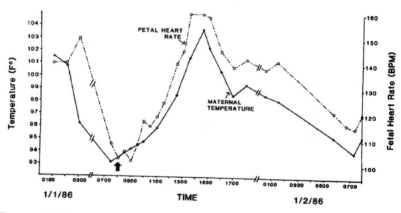

FIGURE 8–2. Fetal heart rate changes are directly related to maternal temperature. From (36)

reached viability (around 25 weeks gestational age), monitoring during cardiac surgery should include FHR. This is especially true during CPB so as to help establish optimal perfusion flow and pressure by aiming to maintain FHR in the normal range of 110–160 bpm.

Impact of Temperature Changes Associated with CPB

Temperature manipulation during CPB affects FHR (34). Typically, hypothermia causes fetal bradycardia whereas maternal hyperthermia results in fetal tachycardia as shown in Figure 8–2 (36). In any individual clinical situation, the cause for fetal bradycardia is difficult to determine, although it may be related to changes in fetal metabolism, changes in the placental vasculature, or fetal distress. For the mother who undergoes hypothermic CPB, a decrease in FHR should be expected. As discussed later in text (in the "Specific CPB Considerations, Hypothermic Versus Normothermic CPB in the Parturient"), whenever possible, normothermia should be maintained during CPB in pregnancy, because fetal asystole, uterine contractions, and decreased placental function and blood flow have been reported during hypothermic CPB.

CPB and Uteroplacental Insufficiency

At the conclusion of CPB, fetal tachycardia with minimal beat-to-beat variability is common. This phenomenon is presumably secondary to fetal acidosis developing from continuous uteroplacental insufficiency throughout CPB. The uteroplacental insufficiency associated with CPB likely has multiple causes. Gaseous, platelet, fibrin, or plastic microemboli may reach the placenta during CPB and, in conjunction with the activation of the complement system and release of humoral mediators like bradykinin, may reduce placental perfusion.

Pulsatile Versus Nonpulsatile CPB

Some studies suggest that nonpulsatile flow present during CPB may induce placental vasoconstriction similar to the known regional alterations in flow in other vascular beds (e.g., cerebral circulation) (37). In a fetal bypass model, nonpulsatile flow was found to inhibit selectively endothelium-dependent vasodilation by comparing the vasoactive effects of acetylcholine (endothelium dependent) and nitroprusside (endothelium independent) (38). Presumably, the absence of sheer stress in the vessel, as occurs with nonpulsatile flow, inhibits endothelial production of nitric oxide. In contrast, pulsatile flow during CPB preserves nitric oxide synthesis in the placental endothelium (39, 40). With the placental vasoconstriction that occurs with nonpulsatile CPB, higher flows and increased mean arterial pressures *may* be necessary to offset the adverse effects of nonpulsatility on placenta circulation.

THE MYOMETRIUM DURING CPB

Effect of Temperature on the Myometrium

When the uterus contracts, placental vascular resistance increases, placental perfusion decreases, and if complete uterine relaxation does not occur, subsequent fetal hypoxia ensues. Both the cooling and rewarming phases of CPB are associated with sustained uterine contractions

(23). The onset of sustained contractions during CPB can lead to fetal distress and possible fetal death. Normothermic (vs. hypothermic) CPB improves fetal survival probably by preventing the contractions associated with temperature change (24).

Effect of Hemodilution

Hemodilution at the initiation of CPB results in the dilution of progesterone levels, which may lead to increased excitability of the uterine muscle (28, 41). This effect may be offset by increased placental blood flow related to decreased blood viscosity (42).

Tocolytics

Progesterone, indomethacin, nitroglycerin, intravenous ethanol, magnesium sulfate, and β_2-sympathomimetics (ritodrine, terbutaline) are capable of decreasing uterine contractions (28, 35, 41, 43). The potent inhalational anesthetics (such as desflurane) also suppress uterine contractions in a dose-dependent manner (44). Although the suppression of uterine contractions during CPB is desirable, the routine, prophylactic use of tocolytics, especially the β_2-sympathomimetic agents, during CPB surgery cannot be recommended because of possible deleterious cardiac effects, particularly in patients with underlying cardiac disease (45, 46). In general, uterine contractions initially should be treated by increasing perfusion pressure and flow, then by increasing the potent volatile anesthetic agent to reduce uterine tone, and finally with cautious titration of a tocolytic agent such as magnesium, ritodrine, or terbutaline, taking into account the known risks associated with its use. Because uterine contractions have an impact on fetal outcome, monitoring of contractions is an important aspect of the management of patients undergoing CPB, particularly those likely to require titration of tocolytic agents to suppress uterine contractions.

OBSTETRIC MONITORING DURING CPB

Monitoring FHR

FHR monitoring should be used in the pregnant woman undergoing CPB when the fetus has reached an age when viability may reasonably be expected, typically after the 25th week of gestation. Multiple case reports have described fetal distress detected and corrected with FHR monitoring during CPB (32, 35, 47). Typically, FHR monitoring is performed with an external Doppler ultrasound transducer that is affixed to the parturient's abdomen. Fetal movement, usually minimal during general anesthesia, can result in loss of the FHR signal and may require that the transducer position be adjusted to achieve a good signal. Less optimal alternatives to continuous FHR monitoring include intermittent auscultation performed by obstetric personnel or ultrasonography to visualize the fetal heart and determine FHR. The availability of obstetric ultrasound equipment and an experienced operator who can focus attention on the well-being of the fetus is desirable in these situations. A decrease or loss of FHR as determined by Doppler, intermittent auscultation, and/or ultrasonography should be treated urgently by increasing CPB flow and pressure. FHR monitoring should be continued into the postoperative period.

Uterine Contractions

A tocodynamometer should also be placed on the abdomen to detect uterine contractions. During periods of reduced flow, cooling, and rewarming, uterine activity can be expected (23). As already mentioned, uterine contractions increase placental vascular resistance and can create temporary states of fetal oxygen deficiency. If this deficiency is prolonged, then fetal acidosis can ensue. Excessive uterine contractions can result in or even predict fetal death (21). Therefore, if consistent uterine contractions or prolonged tetany of the uterus are detected, prompt treatment is warranted. The treatment should include increasing CPB flow and pressure and administering a potent inhalational anesthetic, and consideration should be given to the use of other tocolytics (see the section "The Myometrium during CPB"). Tocodynamometry should be continued into the postoperative period. The combination of FHR and uterine contraction monitoring may be incorporated into a single device, the cardiotocograph.

SPECIFIC CPB CONSIDERATIONS

Pulsatile Versus Nonpulsatile Perfusion

When compared with nonpulsatile flow, pulsatile flow significantly improves blood flow to vital organs like the brain, heart, liver, and kidneys (48). Pulsatile flow during CPB also has been associated with many beneficial hormonal effects like lower cortisol, catecholamine, renin, and thromboxane levels and an overall reduction in the systemic inflammatory response syndrome (48). However, in randomized clinical trials, there is little evidence that pulsatile perfusion results in improved outcome as compared with nonpulsatile flow. One randomized trial (49) found an improvement in total mortality and myocardial infarction rate with pulsatile perfusion. However, there are no clinical data to show that pulsatile perfusion reduces the incidence of stroke or renal failure (50). In one randomized controlled trial, pulsatile perfusion was associated with increased hemolysis (51). It is not surprising then, that despite laboratory data showing enhanced organ perfusion, improved oxygen delivery, and decreased myocardial lactate production, pulsatile CPB is applied rarely clinically.

In the pregnant patient, the benefits of pulsatile flow may be more important than they are in nonpregnant patients. In a lamb model using fetal bypass, nonpulsatile flow perfusion has been shown to induce placental vasoconstriction and an increase in placental vascular resistance (52). As discussed earlier, nonpulsatile flow and the absence of sheer stress on the vessel inhibit the placental endothelium's ability to synthesize nitric oxide (38). These same investigators also demonstrated that the levels of endothelin-1, a potent vasoconstrictor, were significantly higher in the nonpulsatile group after 60 minutes of CPB (38). Pulsatile flow also has been shown to maintain placental perfusion by decreasing the activation of the fetal renin–angiotensin–aldosterone axis, decreasing vasoconstriction of the fetal placental vasculature (39).

Despite these proposed benefits of pulsatile CPB, nonpulsatile CPB perfusion is the standard of care at most institutions. Pulsatile flow has been attempted in human parturients. Different techniques for achieving pulsatility have been described. In one example, a roller pump was used in a pulsed mode to produce a maternal arterial pulse pressure of about 35 mm Hg (53). Pulsatile flow also has been produced with an intraaortic balloon pump (IABP) during the bypass period (54). The use of a balloon pump may not be optimal for parturients because the IABP may not have the same advantages as it does in the nonpregnant patients. Although the IABP provides adequate pulsatility to the vessels of the aortic arch (structures receiving their blood supply from vessels proximal to the intraaortic balloon), distal vessels such as the internal iliac arteries, which supply the uterine arteries, are likely to experience diminished diastolic pressure augmentation. A similar effect may be expected for renal and splanchnic blood flow when the IABP is used; however, in a small prospective randomized clinical trial of 40 patients, continuing to maintain pulsatile flow during CPB with an IABP was associated with improved creatinine clearance and lower liver enzymes (55).

In summary, despite reports of enhanced organ perfusion, improved oxygen delivery, and decreased myocardial lactate production with pulsatile perfusion, there are few clinical outcome data supporting the use of pulsatile flow during CPB. In addition, achieving pulsatile perfusion is technically more difficult and also may be associated with some adverse effects, including hemolysis. At this time, therefore, pulsatile perfusion is not recommended.

Hypothermic Versus Normothermic CPB in the Parturient

Hypothermic CPB as well as deep hypothermic circulatory arrest have been described in the parturient undergoing cardiac surgery without fetal morbidity or mortality (45, 56). Systemic hypothermia during CPB is used for organ (especially brain and heart) protection because it reduces tissue metabolic rate. For example, cerebral oxygen consumption decreases by a factor of 2.5 for each 10° C drop in temperature (37). Although hypothermia also decreases fetal oxygen requirements, it is likely that subjecting the parturient to hypothermia does have some potentially harmful effects, including fetal bradycardia and perhaps asystole, uterine contractions, reduced placental blood flow, and alterations in placental function.

As maternal temperature decreases, FHR also decreases as demonstrated in Figure 8–2. During hypothermic CPB, attempts at increasing FHR to the normal range (110–160 bpm) by increasing CPB flow may not be successful as described in one case report in which the FHR was 50bpm. In spite of increasing flow, the FHR in this case increased only after rewarming. Two case reports describe the loss of fetal heart tones and presumed fetal asystole during hypothermia that were detected again after completion of the surgical procedure (56, 57).

Much of the information we have about the impact of hypothermia on placental and fetal blood flow is based on individual case studies or limited animal investigations. One study found that the placenta acts as a poor oxygenator during hypothermic CPB. In a study comparing hypothermic to normothermic conditions, eight fetal ewes were placed on CPB with the placenta functioning as the oxygenator (58). In four fetal ewes, perfusion was performed at 37° C at various flow rates, and in the other ewes perfusion temperature was reduced to 25° C at various flow rates. The significantly lower fetal oxygenation in the hypothermic ewes could not be explained by the lower pCO_2.

Hypothermia also has been shown to decrease umbilical blood flow velocity in the human fetus. Goldstein and colleagues (34) measured umbilical artery flow velocity with transvaginal ultrasonography during hypothermic (around 30° C) CPB in a patient with severe mitral regurgitation at 15 weeks gestation (34). Diastolic uterine artery blood flow disappeared 10 minutes after initiation of CPB. This disappearance persisted for 40 minutes, and returned only after patient rewarming was instituted. A graphic of their findings is shown in Figure 8–3. Because the diastolic flow returned after rewarming but before the end of CPB, Goldstein and colleagues related the decrease in UBF to hypothermia, independent of the effects of nonpulsatile CPB alone.

The most significant findings related to the potential beneficial effects of normothermia during CPB in pregnancy come from a review of 69 case

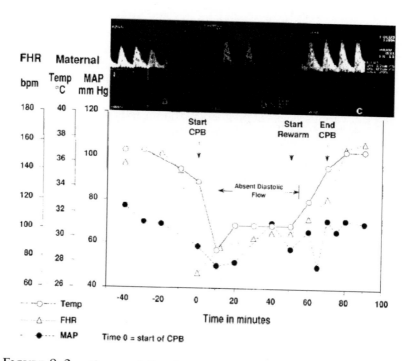

FIGURE 8–3. Absence of diastolic uterine artery blood flow as related to temperature during CPB. From (34; p. 1117)

reports from 1958 through 1992 of parturients needing cardiovascular surgery with CPB (24). Review of the 40 most recent cases in this series found that, although hypothermic CPB had no effect on maternal mortality, it was associated with a fetal mortality rate of 24%. By comparison, in the normothermic CPB group, there was no fetal loss. Hypothermic perfusion also provoked decreased placental blood flow, fetal asystole, and uterine contractions in several patients. Uterine contractions have been described during the cooling and the rewarming phases in other studies as well and may have contributed to the worse outcomes (23).

In summary, hypothermia should be avoided when CPB is used in parturients for the following reasons: placental blood flow is decreased, placental oxygen transfer is adversely affected, uterine contractions and irritability are increased, fetal bradycardia and asystole may occur, and increased fetal mortality has been described.

CPB Flow and Perfusion Pressure

The etiology of placental dysfunction after fetal CPB is probably mediated by reductions in placental nitric oxide concentrations leading to increases in placental vascular resistance and worsening placental gas exchange (60). In fetal bypass models, increased perfusion flow rates improve placental perfusion and function (58, 59). In humans there are multiple case reports suggesting a similar conclusion based on the finding that fetal bradycardia during CPB is reversed by increasing perfusion flow and pressure. In summarizing data from 69 case reports of parturients undergoing CPB at various stages of pregnancy, Pomini and colleagues (24) state that "pump flow and mean arterial pressure during CPB seem to be the most important parameters that influence fetal oxygenation."

Although it is difficult to recommend a specific perfusion flow rate and/or pressure for the optimal conduct of CPB in the parturient, some increase in baseline perfusion flow must be instituted. The increased perfusion flow rate should take into account the gestational age of the fetus and the ease of achieving higher flow rates with the standard circuitry employed in conventional CPB. Cardiac output is 40% above baseline by gestational week 26, which equates to a cardiac index of approximately 3.4 $L \cdot min^{-1} \cdot m^2$. Based on clinical experience, during CPB for the parturient, a cardiac index >2.4 $L \cdot min^{-1} \cdot m^2$ and a mean arterial pressure >70 mm Hg are recommended, particularly as the parturient reaches the end of the second trimester (57). One case report describes fetal bradycardia occurring at a flow index of 2.8 $L \cdot min^{-1} \cdot m^2$, which improved only after increasing the flow to 4.6 $L \cdot min^{-1} \cdot m^2$ (35).

Maternal Acid–Base Balance

During pregnancy, maternal $PaCO_2$ decreases to 30 mm Hg by week 12, bicarbonate concentration decreases to about 20 meq/L, the base excess decreases to –2 to –3 meq/L, and the blood pH increases by 0.02–0.06 units as summarized in Table 8–2 (13). The fetus cannot respond to acid–base changes with the normal respiratory or metabolic mechanisms typical in the mother or even the neonate. Normally, the fetal pH is 0.1 units lower than that of the mother. Maternal acidosis can result in fetal acidosis, and because of the fetus's inability to compensate for acidemia by compensatory hyperventilation or by renal responses like the adult, the maternal pH should be kept as close to 7.44 as possible. In sheep, it has been demonstrated that the hypocapnia and alkalemia caused by maternal hyperventilation decreases fetal oxygenation (61).

It seems prudent, therefore, that the maternal $PaCO_2$ should be kept as close to 30 mm Hg as possible. Arterial pCO_2 during CPB can easily be maintained at this level by adjusting fresh gas flow rate into the membrane oxygenator. Arterial PO_2 can be modified by adjusting FO_2 in the gases flowing to the membrane oxygenator. There are few data to guide decision making about the optimal PaO_2 during CPB; conventionally, an arterial PO_2 of 150 mm Hg is the goal.

Myocardial Protection

Infusion of a cardioplegic solution into the coronary circulation is used to cause diastolic arrest of the heart and protect the myocardium during a period of cardiac ischemia while using CPB to perfuse the rest of the body. Fetal bradycardia has been reported with the administration of cold cardioplegic solution—in this instance, FHR returned to normal with increased perfusion and temperature (62). If CPB is maintained with high perfusion flow and normothermia, then repeated administration of cardioplegic solution may be needed (63). Similarly, increased maternal potassium levels can result from repeated doses of cardioplegic solution containing high potassium concentrations. In the absence of specific data, precautions should be taken to avoid hypothermia or hyperkalemia resulting from the use of cold hyperkalemic cardioplegic solutions. Avoidance of such hypothermia and hyperkalemia can be achieved by completing the cardiac surgical repair with the shortest period of cardiac ischemia (aortic cross-clamp time) and by using lower concentrations of potassium in the cardioplegic solution when subsequent administration is necessary. Perfusion temperature and serum potassium are easily monitored by continuous in-line analysis of these parameters.

CPB Prime

The fluid used for priming the CPB circuit is similar to that of plasma, except that in most cases mannitol is added for its osmotic diuretic effect. Passive transfer of mannitol (molecular weight 182; similar to glucose) across the placenta is low, reflecting a barrier to diffusion (64). This barrier leads to a concentration gradient for mannitol. In theory, as the osmotic pressure of the maternal blood increases, water would be pulled from the fetal into the maternal circulation. One report suggests omitting mannitol in the CPB prime to decrease the risk of hemoconcentrating fetal blood (54). In contrast, maternal hemodilution resulting from CPB may cause overhydration of the fetus. One case of fetal hydrocephalus and hydrops detected after CPB at 19 weeks gestation has been reported (29). Further investigation is needed regarding the use of mannitol and the effects of hemodilution resulting from variations in the CPB priming solution.

Anticoagulation and Hematologic Considerations

The coagulation and fibrinolytic pathways are amplified in pregnancy. The changes in coagulation and fibrinolytic parameters associated with pregnancy are summarized in Table 8–3. Platelet turnover is increased,

TABLE 8–3. Changes in coagulation and fibrinolytic parameters at term gestation, compared to nonpregnant women

Increased factor concentrations
Factor I (fibrinogen)
Factor VII (proconvertin)
Factor VIII (antihemophilic factor)
Factor IX (Christmas factor)
Factor X (Stuart-Prower factor)
Factor XII (Hageman factor)

Unchanged factor concentrations
Factor II (prothrombin)
Factor V (proaccelerin)

Decreased factor concentrations
Factor XI (thromboplastin antecedent)
Factor XIII (fibrin-stabilizing factor)
Prothrombin time: shortened 20%
Partial thromboplastin time: shortened 20%
Thromboelastography: hypercoagulable
Fibrinopeptide A: increased
Antithrombin III: decreased
Platelet count: no change or decreased
Bleeding time: no change
Fibrin degradation products: increased
Plasminogen: increased

From (14), p 22.

and in 7.6% of otherwise normal parturients platelet counts are $<150,000/mm^3$ at term (65).

Heparin and protamine, FDA Pregnancy Category C medications, do not cross the placenta and have posed little risk to the fetus when used for CPB. Antithrombin III concentrations are decreased in pregnancy, and many parturients with cardiac disease will be on chronic subcutaneous heparin during their pregnancy. As a result, heparin resistance should be expected and management adjusted to address it. After heparin administration, the activated clotting time (ACT) must be checked prior to the initiation of CPB. Heparin dosing prior to CPB, typically 3 mg/kg, should remain the same as in the nonpregnant patient, on a milligram per kilogram body weight basis. If the ACT is less than expected after heparin administration, then heparin resistance should be suspected and treatment with antithrombin III instituted.

The use of antifibrinolytic agents to reduce blood loss in cardiac surgery during pregnancy is uncertain. Because pregnancy is associated with a physiologic enhancement in clotting, the parturient likely relies upon fibrinolysis to prevent adverse thrombotic events such as placental infarction or deep venous thrombosis formation. In a retrospective analysis of 256 pregnant patients with various bleeding disorders who were treated with tranexamic acid, no relationship between tranexamic acid use and thromboembolism could be identified (66). Nevertheless, on balance, antifibrinolytic agents should not be used in pregnancy unless a specific bleeding disorder is identified suggesting a likely benefit.

Consideration should be given to maintaining the physiologic anemia of pregnancy (hemoglobin 11.6 g/dL or hematocrit 35.5%) during and after CPB. It is thought that the decreased blood viscosity resulting from the physiologic hemodilution of pregnancy helps maintain uteroplacental perfusion. In one study (67), an elevation of maternal hematocrit was associated with placental infarction. However, hemodilution to a hematocrit of 21%, as may occur with CPB, may reduce oxygen carriage to the fetus. The ideal hematocrit for CPB in the parturient is not known. Maintaining a hematocrit >25% is a reasonable goal to moderate the need for blood transfusion while avoiding fetal hypoxemia.

GENERAL CONSIDERATIONS FOR THE PARTURIENT DURING ANESTHESIA AND SURGERY

Uterine Displacement

After about 20 weeks gestation, the parturient should be positioned in the left lateral recumbent position during CPB. The supine position without any lateral tilt results in aortocaval compression and impairment of uteroplacental blood flow as shown in Figure 8–4 (68). This phenomenon is exaggerated during periods of hypotension, so it is critical to avoid aortocaval compression at all times during the procedure.

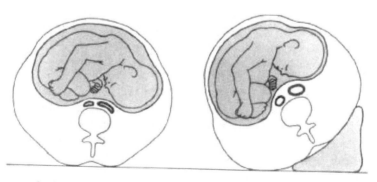

FIGURE 8–4. Aortocaval decompression with left lateral tilt. From (68)

Hypoxemia and Endotracheal Intubation

Anesthesiologists also must be aware that parturients have increased rates of failed intubation (15, 69). Edema of the airway structures progresses during pregnancy and may impede the anesthesiologist's laryngoscopic view. The reduction in FRC and an increased oxygen consumption that occurs with pregnancy decrease apnea time compared with the nonpregnant state (70). Therefore, careful attention should be paid to preoxygenation and rapid control of the airway with induction of anesthesia in the pregnant patient.

Preeclampsia

Patients with preeclampsia or eclampsia are exquisitely sensitive to catecholamines from impaired endothelial function and impaired nitric oxide production. Malignant hypertension, as may result from an inadequate depth of anesthesia at the time of laryngoscopy, risks hemorrhagic stroke and must be avoided. Anesthetic depth during surgery and careful titration of sympathomimetic agents are necessary to avoid hypertensive crises. The anesthetic implications in preeclampsia and eclampsia are reviewed in detail elsewhere (71, 72).

PHARMACOLOGIC CONSIDERATIONS

Anesthetic Agents

The major risks of surgery during pregnancy are preterm labor, low-birth-weight babies, or fetal loss (25). It is likely that the major source of these fetal hazards is the parturient's illness and is not directly related to the anesthetic agent. Although no clinical studies have established a link between anesthetic drugs and subsequent fetal defects (25, 73, 74), laboratory studies suggest that some anesthetic drugs should be used with caution or avoided entirely during pregnancy. Anesthesiologists should be aware of animal studies in which anesthetic agents may have caused teratogenicity, fetal loss, or preterm labor and the timing of the surgery relative to these risks.

Nitrous Oxide
Nitrous oxide inactivates methionine synthetase thereby inhibiting, in turn, the synthesis of the nucleoside thymidine, DNA, and cell division (75). Although no human birth defects have been linked to nitrous oxide, female dental assistants, working in dental offices and administering nitrous oxide without scavenging equipment, have increased rates of fetal loss (76). Interestingly, although nitrous oxide exhibits teratogenic

effects in mice, the coadministration of halothane or isoflurane with nitrous oxide offsets this teratogenic effect without reversing methionine synthetase inactivation (77). In a large retrospective clinical study, nitrous oxide was not associated with an increased risk of fetal defect or loss (25). These data suggest that a short exposure to nitrous oxide during pregnancy is harmless.

Benzodiazepines

Benzodiazepines used to be avoided in the first trimester of pregnancy because of a reported association with fetal oral cleft palates (78). This reported association has been disproven (79, 80), and experts no longer believe that benzodiazepines are contraindicated in the parturient (81, 82). Midazolam, by virtue of its ease of administration and shorter duration, is preferred over diazepam or lorazepam in the parturient.

Ketamine

Ketamine at doses >1.5 mg/kg has been shown to increase uterine tone by up to 40% during the first and second trimesters (83). This effect seems to be absent during the third trimester. Ketamine should be avoided in the preeclamptic parturient because it may increase the systemic and pulmonary arterial pressures.

Sympathomimetic Agents

During a normal healthy pregnancy, a woman demonstrates a reduction in sensitivity to vasoconstricting agents. Angiotensin II, norepinephrine, and phenylephrine infusions all illustrate attenuated systemic pressor responses in the gravid ewe (84).

Ephedrine

Ephedrine historically has been considered the vasopressor of choice in pregnancy to treat hypotension associated with neuraxial anesthesia. Likewise, it is probably safe to use during cardiac surgery in the parturient, but may be less effective than direct acting sympathomimetics.

Phenylephrine

Possible increases in uterine vascular resistance with phenylephrine as demonstrated in animal studies limited its use in the parturient for many years. However, in a review of seven randomized trials comparing ephedrine with phenylephrine to manage hypotension during spinal anesthesia for elective cesarean delivery, there was no decrease in fetal pH or neonatal Apgar scores with the use of phenylephrine (85). In fact, one study showed phenylephrine produced greater (better) fetal pH measurements than ephedrine did, although the difference was clinically insignificant (86). Similarly, it is likely that phenylephrine can be used safely to maintain perfusion pressure during CPB. However, as in conventional CPB, when an increase in mean arterial pressure is desired, increases in perfusion flow will provide greater uteroplacental blood flow than will increases obtained with phenylephrine.

Inotropic and Antiarrhythmic Agents

Digoxin

Although used less commonly now than in the past, digoxin is still administered to some patients with cardiac disease requiring CPB. Rates of fetal anomalies were not increased in 142 parturients who took digoxin throughout the first trimester (87). When digoxin is given to the parturient, the digoxin level should be monitored carefully throughout pregnancy because as plasma volume increases, plasma levels may become subtherapeutic. Furthermore, digoxin toxicity could lead to fetal death.

Isoproterenol

In the Collaborative Perinatal Project, 31 parturients who were treated with isoproterenol during the first trimester did not have an increase in fetal malformations (88). There are also no reports of inotropic agents such as dopamine or dobutamine causing teratogenicity.

Amiodarone

Amiodarone administration is associated with a number of side effects. During pregnancy the concerns are similar to those for the nonpregnant patient, although they affect both the mother and the newborn. A review of the side effects of amiodarone in 64 parturients found hypothyroidism in 17% of the neonates, hyperthyroidism in 3%, and goiter in 3%. In addition to the fetal thyroid effects, concerns were raised about mild neurodevelopmental alterations in these neonates (89). A summary of these data and those on other antiarrhythmic agents, as well as recommendations for their use during pregnancy, can be found in Table 8–4.

β-Adrenergic Receptor Antagonists

There is no evidence that any of the β-adrenergic receptor antagonists are teratogenic. Atenolol use has been associated with lesser neonatal birth weights (90). In a randomized, double-blind controlled trial of labetalol versus placebo in pregnancy-induced hypertension, there was no increase in fetal malformations in the group treated with labetalol (91). Of note, β-adrenergic receptor antagonists will cross the placenta; this will result in a decrease in FHR and variability. When assessing fetal status, the anes-

TABLE 8–4. Antiarrhythmic therapy during pregnancy

	FDA	Pregnancy	Lactation	Remarks	Use
Class IA					
Quinidine	C	+	+	First Choice IA	SVT
Procainamide	C	+	+		SVT/VT
Disopyramide	C	?	?		SVT
Class IB					
Lidocaine	B	+	+		VT
Class IC					
Flecainide	C	?	?		SVT
Propafenone	C	?	?		SVT
Class II					
Propranolol	C	+	+		SVT/VT
Metoprolol	C	+	+		SVT/VT
Class III					
Satalol	B	+	+/–	High dose in breast milk	SVT/VT
Amiodarone	D	+/–	–	Only use if others fail	SVT/VT
Class IV					
Verapamil	C	+	+	First Choice IV	SVT
Diltiazem	C	–	?		SVT
Digoxin	C	+	+	Toxicity may cause fetal death	SVT
Adenosine	C	+	+		SVT

From (10), p. 185.

thesiologist should be aware of these effects of the β-antagonists, because changes in FHR and variability will not necessarily reflect fetal distress.

Vasodilating Agents

Sodium nitroprusside and nitroglycerin are considered safe in pregnancy. In a gravid ewe study, both agents produced no significant changes in UBF or uterine vascular conductance (UVC) when infused into a normotensive ewe despite significant decreases in mean aortic pressure (92). This study also demonstrated that these agents counteract the uterine artery–vasoconstricting effects of alpha-stimulation. When norepinephrine was given to the pregnant ewes in the presence of these agents, UBF and UVC were higher whereas mean aortic pressure was lower than when norepinephrine was given alone. In other words, during periods of alpha-stimulation, sodium nitroprusside and nitroglycerin do not produce vasodilation that results in shunting of blood away from the fetus, but instead produce uterine artery vasodilation that improves placental blood flow. Pregnant patients who receive nitroprusside should be monitored for cyanide and thiocyanate toxicity. Just as cyanide levels can increase in the parturient when sodium nitroprusside infusion is continued at length, these levels can increase in the fetus as well. Gravid ewe studies show that this increase can result in fetal demise (93).

CONCLUSION

CPB during pregnancy is safe for the parturient but poses significant risk to the fetus. If possible, delaying the surgery until after delivery is best for the neonate, but can result in increased morbidity and mortality for the mother. High flow, normothermic, pulsatile CPB of the shortest length possible is likely to produce the best outcome for the fetus. The usual anesthetic precautions for a parturient should be undertaken. The anesthesiologist must be aware of and prepared to address difficulties with securing the parturient's airway, must avoid hypoxia because of the shorter safe apneic period, and must take care in positioning the parturient with a left lateral tilt to avoid aortocaval compression. If the fetus is of viable age, FHR and uterine activity should be monitored throughout CPB. The anesthesiologist should be prepared to treat fetal bradycardia by increasing perfusion flow and pressure. Uterine contractions should be treated promptly by increasing the administration of the potent inhalational anesthetics and by administering other tocolytics as necessary. Fetal and uterine monitoring should be continued postoperatively. The acid–base status of the parturient should be maintained according to the normal values of pregnancy.

References

1. Brock RC: Valvotomy in pregnancy. Proc Roy Soc Med 1952; 45:538
2. Cooley DA, Chapman DW: Mitral commissurotomy during pregnancy. JAMA 1952; 150:1113–4
3. Pavankumar P, Venugopal P, Kaul U, et al.: Closed mitral valvotomy during pregnancy: a 20-year experience. Scand Cardiovasc J 1988; 22:11–5
4. Vosloo S, Reichart B: The feasibility of closed mitral valvotomy in pregnancy. J Thorac Cardiovasc Surg 1987; 93:675–9
5. Abid A, Abid F, Zargouni N, Khayati A: Closed mitral valvotomy in pregnancy—a study of seven cases. Int J Cardiol 1990; 26:319–21
6. Dubourg G, Broustet H, Bricaud H, Fontan F, Tarieux M, Fontanille P: Correction complete d'une triade de Fallot, en circulation extra-corporelle, chez une femme enceinte. Arch Mal Coeur Vaiss 1959; 52:1389–92

7. Kultursay H, Turkoglu C, Akin M, Payzin S, Soydas C, Akilli A: Mitral balloon valvuloplasty with transesophageal echocardiography without using fluoroscopy. Cathet Cardiovasc Diagn 1992; 27:317–21

8. Trehan V, Mukhopadhyay S, Nigam A, et al.: Mitral valvuloplasty by Inoue balloon under transthoracic echocardiographic guidance. J Am Soc Echocardiogr 2005; 18:964–9

9. Spatling L, Fallenstein F, Huch A, Huch R, Rooth G: The variability of cardiopulmonary adaptation to pregnancy at rest and during exercise. Br J Obstet Gynaecol 1992; 99:1–40

10. Abbas AE, Lester SJ, Connolly H: Pregnancy and the cardiovascular system. Int J Cardiol 2005; 98:179–89

11. Alaily AB, Carr KB: Pulmonary ventilation in pregnancy. BJOG 1978; 85:518–24

12. Templeton A, Kelman GR: Maternal blood-gases, (P AO2-P aO2), physiological shunt and VD/VT in normal pregnancy. Br J Anaesth 1976; 48:1001–4

13. Machida H: Influence of progesterone on arterial blood and CSF acid-base balance in women. J Appl Physiol 1981; 51:1433–6

14. Chestnut DH: Obstetric anesthesia : principles and practice, 3rd Edition. Philadelphia, PA, Mosby/Elsevier, 2004.

15. Lyons G: Six years' experience in a teaching maternity unit. Anaesthesia 1985; 40:759–62

16. Samsoon GLT, Young JRB: Difficult tracheal intubation: a retrospective study. Anaesthesia 1987; 42:487–90

17. Siu SC, Sermer M, Colman JM, et al.: Prospective multicenter study of pregnancy outcomes in women with heart disease. Circulation 2001; 104(5):515–21

18. Mandel W, Evans EW, Walford RL: Dissecting aortic aneurysm during pregnancy. N Engl J Med 1954; 251:1059–61

19. Weiss BM, von Segesser LK, Alon E, Seifert B, Turina MI: Outcome of cardiovascular surgery and pregnancy: a systematic review of the period 1984–1996. Am J Obstet Gynecol 1998; 179:1643

20. Zitnik RS, Brandenburg RO, Sheldon R, Wallace RB: Pregnancy and open-heart surgery. Circulation 1969; 39:257–62

21. Bernal JM, Miralles PJ: Cardiac surgery with cardiopulmonary bypass during pregnancy. Obstet Gynecol Surv 1986; 41:1–6

22. Strickland RA, Oliver WC, Chantigian RC, Ney JA, Danielson GK: Anesthesia, cardiopulmonary bypass, and the pregnant patient. Mayo Clin Proc 1991; 66(4):411–29

23. Becker RM: Intracardiac surgery in pregnant women. Ann Thorac Surg 1983; 36:453–8

24. Pomini F, Mercogliano D, Cavalletti C, Caruso A, Pomini P: Cardiopulmonary bypass in pregnancy. Ann Thorac Surg 1996; 61:259–68

25. Mazze RI, Kallen B: Reproductive outcome after anesthesia and operation during pregnancy: a registry study of 5405 cases. Am J Obstet Gynecol 1989; 161:1178–85

26. Leyse R, Ofstun M, Dillard DH, Merendino KA: Congenital aortic stenosis in pregnancy, corrected by extracorporeal circulation, offering a viable male infant at term but with anomalies eventuating in his death at four months of age—report of a case. JAMA 1961; 176:1009–12

27. Lapiedra OJ, Bernal JM, Ninot S, Gonzalez I, Pastor E, Miralles PJ: Open heart surgery for thrombosis of a prosthetic mitral valve during pregnancy. Fetal hydrocephalus. J Cardiovasc Surg (Torino) 1986; 27:217–20

28. Parry AJ, Westaby S: Cardiopulmonary bypass during pregnancy. Ann Thorac Surg 1996; 61(6):1865–9

29. Khandelwal M, Rasanen J, Ludormirski A, Addonizio P, Reece EA: Evaluation of fetal and uterine hemodynamics during maternal cardiopulmonary bypass. Obstet Gynecol 1996; 88 (4 Pt 2):667–71

30. Salazar E, Espinola N, Molina FJ, Reyes A, Barragan R: Heart surgery with cardiopulmonary bypass in pregnant women. Arch Cardiol Mex 2001; 71:20–7

31. Bilardo CM, Nicolaides KH, Campbell S: Doppler measurements of fetal and uteroplacental circulations: relationship with umbilical venous blood gases measured at cordocentesis. Am J Obstet Gynecol 1990; 162:115–20

32. Koh KS, Friesen RM, Livingstone RA, Peddle LJ: Fetal monitoring during maternal cardiac surgery with cardiopulmonary bypass. CMAJ 1975; 112:1102–4

33. Levy DL, Warriner RA, 3rd, Burgess GE, 3rd: Fetal response to cardiopulmonary bypass. Obstet Gynecol 1980; 56:112–5

34. Goldstein I, Jakobi P, Gutterman E, Milo S: Umbilical artery flow velocity during maternal cardiopulmonary bypass. Ann Thorac Surg 1995; 60:1116–8

35. Werch A, Lambert HM, Cooley D, Reed CC: Fetal monitoring and maternal open heart surgery. South Med J 1977; 70:1024

36. Jadhon ME, Main EK: Fetal bradycardia associated with maternal hypothermia. Obstet Gynecol 1988; 72:496

37. Murkin JM, Farrar JK, Tweed WA, McKenzie FN, Guiraudon G: Cerebral autoregulation and flow/metabolism coupling during cardiopulmonary bypass: the influence of PaCO2. Anesth Analg 1987; 66:825–32

38. Reddy VM, McElhinney DB, Rajasinghe HA, et al.: Role of the endothelium in placental dysfunction after fetal cardiac bypass. J Thorac Cardiovasc Surg 1999; 117(2):343–51

39. Vedrinne C, Tronc F, Martinot S, et al.: Better preservation of endothelial function and decreased activation of the fetal renin-angiotensin pathway with the use of pulsatile flow during experimental fetal bypass. J Thorac Cardiovasc Surg. 2000; 120(4):770–7

40. Champsaur G, Vedrinne C, Martinot S, et al.: Flow-induced release of endothelium-derived relaxing factor during pulsatile bypass: experimental study in the fetal lamb. J Thorac Cardiovasc Surg. 1997; 114(5):738–44; discussion 744–5

41. Korsten HH, Van Zundert AA, Mooij PN, De Jong PA, Bavinck JH: Emergency aortic valve replacement in the 24th-week of pregnancy. Acta Anaesthesiol Belg 1989; 40:201–5

42. Crino JP, Harris AP, Parisi VM, Johnson TRB: Effect of rapid intravenous crystalloid infusion on uteroplacental blood flow and placental implantation-site oxygen delivery in the pregnant ewe. Am J Obstet Gynecol 1993; 168:1603–9

43. Karahan N, Öztürk T, Yetkin U, Yilik L, Baloglu A, Gürbüz A: Managing severe heart failure in a pregnant patient undergoing cardiopulmonary bypass: case report and review of the literature. J Cardiothorac Vasc Anesth 2004; 18:339–43

44. Yoo KY, Lee JC, Yoon MH, et al.: The effects of volatile anesthetics on spontaneous contractility of isolated human pregnant uterine muscle: a comparison among sevoflurane, desflurane, isoflurane, and halothane. Anesth Analg 2006; 103:443

45. Kawkabani N, Kawas N, Baraka A, Vogel T, Mangano CM: Severe fetal bradycardia in a pregnant woman undergoing hypothermic cardiopulmonary bypass. J Cardiothorac Vasc Anesth 1999; 13:346–9

46. Chambers CE, Clark SL: Cardiac surgery during pregnancy. Clin Obstet Gynecol 1994; 37:316–23

47. Lamb MP, Ross K, Johnstone AM, Manners JM: Fetal heart monitoring during open heart surgery. Two case reports. Br J Obstet Gynaecol 1981; 88:669–74

48. Ji B, Ündar A: An evaluation of the benefits of pulsatile versus non-pulsatile perfusion during cardiopulmonary bypass procedures in pediatric and adult cardiac patients. ASAIO J 2006; 52:357

49. Murkin JM, Martzke JS, Buchan AM, Bentley C, Wong CJ:. A randomized study of the influence of perfusion technique and pH management strategy in 316 patients undergoing coronary artery bypass surgery: I. Mortality and cardiovascular morbidity. J Thorac Cardiovasc Surg 1995; 110:340–8

50. Abdullah A, Alghamdi DAL: Pulsatile versus nonpulsatile cardiopulmonary bypass flow: an evidence-based approach. J Card Surg 2006; 21:347–54
51. Zumbro GL, Jr.: A prospective evaluation of the pulsatile assist device. Ann Thorac Surg 1979; 28:269–73
52. Champsaur G, Parisot P, Martinot S, et al.: Pulsatility improves hemodynamics during fetal bypass. Experimental comparative study of pulsatile versus steady flow. Circulation 1994; 90(5 Pt 2):II47–50
53. Tripp HF, Stiegel RM, Coyle JP: The use of pulsatile perfusion during aortic valve replacement in pregnancy. Ann Thorac Surg 1999; 67(4):1169–71.
54. Willcox TW, Stone P, Milsom FP, Connell H: Cardiopulmonary bypass in pregnancy: possible new role for the intra-aortic balloon pump. J Extra Corpor Technol 2005; 37:189–91
55. Onorati F, Cristodoro L, Mastroroberto P, et al.: Should we discontinue intraaortic balloon during cardioplegic arrest? Splanchnic function results of a prospective randomized trial. Ann Thorac Surg 2005; 80:2221–8
56. Buffolo E, Palma JH, Gomes WJ, et al.: Successful use of deep hypothermic circulatory arrest in pregnancy. Ann Thorac Surg 1994; 58:1532–4
57. Mahli A, Izdes S, Coskun D: Cardiac operations during pregnancy: review of factors influencing fetal outcome. Ann Thorac Surg 2000; 69:1622–6
58. Hawkins JA, Paape KL, Adkins TP, Shaddy RE, Gay WA, Jr.: Extracorporeal circulation in the fetal lamb. Effects of hypothermia and perfusion rate. J Cardiovasc Surg (Torino) 1991; 32:295–300
59. Hawkins JA, Clark SM, Shaddy RE, Gay WA, Jr.: Fetal cardiac bypass: improved placental function with moderately high flow rates. Ann Thorac Surg 1994; 57:293–6
60. Lam C, Baker RS, McNamara J, et al.: Role of nitric oxide pathway in placental dysfunction following fetal bypass. Ann Thorac Surg 2007; 84:917–25
61. Levinson G, Shnider SM, DeLorimier AA, Steffenson JL: Effects of maternal hyperventilation on uterine blood flow and fetal oxygenation and acid base status. Anesthesiology 1974; 40:340–7
62. Garry D, Leikin E, Fleisher AG, Tejani N: Acute myocardial infarction in pregnancy with subsequent medical and surgical management. Obstet Gynecol 1996; 87:802
63. Lichtenstein SV: Warm heart surgery. J Thorac Cardiovasc Surg 1991; 101:269–74

64. Bain MD, Copas DK, Landon MJ, Stacey TE: In vivo permeability of the human placenta to inulin and mannitol. J Physiol 1988; 399:313–9
65. Burrows RF, Kelton JG: Thrombocytopenia at delivery: a prospective survey of 6715 deliveries. Am J Obstet Gynecol 1990; 162:731–4
66. Lindoff C, Rybo G, AStedt B. Treatment with tranexamic acid during pregnancy, and the risk of thrombo-embolic complications. Thromb Haemost 1993; 70:238–40
67. Naeye RL: Placental infarction leading to fetal or neonatal death. A prospective study. acogjnl 1977; 50:583–8
68. Camann WR, Ostheimer GW: Physiological adaptations during pregnancy. Int Anesthesiol Clin 1990; 28:2–10
69. Hawthorne L, Wilson R, Lyons G, Dresner M: Failed intubation revisited: 17-yr experience in a teaching maternity unit. Br J Anaesth 1996; 76:680–4
70. Archer GW, Marx GF: Arterial oxygen tension during apnoea in parturient women. Br J Anaesth 1974; 46:358–60
71. Von Dadelszen P, Menzies J, Gilgoff S, et al.: Evidence-based management for preeclampsia. Front Biosci 2007; 12:2876–89
72. Connell H, Dalgleish JG, Downing JW: General anaesthesia in mothers with severe pre-eclampsia/eclampsia. Br J Anaesth 1987; 59:1375–80
73. Shnider SM, Webster GM: Maternal and fetal hazards of surgery during pregnancy. Am J Obstet Gynecol 1965; 92:891–900
74. Duncan PG, Pope WD, Cohen MM, Greer N: Fetal risk of anesthesia and surgery during pregnancy. Anesthesiology 1986; 64:790–4
75. Koblin DD, Watson JE, Deady JE, Stokstad ELR, Eger EI: Inactivation of methionine synthetase by nitrous oxide in mice. Anesthesiology 1981; 54:318–24
76. Rowland AS, Baird DD, Shore DL, Weinberg CR, Savitz DA, Wilcox AJ: Nitrous oxide and spontaneous abortion in female dental assistants. Am J Epidemiol 1995; 141:531–8
77. Mazze RI, Fujinaga M, Baden JM: Halothane prevents nitrous oxide teratogenicity in Sprague-Dawley rats; folinic acid does not. Teratology 1988; 38:121–7
78. Saxen I: Associations between oral clefts and drugs taken during pregnancy. Int J Epidemiol 1975; 4:37–44
79. Dolovich LR, Addis A, Vaillancourt JM, Power JD, Koren G, Einarson TR: Benzodiazepine use in pregnancy and major malformations or oral cleft: meta-analysis of cohort and case-control studies. BMJ 1998; 317:839–43
80. Ornoy A, Arnon J, Shechtman S, Moerman L, Lukashova I: Is benzodiazepine use during pregnancy really teratogenic? Reprod Toxicol 1998; 12:511–5

81. Koren G, Pastuszak A, Ito S: Drugs in pregnancy. N Engl J Med 1998; 338:1128–37

82. Rosen MA: Management of anesthesia for the pregnant surgical patient. Anesthesiology 1999; 91:1159–63

83. Oats JN, Vasey DP, Waldron BA: Effects of ketamine on the pregnant uterus. Br J Anaesth 1979; 51:1163–6

84. Magness RR, Rosenfeld CR: Systemic and uterine responses to alpha-adrenergic stimulation in pregnant and nonpregnant ewes. Am J Obstet Gynecol 1986; 155:897–904

85. Lee A, Ngan Kee WD, Gin T: A quantitative, systematic review of randomized controlled trials of ephedrine versus phenylephrine for the management of hypotension during spinal anesthesia for cesarean delivery. Anesth Analg 2002; 94:920–6

86. Thomas DG, Robson SC, Redfern N, Hughes D, Boys RJ: Randomized trial of bolus phenylephrine or ephedrine for maintenance of arterial pressure during spinal anaesthesia for Caesarean section. Br J Anaesth 1996; 76:61–5

87. Aselton P, Jick H, Milunsky A, Hunter JR, Stergachis A: First-trimester drug use and congenital disorders. Obstet Gynecol 1985; 65:451–5

88. Heinonen OP, Slone D, Shapiro S: Birth defects and drugs in pregnancy. Littleton, MA, Publishing Sciences Group, 1977

89. Bartalena L, Bogazzi F, Braverman LE, Martino E: Effects of amiodarone administration during pregnancy on neonatal thyroid function and subsequent neurodevelopment. J Endocrinol Invest 2001; 24:116–30

90. Lydakis C, Lip GYH, Beevers DG: Atenolol and fetal growth in pregnancies complicated by hypertension. Am J Hypertens 1999; 12:541

91. Pickles CJ, Symonds EM, Pipkin FB: The fetal outcome in a randomized double-blind controlled trial of labetalol versus placebo in pregnancy-induced hypertension. BJOG 1989; 96:38–43

92. Wheeler AS, James FM, Meis PJ, et al.: Effects of nitroglycerin and nitroprusside on the uterine vasculature of gravid ewes. Anesthesiology 1980; 52:390–4

93. Naulty J, Cefalo RC, Lewis PE: Fetal toxicity of nitroprusside in the pregnant ewe. Am J Obstet Gynecol 1981; 139:708–11

Jutta Novalija, MD, PhD
Thomas J. Ebert, MD, PhD

Anesthetic Management of the Extremely Obese Patient Undergoing
9 | Cardiovascular Surgery

INTRODUCTION

Obesity is a serious problem in the United States. Its incidence has increased from 8% to 30% since 1994 and is now considered to be a national epidemic. The prevalence of obesity and extreme obesity continues to grow. The ramifications of obesity are related not only to its impact on clinical management of the obesity and its sequelae, but also to its impact on life expectancy. The morbidly obese (MO) patient has only a one in seven chance of a having a normal life expectancy (1).

The definition of obesity has undergone refinement over the past few years. The National Institutes of Health guidelines published in 2003 use body mass index (BMI; kg/m^2) to categorize obesity into three classes: class I, BMI of 30–34.9 kg/m^2; class II, BMI of 35–39.9 kg/m^2; and class 3, extreme (morbid) obesity, BMI of $\geq$ 40 kg/m^2 (2). There is now a measurable and increasing proportion of the population (2%–3%) in the MO group (1).

Not only is obesity increasing, but the associated medical problems are also escalating. They are having significant impact on the surgical population and are creating significant perioperative management challenges for the anesthesiologist. For example, coronary artery disease (CAD) and cardiac dysfunction are common in MO patients. As a result, the demand for cardiac surgical procedures in MO patients is increasing. The increase of obesity in adolescents and young adults has correlated with increasing numbers of obese patients requiring coronary

Medically Challenging Patients Undergoing Cardiothoracic Surgery, edited by Neal H. Cohen, MD, MPH, MS, Lippincott Williams & Wilkins, Baltimore © 2009.

revascularization procedures, many at younger ages (3). Anesthesia providers must understand the clinical consequences of obesity, its effects on organ function, and anesthetic management. By doing so, we can more safely address these challenges and manage patients to minimize morbidity and mortality for these patients.

MORBIDITY AND MORTALITY

The risks associated with cardiac surgery in the MO patient and the necessary resources to deliver the required care continue to be refined (2, 4). As obese patients make up a larger percentage of the surgical population, there is an associated increase in the use of a number of critical resources. For example, this patient population has more comorbidities for which more extensive evaluation and management are required. This patient population has a higher incidence of glucose intolerance, diabetes, insulin resistance, hypertension, hyperlipidemia, renal and CAD, stroke, osteoarthritis, and obstructive sleep apnea (OSA). The frequency and severity of comorbid conditions are directly proportional to the weight of the patient. The obese patients often have longer operating room times, in part because of the challenges associated with the anesthetic management and the surgical procedure and in part because of the increased need for intensive care unit (ICU) care, longer lengths of hospital stay, and higher incidence of postoperative complications.

The prevalence of comorbid conditions in extremely obese patients has led to the presumption that the degree of obesity would be a risk factor for adverse perioperative outcome in patients undergoing cardiac surgery. However, at this point only the risks of heightened postoperative complications associated with cardiac surgery have been documented (Figure 9–1). Prabhakar and colleagues (5) found that the incidence of renal failure after cardiac surgery increased markedly with increasing BMI (relative risk = 1.58 in the moderately obese and 1.92 in the extremely obese). This finding may be caused by the higher incidence of hypertension and diabetes in these extremely obese patients. Prolonged periods of postoperative ventilation and increased length of hospital stay were noted in the extremely obese group. Data from a large study comprising 11,101 patients from the Northern New England Cardiovascular Disease Study Group found that obesity was associated with an increased number of sternal wound infections (6). The relative risk of deep sternal infection was 2.22 (95% confidence interval [CI], 2.01–2.44) in moderately obese patients and rose to an odds ratio (OR) of 3.15 (95% CI, 2.79–3.55) in extremely obese patients. A 12-year database (1993–2005) was recently evaluated for cardiac surgical outcomes in the extremely obese patient. Data from 57 cardiac surgical patients

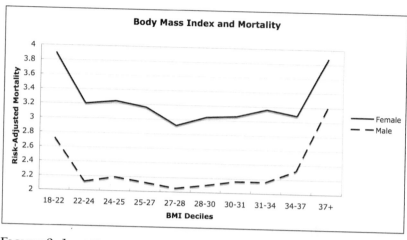

FIGURE 9–1. Effect of body mass index (BMI) on mortality by gender shows a consistently higher risk for females across all levels of BMI and the increase in mortality at the extremes of BMI. From Prabhakar et al. (5).

with BMI values >50 kg/m² were summarized (7). The retrospective evaluation reported prolonged ICU and hospital stay, prolonged intubation, and increased wound infections. It was also noted that a disproportionately high number of these patients (half) underwent cardiac surgery under nonelective circumstances. This finding may reflect the reluctance on the part of cardiac surgeons to accept the extremely obese patient for elective procedures (2).

Increased BMI also has been linked with postoperative arrhythmias (8). Although multiple factors, including age, type of surgery, and low ejection fraction, have been identified as risk factors, morbid obesity was found to be independently associated with an increased risk for atrial fibrillation (9). No clear mechanistic pathways have been identified, although some publications have suggested that there is a higher incidence of cardiomegaly in obese patients, resulting in dilation of the atria and subsequent arrhythmias. Although our understanding of the adverse outcomes associated with cardiac surgery in the obese patient has improved, it remains unclear whether modifications in anesthetic management will impact them.

Despite the documented higher rate of complications in the obese patient undergoing cardiac surgery, controversy remains as to whether mortality is increased. Several studies do suggest that mortality is increased. For example, in a retrospective examination of the Society of Thoracic Surgeons database, evaluating 559,004 patients, an increase of the operative risk for patients with BMI >35 was noted (5). Moderate obesity (BMI = 35–39.9) was associated with a slight but statistically significant risk-adjusted increase in mortality (OR, 1.21; 95% CI, 1.13–1.29) compared to normal or mild obesity. Those with extreme obesity had nearly a 50% increase in risk-adjusted mortality (OR, 1.58; 95% CI, 1.45–1.73). This result is consistent with an evaluation from multiple Department of Veterans Affairs (VA) hospitals over a 14-year period that found a significant increased mortality at the extremes of weight (10). In contrast, a number of earlier studies found that obesity is not a risk factor for operative mortality after coronary artery bypass graft surgery (4, 6, 11–18).

PULMONARY AND AIRWAY PATHOPHYSIOLOGY IN OBESITY

Many obese patients have significant alternations in the airway and/or pulmonary function. Obstruction of the airway by the abundant soft tissue in the upper airway in obese patients can produce hypoxemia and hypercapnia during sedation or anesthetic induction (19, 20). Recently, neck circumference >43 cm has been demonstrated to be a stronger predicator than obesity of difficult intubation (21). Pulmonary function abnormalities occur, often related specifically to body habitus and weight. Functional residual capacity (FRC) is often reduced in these patients secondary to body habitus (large torso and abdomen impairing diaphragmatic excursion), severely shortening the period of time before desaturation in the event of apnea or hypoventilation (Figure 9–2).

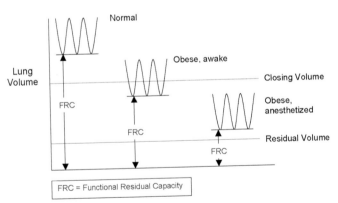

FIGURE 9–2. Effects of obesity and anesthesia on functional residual capacity (FRC). Closing volume represents the lung volume at which the alveoli begin to collapse, adding to ventilation/perfusion mismatching. The reduced FRC with obesity limits the oxygen reserve during times of apnea.

Obstructive Sleep Apnea

An increase in BMI by about two units (e.g., 27–29 kg/m^2) increases the likelihood of coexisting OSA by a factor of 4 (22). Whereas the prevalence of OSA in the general U.S. population is 2% in women and 4% in men, it is 3%–25% and 40%–78% in MO women and men, respectively (22–27). OSA in obese patients is usually a consequence of the airway narrowing from abundant peripharyngeal adipose tissue and an abnormal decrease in upper airway muscle tone, particularly during rapid eye movement (REM) sleep. Patients with OSA are known to be more susceptible to the depressant effects of narcotics and anxiolytics, perhaps because of reduced muscle tone of the airway. They also are more likely to be difficult to mask ventilate; laryngoscopy is also more difficult in many obese patients (28–30). OSA in the obese patient generally improves after weight reduction (23), but because of the often urgent or emergent nature of cardiac surgery in this patient population, preoperative planning for weight reduction has limited feasibility.

In the United States, sleep apnea is undiagnosed in 80%–90% of sufferers. Useful information can often be elicited from the patient's roommate or sleeping partner. Historical information presumptive of sleep apnea includes habitual snoring, interrupted breathing during sleep (apneic spells followed by short gasps, grunts, or resuscitative snorting), impaired daytime performance, morning headache, and irritability. The presence and severity of OSA in obese patients cannot be reliably predicted by BMI, neck circumference, pulmonary function tests, daytime room-air arterial blood gasses, or questionnaires to detect and quantify sleep-related complaints (or any combination of these factors) (31–36). Although history is suggestive of OSA, the definitive diagnostic test for it is made using polysomnography.

OSA patients may benefit from continuous positive airway pressure (CPAP) and, in some circumstances, by elective tracheostomy. The American Society of Anesthesiologists has recently published guidelines for the perioperative care of the patients with OSA (37). Most of the recommendations are not scientifically based, but rather are based on expert opinion.

Obesity Hypoventilation Syndrome

Obesity hypoventilation syndrome (OHS), an extreme disorder seen in some obese patients, was described in 1955 and labeled the Pickwickian syndrome in 1956 because these patients seemed to resemble an obese character (the messenger boy, Joe) in Charles Dickens's *The Pickwick Papers*. The disorder is characterized by alveolar hypoventilation, chronic hypercapnia and hypoxia, hypersomnolence, polycythemia, and right ventricular failure. Pulmonary function tests reveal reduced inspiratory and expiratory volumes, and chest radiography displays evidence of pulmonary congestion and right-heart enlargement. The diagnosis of OHS is made based on exclusion of other causes of respiratory failure in conjunction with the above-described clinical picture.

Other factors beyond obesity must be part of the pathophysiology of OHS because body weight alone does not correlate with daytime hypercapnia. The normal response to hypercapnia and hypoxia is increased minute ventilation. This response is impaired in patients suffering from OHS, but not impaired in patients who are only obese. CPAP does not reverse the hypercarbia for patients with OHS. Nasal intermittent positive pressure ventilation applied during sleep has been shown to reset, at least partially, the carbon dioxide response curve (38). Observational data show improvement in ventilation with reduction in total body weight (TBW) along with administration of progesterone, a known respiratory stimulant (39, 40). These data suggest that the cause of OHS involves both peripheral (obesity) and central processes. Treatment includes abstinence from respiratory depressants, improving airway patency, and administration of respiratory stimulants (39–45).

CARDIOVASCULAR PATHOPHYSIOLOGY IN OBESITY

The obese patient's cardiovascular system responds to the increased oxygen demand from the extra body tissue by increasing absolute blood volume, whereas the relative blood volume per kilogram decreases (from 86 to 47 mL/kg) (46). The decrease in blood volume per kilogram may be expected because the added weight is mostly adipose tissue, which is poorly perfused. The cardiovascular system responds to the increased oxygen demand by increasing the cardiac output predominantly through increased stroke volume, as the heart rate remains unchanged. Splanchnic blood flow is slightly increased and renal blood flow slightly reduced in obesity. Otherwise, cardiac output is similarly distributed to various organs among normal and obese persons. It should be noted that cardiac output, when indexed for body surface area, is not different between obese and nonobese individuals (47, 48). As a result, obesity should not complicate the interpretation of hemodynamic data (49).

The adaptation to obesity appears to be effective because the arteriovenous oxygen difference is normal; however, there is good evidence that ventricular performance is impaired. The ratio of eft ventricular stroke work index to left ventricular end-diastolic pressure is reduced and is negatively correlated with the degree of obesity. The obesity-related increase in stroke volume results in increased end-diastolic volume and pressure, leading to eccentric hypertrophy of the ventricle in the absence of hypertension. If the patient develops hypertension—a common comorbidity of obesity—concentric hypertrophy will develop along with an increase in systemic vascular resistance compared to the effects of hypertension in nonobese patients. Either of these two mechanisms results in increased left ventricular stroke work. In mild to moderately obese patients, the degree of left ventricular enlargement and wall thickening correlates with the amount of obesity, whereas the decrement in cardiac performance is related to its duration (50). Hypertension superimposed on obesity acts synergistically to increase the risk for cardiac failure (46, 47, 51, 52).

Hemodynamic Monitoring

Oscillometric measurement of noninvasive blood pressure by automated cuffs or by direct auscultation often underestimates arterial blood pressure in the extremely obese patient. Although standard of care for cardiac surgery, direct intraarterial blood pressure monitoring should be strongly considered even in noncardiac procedures. Unfortunately, obese patients often present a challenge when it comes to placing the necessary arterial and venous access, as normal anatomical landmarks and pulses traditionally used to guide placement are often obscured. In adults, use of two-dimensional ultrasound guidance for cannulation of the internal jugular and femoral veins unequivocally decreases the risk of failed catheter placement, improves first-pass success, and facilitates faster placement compared with the landmark method (53). Recent data support the use of real time, continuous, ultrasound guidance for all central venous cannulations, and this may be even more important in obese patients.

Obese patients have higher resting cardiac filling pressures (51) that may increase further when the patient is supine (54). As a result, these patients are at higher risk for pulmonary edema. Because the physical examination in the obese patient is challenging, and subtle changes in cardiac output or filling pressures may be difficult to identify, invasive hemodynamic monitoring with a pulmonary artery catheter may be of benefit in some obese patients. Transesophageal echocardiography may also facilitate assessment of intravascular volume and changes in myocardial function, particularly during cardiac surgery.

PHARMACOKINETIC ALTERATIONS ASSOCIATED WITH OBESITY

Obese persons may metabolize lipophilic drugs to a greater degree (and for longer periods) than their nonobese counterparts may. One would assume that responses to drugs stored in fat (e.g., narcotics, barbiturates, volatile anesthetics) would be prolonged in obese persons. However, there is no clinically relevant evidence that use of the more soluble anesthetics delays recovery time in obese patients (55–57).

The dose requirements for drugs used to provide analgesia and to produce sedation and/or hypnosis are altered by significant overweight status (BMI > 27.5). Increased body fat increases the volume of distribution of sufentanil and slows its elimination. In one study, the elimination half-life of sufentanil was 208 minutes for eight mildly obese patients (mean weight, 94 kg) versus 135 minutes for eight controls (mean weight, 70 kg) (58). Muscle relaxants with weak to moderate lipophilicity, such as vecuronium and rocuronium, are distributed mainly to lean tissues, so dosing of neuromuscular blockers to ideal body weight (IBW) is preferred (as opposed to TBW). Rocuronium dosed at 0.6 mg/kg (2 × 95% effective dose) to IBW had a duration of ~30 minutes whereas dosing to TBW had a duration of ~60 minutes with an increased variability of the duration as well (59). A dose of cisatracurium at 0.2 mg/kg to IBW lasted ~45 minutes but was ~90 minutes in duration when dosed to TBW (60). Succinylcholine has proved to be effective at either IBW or TBW, but resulted in significantly better intubating conditions when TBW dosing is employed in MO patients (61).

PERIOPERATIVE ANESTHETIC MANAGEMENT

The anesthetic induction period is far more complex in the extremely obese patient than it is for the lean patient. A variety of factors should be considered, including the physiologic impact of changes in position of the patient, methods to optimize preoxygenation during induction, selection of the most appropriate induction agent(s), airway management techniques and devices, and approaches to ventilatory management.

Positioning

Proper positioning of the extremely obese patient requires careful consideration. In general, the patient should be supported behind the upper back and head to achieve the anatomical position in which the head is above the horizontal plane of the upper chest ("ramping up") or in which a horizontal plane between the sternal notch and the external auditory meatus is established (62). This positioning improves not only pulmonary mechanics, but the alignment from mouth to glottic opening. The ramping up of patients should not be subtle—rather it should be extreme. Because of the rapid desaturation common in the obese patient, there is no time or available manpower to further reposition a patient after induction if intubation fails.

Preoxygenation

The rapid desaturation of blood oxygen tension during the apneic period of anesthetic induction can be modified through improved preoxygenation. This increase in the pulmonary oxygen capacity is vitally important because the extremely obese patient has a reduced FRC, often falling below the closing capacity of the small airways, leading to atelectasis, increased intrapulmonary shunting, and impaired oxygenation. FRC is further reduced in the supine position and after induction of anesthesia (Figure 9–2) (63). Conventional techniques to denitrogenate the lungs apply, including at least 3 minutes of breathing 100% oxygen or five vital capacity breaths of 100% oxygen. However, CPAP or pressure support can be used to preoxygenate the obese patient through a tight-fitting face mask, because it will improve FRC and should prolong the time before significant desaturation occurs (64). Preoxgenating the obese patient in the 25-degree head-up tilt position can achieve a similar gain of nearly 1 minute of time before significant desaturation occurs (65). If proper ramping up of the patient has taken place and the bed is tilted upright, the patient's head might be at the level of the head of the anesthesia provider. To optimize airway management associated with this change in position, the anesthesia provider may need to stand on a step stool until the patient's head can be safely lowered to the supine position to complete the induction of anesthesia.

Mask Ventilation and Intubation

A BMI >26 kg/m^2 results in a threefold increase in difficult ventilation via mask (28). The five independent risk factors for difficult mask ventilation are age >55 years, BMI >26 kg/m^2, lack of teeth, presence of beard, and history of snoring (28).

Preoperative identification of the patient with a potentially difficult airway is the first step in preventing an adverse outcome. Several investigators have suggested that the difficult intubation rate is higher in the extremely obese patient, from two- to tenfold (19, 20), although this finding is not consistent in all studies. One study performed in the extremely obese population was able to demonstrate only two correlates of difficult intubation: Mallampati score >3 and neck circumference >40 cm. Neither absolute weight nor increasing BMI were associated with difficult intubation (66). One explanation for the discrepancies in findings from one study to another may be related to the lack of consistency in the interpretation of "difficult intubation." In a recent study by Gonzalez and colleagues (21), the intubation difficulty scale score was used to standardize the assessments (Table 9–1). They confirmed an association between BMI and problematic intubations and found thyromental dis-

TABLE 9–1. Comparison of demographic data in normal and difficult to intubate patients

	Difficult intubation	Normal intubation
BMI	46 ± 12*	34 ± 3
Neck circumference	47 ± 4*	40 ± 4
Mallampati score >3	67%*	13%
Thyromental distance	10 ± 3*	8 ± 3
Sternomental distance	17 ± 5	14 ± 4

* Significantly different from normal intubation group, $p < .05$.
Adapted from Gonzalez et al. (21).

tance, increasing neck circumference (>43 cm), and Mallampati score >3 to be predictors of difficult intubation (21).

Of the many important considerations in managing the difficult airway is the decision to manage the airway while the patient is awake or after induction of anesthesia. Historically, the successful intubation of the extremely obese patient with the suspected difficult airway was approached with an awake, fiberoptic technique. However, an awake intubation carries risks for the patient with unstable angina and documented CAD. Performing an awake intubation and at the same time avoiding tachycardia, hypertension, and myocardial ischemia is a challenge. Such management requires technical skill, pharmacologic expertise, and often an extra set of hands (67).

In contrast, recent studies have described the highly successful use of alternate airway devices like the intubating laryngeal mask airway (ILMA). In MO patients, successful tracheal intubation was achieved 96% of the time on first attempt to insert the device (68). In a separate report, a comparison was made of the success of intubating the trachea with the ILMA in a MO group versus a lean control group (69). There were several important findings from this report. The first was that 100% of the patients were successfully ventilated through the ILMA device prior to intubation of the trachea. The use of the device prevented airway collapse after induction and facilitated ventilation in extremely obese patients. Second, the study confirmed the 96% success rate of intubating the trachea through this device. A number of other airway devices are now available that might aid intubation of the extremely obese patient. These would include video laryngoscopes, although their ability to improve intubation success in the extremely obese patient awaits prospective evaluation.

Anesthetic Induction

During anesthetic induction for patients scheduled for cardiac surgery, not only must the airway be established, but while doing so it is also critically important to avoid tachycardia and hypertension in this patient population. Rapid sequence induction (RSI) is frequently employed because many anesthesiologists consider extremely obese patients to be at risk for acid aspiration syndrome. However, acid aspiration syndrome has been reported as a rare event, occurring in 1:3216 anesthetics (70), and not uniquely associated with obesity. When aspiration occurred, it was associated with gagging and vomiting in one third of the cases and might have been avoided by deeper sedation and/or hypnosis on induction. Historically, obese patients were thought to be at increased risk for acid aspiration syndrome because 70% were reported to have a gastric pH <2.5 and/or residual gastric fluid volume of ≥25 mL after fasting compared to only 5% of nonobese individuals (71). More recently, Harter and colleagues (72) found a substantially lower incidence of combined high gastric volume and low pH in fasted, obese patients compared with lean patients, and a very favorable response to oral sodium citrate. The rate of gastric emptying appears to be similar in obese and nonobese patients (73).

Whether or not one believes that extremely obese patients should be considered "full stomach" despite fasting, the use of cricoid pressure should be considered. Properly applied pressure should compress the esophagus against the vertebral body. The protection afforded by cricoid pressure, however, is questionable. In an observational study using magnetic resonance imaging, the cricopharyngeal muscle rather than the esophagus was lying posterior to the cricoid in 18 of 19 participants. During cricoid pressure, the esophagus was displaced laterally in 90% of the participants (74). They also found that the airway was displaced in 67% of patients with cricoid pressure and the diameter of the airway was compressed at least 1 mm in 81%. Considering that the esophagus is usually 10 mm below the cricoid and often displaced laterally, it is not surprising that cricoid pressure has not been documented to prevent aspiration. Thus, in an elective, fasted, obese patient with a thick neck, the value of RSI in combination with cricoid pressure to reduce the risk of regurgitation and aspiration is debatable. Furthermore, committing to early paralysis for successful RSI seems unsafe and may be outweighed by the safety of controlled induction and confirmation of a patent airway by mask or via an ILMA before paralysis.

The choice of one volatile anesthetic over another seems irrelevant in the extremely obese patient scheduled for cardiac surgery. All volatile anesthetics have the ability to provide cardioprotection from ischemic injury (75). In some centers where extubation prior to transfer to the postanesthesia care unit might be desired, either of the two newer volatile anesthetics, desflurane and sevoflurane, may result in more rapid awakening in the obese patient (56). However, it is more likely that a fast track extubation protocol would involve extubation not "on the table," but within 6 hours of surgery. The specific volatile anesthetic may have little or no impact on time to extubation, if carefully titrated. In contrast, unrelated to anesthetic agent, the incidence of failure at early extubation is increased in the obese cardiac surgical patient (76). As a result, the early extubation strategy must be carefully considered in the obese patient and, when the patient is successfully extubated, ongoing monitoring of the airway and gas exchange must be provided.

Mode of Mechanical Ventilation

Volume-controlled ventilation is most commonly used to ventilate the obese patient. For most patients, a constant flow is delivered at a target tidal volume to establish a desired minute ventilation. Obesity can result in reduced lung compliance, reduced chest wall compliance, and (often) higher airway pressure levels during volume-controlled ventilation. In addition, the selection of the most appropriate tidal volume may be challenging, but should take into account the risks associated with larger tidal volume ventilation, particularly when the mean airway pressure is high. Recently, pressure-controlled ventilation has been demonstrated to be an effective mode of ventilation for obese patients undergoing laparoscopic surgery (77). Pressure-controlled ventilation generates higher instantaneous flow peaks and allows a better alveolar recruitment to improve oxygenation without some of the side effects of volume ventilatory modes. At the present time, however, no single mode of ventilation has been demonstrated to be superior in the obese patient population.

Glucose Regulation

Recent evidence that diabetes and hyperglycemia alone increase perioperative risk in the cardiac surgical patient population is compelling. In a randomized, prospective controlled trial, patients in the ICU on mechanical ventilation received either intensive insulin therapy (maintaining glucose levels between 80 and 110 mg/dL) or conventional treatment (insulin therapy of glucose levels >215 mg/dL) (78). The mortality in the conventional group was 8% versus 4.6% in the intensive therapy group. Intensive insulin therapy reduced overall in-hospital mortality, bloodstream infections, acute renal failure requiring dialysis, and the number of blood transfusions. Similar findings have been reported with continuous insulin administration in a retrospective study of 3554 diabetic patients after coronary artery bypass graft surgery (79). The mortality was 2.5% for continuous intravenous infusion of insulin versus

5.3% for subcutaneous administration. The authors of the study noted that the glucose control was tighter in the continuous insulin group than in the bolus administration group. In a prospective study of 200 diabetic patients undergoing cardiac surgery, tight perioperative glycemic control was targeted to a glucose level <140 mg/dL (80). Poor glucose control was noted in 18% of patients with glucose levels >200 mg/dL. The poor control group was more likely to develop severe postoperative morbidities (37% vs. 10%), including adverse cardiovascular, respiratory, renal, neural, and infectious outcomes. At the same time, it is critical to monitor the glucose closely to prevent hypoglycemia, which could also seriously impact postoperative recovery. The reason for the improved outcome with tighter glucose control is multifactorial. Hyperglycemia is known to abolish the cardioprotective effects of volatile anesthetics (81). This may explain in part the worsened outcome in patients with high blood glucose during and after surgery.

Pulmonary Hypertension

Pulmonary hypertension (PH) is a common problem in obese patients scheduled for cardiac surgery. It is defined as a mean pulmonary artery pressure ≥25 mm Hg at rest or >30 mm Hg with exercise. Alternatively, PH can be defined by a pulmonary vascular resistance >2–3 Wood units or >200–300 dyne/s/cm^5. As discussed earlier in this chapter, OSA and OHS are comorbidities in patients with morbid obesity and may account for the increased incidence of PH and subsequent right-heart dysfunction in the obese patient (44, 45, 82–84).

PH in patients undergoing cardiac surgery is associated with increased mortality and morbidity rates (85). The specific additional risk in the MO patient is not as clearly described. In MO patients, the cardiac anesthesiologist has to be particularly careful to avoid oversedation, hypercarbia, and sympathetic stimulation, because the patients are more sensitive to some of these adverse effects that will worsen the preexisting PH. Cardiopulmonary bypass (CPB) induces pulmonary endothelial cell injury and pulmonary dysfunction, probably caused by hypoperfusion of the lungs during CPB or activation of the systemic inflammatory response, which exacerbates the reactivity of the pulmonary vascular bed (86–93).

The treatment of PH always has been challenging but can be even more difficult in the MO patient. Most intravenous agents that dilate the pulmonary vasculature, such as dobutamine, nitroglycerin, milrinone, sodium nitroprusside, and calcium channel antagonists, can cause systemic hypotension. Volume resuscitation and mechanical ventilation may worsen hemodynamics and lead to right ventricular failure. The administration of vasoactive drugs by inhalation to limit vasodilation to the pulmonary circulation has improved the management of PH in cardiac surgery patients. The two inhaled agents that have been investigated in this respect are inhaled nitric oxide and prostacyclin. The perioperative use of inhaled nitric oxide should be considered in the MO patient with PH.

Postoperative Management

Postoperative management of any patient undergoing cardiac surgery includes careful attention to pain management, gas exchange, administration of drugs to optimize cardiac function, and intensive glucose control. These same goals may be even more important for the postoperative management of the obese patient. Pain management is important for any patient who undergoes cardiac surgery, but it may be even more important in the obese patient. When most analgesics and sedatives are used to treat postoperative pain, their respiratory effects must be carefully monitored. For some patients, thoracic epidural analgesia may be indicated, although the concerns about coagulopathy compromise the routine use of this approach to pain control. Dexmedetomidine has been used to provide analgesia and sedation in the obese patient, particularly during transfer to the ICU and weaning from mechanical ventilation because it does not compromise ventilatory drive (94, 95). Avoiding respiratory depressant drugs may prove particularly advantageous in the extremely obese patient, in whom sleep apnea is more prevalent and respiratory drive may be important. A loading dose of 1 µg/kg lean body weight over 10 minutes at sternal wire placement followed by an infusion of 0.2–0.7 µg/kg/h can reduce postoperative morphine needs by ~50%. Dexmedetomidine is associated with a lower heart rate as well, although it must be administered with caution, because it has the potential for hemodynamically significant bradycardia, especially after the loading dose. Because dexmedetomidine can activate vascular alpha$_2$-receptors, transient hypertension and reflex bradycardia can occur when this drug is rapidly administered. In addition, in patients with heart failure and high basal sympathetic tone, the sympatholytic effect of dexmedetomidine can result in significant decreases in blood pressure that may require therapeutic countermeasures.

CONCLUSION

The rise of obesity in the general population will be mirrored in the surgical population, especially in the cardiac surgical population because of the increased incidence of cardiac disease in this population of patients. These patients have significant associated medical conditions that must be taken into account in optimizing their care. The anesthesiologist must be aware of the associated risks and the host of complications that occur in obese patients in the perioperative period.

The anesthetic management of the extremely obese patient requires a focus on a number of issues beginning with a careful preoperative evaluation and assessment of preexisting disease processes that might impact the management plan. Special attention should be paid to whether the patient has sleep apnea or alternations in ventilation. Airway management must be approached with care. Careful attention to patient positioning is essential to aid in airway management. The common misperception that all extremely obese patients are "full stomach" has been challenged. New approaches to optimizing oxygenation during induction to lessen the rapidity of oxygen desaturation during apnea are important, particularly because the patient may have unanticipated difficulty with tracheal intubation. Promising results have been demonstrated with the use of the ILMA to facilitate ventilation and tracheal tube placement in the obese patient. Postoperative management also must be modified for the obese patient undergoing cardiac surgery. Early extubation may fail more often in obese patients. A number of approaches to pain management can be used, as long as the patient is carefully monitored to ensure that gas exchange and hemodynamics are not compromised. Intensive glucose control has documented benefits in this patient population. In addition, the use of dexmedetomidine may be appropriate for selected patients as part of postoperative management, particularly during weaning from mechanical ventilation. Careful planning and coordination of the entire perioperative period is essential for these patients, because they are at risk for prolonged ICU and hospital stay.

References

1. Mokdad AH, Ford ES, Bowman BA, et al.: Prevalence of obesity, diabetes, and obesity-related health risk factors, 2001. JAMA 2003; 289:76–9.
2. Villavicencio MA, Sundt TM, 3rd, Daly RC, et al.: Cardiac surgery in patients with body mass index of 50 or greater. Ann Thorac Surg 2007; 83:1403–11.
3. Habib RH, Zacharias A, Schwann TA, et al.: Effects of obesity and small body size on operative and long-term outcomes of coronary artery bypass surgery: a propensity-matched analysis. Ann Thorac Surg 2005; 79:1976–86.
4. Kuduvalli M, Grayson AD, Oo AY, et al.: Risk of morbidity and in-hospital mortality in obese patients undergoing coronary artery bypass surgery. Eur J Cardiothorac Surg 2002; 22:787–93.

5. Prabhakar G, Haan CK, Peterson ED, et al.: The risks of moderate and extreme obesity for coronary artery bypass grafting outcomes: a study from the Society of Thoracic Surgeons' database. Ann Thorac Surg 2002; 74:1125–30; discussion 30–1.
6. Birkmeyer NJ, Charlesworth DC, Hernandez F, et al.: Obesity and risk of adverse outcomes associated with coronary artery bypass surgery. Northern New England Cardiovascular Disease Study Group. Circulation 1998; 97:1689–94.
7. Wigfield CH, Lindsey JD, Munoz A, et al.: Is extreme obesity a risk factor for cardiac surgery? An analysis of patients with a BMI > or = 40. Eur J Cardiothorac Surg 2006; 29:434–40.
8. Moulton MJ, Creswell LL, Mackey ME, et al.: Obesity is not a risk factor for significant adverse outcomes after cardiac surgery. Circulation 1996; 94:II87–92.
9. Echahidi N, Mohty D, Pibarot P, et al.: Obesity and metabolic syndrome are independent risk factors for atrial fibrillation after coronary artery bypass graft surgery. Circulation 2007; 116:I213–9.
10. Wagner BD, Grunwald GK, Rumsfeld JS, et al.: Relationship of body mass index with outcomes after coronary artery bypass graft surgery. Ann Thorac Surg 2007; 84:10–6.
11. Schwann TA, Habib RH, Zacharias A, et al.: Effects of body size on operative, intermediate, and long-term outcomes after coronary artery bypass operation. Ann Thorac Surg 2001; 71:521–30; discussion 30–1.
12. Syrakas CA, Neumaier-Prauser P, Angelis I, et al.: Is extreme obesity a risk factor for increased in-hospital mortality and postoperative morbidity after cardiac surgery? Results of 2251 obese patients with BMI of 30 to 50. Thorac Cardiovasc Surg 2007; 55:491–3.
13. Rockx MA, Fox SA, Stitt LW, et al.: Is obesity a predictor of mortality, morbidity and readmission after cardiac surgery? Can J Surg 2004; 47:34–8.
14. Rohs T, Jr., Polanski P, Just SC, et al.: Early complications and long-term survival in severely obese coronary bypass patients. Am Surg 1995; 61:949–53.
15. Engelman DT, Adams DH, Byrne JG, et al.: Impact of body mass index and albumin on morbidity and mortality after cardiac surgery. J Thorac Cardiovasc Surg 1999; 118:866–73.
16. Jin R, Grunkemeier GL, Furnary AP, Handy JR, Jr.: Is obesity a risk factor for mortality in coronary artery bypass surgery? Circulation 2005; 111:3359–65.
17. Pan W, Hindler K, Lee VV, et al.: Obesity in diabetic patients undergoing coronary artery bypass graft surgery is associated with increased postoperative morbidity. Anesthesiology 2006; 104:441–7.

18. Reeves BC, Ascione R, Chamberlain MH, Angelini GD: Effect of body mass index on early outcomes in patients undergoing coronary artery bypass surgery. J Am Coll Cardiol 2003; 42:668–76.

19. Juvin P, Lavaut E, Dupont H, et al.: Difficult tracheal intubation is more common in obese than in lean patients. Anesth Analg 2003; 97:595–600.

20. Voyagis GS, Kyriakis KP, Dimitriou V, Vrettou I: Value of oropharyngeal Mallampati classification in predicting difficult laryngoscopy among obese patients. Eur J Anaesth 1998; 15:330–4.

21. Gonzalez H, Minville V, Delanoue K, et al.: The importance of increased neck circumference to intubation difficulties in obese patients. Anesth Analg 2008; 106:1132–6, table of contents.

22. Young T, Paulta M, Dempsey J, et al.: The occurrence of sleep-disordered breathing among middle-aged adults. N Engl J Med 1993; 328:1230–5.

23. Rajala R, Partinen M, Sane T, et al.: Obstructive sleep apnoea syndrome in morbidly obese patients. J Intern Med 1991; 230:125–9.

24. Strollo PJ, Jr., Rogers RM: Obstructive sleep apnea. N Engl J Med 1996; 334:99–104.

25. Ferretti A, Giampiccolo P, Cavalli A, et al.: Expiratory flow limitation and orthopnea in massively obese subjects. Chest 2001; 119:1401–8.

26. Vgontzas AN, Tan TL, Bixler EO, et al.: Sleep apnea and sleep disruption in obese patients. Arch Intern Med 1994; 154:1705–11.

27. Resta O, Foschino-Barbaro MP, Legari G, et al.: Sleep-related breathing disorders, loud snoring and excessive daytime sleepiness in obese subjects. Int J Obes Relat Metab Disord 2001; 25:669–75.

28. Langeron O, Masso E, Huraux C, et al.: Prediction of difficult mask ventilation. Anesthesiology 2000; 92:1229–35.

29. Siyam MA, Benhamou D: Difficult endotracheal intubation in patients with sleep apnea syndrome. Anesth Analg 2002; 95:1098–102.

30. Hiremath AS, Hillman DR, James AL, et al.: Relationship between difficult tracheal intubation and obstructive sleep apnoea. Br J Anaesth 1998; 80:606–11.

31. Koenig SM: Pulmonary complications of obesity. Am J Med Sci 2001; 321:249–79.

32. Serafini FM, MacDowell Anderson W, Rosemurgy AS, et al.: Clinical predictors of sleep apnea in patients undergoing bariatric surgery. Obes Surg 2001; 11:28–31.

33. van Kralingen KW, de Kanter W, de Groot GH, et al.: Assessment of sleep complaints and sleep-disordered breathing in a consecutive series of obese patients. Respiration 1999; 66:312–6.

34. Herer B, Roche N, Carton M, et al.: Value of clinical, functional, and oximetric data for the prediction of obstructive sleep apnea in obese patients. Chest 1999; 116:1537–44.
35. van Boxem TJ, de Groot GH: Prevalence and severity of sleep disordered breathing in a group of morbidly obese patients. Neth J Med 1999; 54:202–6.
36. Chung F, Yegneswaran B, Liao P, et al.: STOP questionnaire: a tool to screen patients for obstructive sleep apnea. Anesthesiology 2008; 108:812–21.
37. Gross JB, Bachenberg KL, Benumof JL, et al.: Practice guidelines for the perioperative management of patients with obstructive sleep apnea: a report by the American Society of Anesthesiologists Task Force on Perioperative Management of Patients with Obstructive Sleep Apnea. Anesthesiology 2006; 104:1081–93.
38. Piper AJ, Sullivan CE: Effects of short-term NIPPV in the treatment of patients with severe obstructive sleep apnea and hypercapnia. Chest 1994; 105:434–40.
39. Sugerman HJ, Fairman RP, Baron PL, Kwentus JA: Gastric surgery for respiratory insufficiency of obesity. Chest 1986; 90:81–6.
40. Strohl KP, Hensley MJ, Saunders NA, et al.: Progesterone administration and progressive sleep apneas. JAMA 1981; 245:1230–2.
41. Suratt PM, Wilhoit SC, Hsiao HS, et al.: Compliance of chest wall in obese subjects. J Appl Physiol 1984; 57:403–7.
42. Pillar G, Peled R, Lavie P: Recurrence of sleep apnea without concomitant weight increase 7.5 years after weight reduction surgery. Chest 1994; 106:1702–4.
43. Sugerman HJ, Baron PL, Fairman RP, et al.: Hemodynamic dysfunction in obesity hypoventilation syndrome and the effects of treatment with surgically induced weight loss. Ann Surg 1988; 207:604–13.
44. Kessler R, Chaouat A, Schinkewitch P, et al.: The obesity-hypoventilation syndrome revisited: a prospective study of 34 consecutive cases. Chest 2001; 120:369–76.
45. Leung RS, Bradley TD: Sleep apnea and cardiovascular disease. Am J Respir Crit Care Med 2001; 164:2147–65.
46. Alexander JK, Dennis EW, Smith WG, et al.: Blood volume, cardiac output, and distribution of systemic blood flow in extreme obesity. Cardiovasc Res Cent Bull 1962; 1:39–44.
47. Alpert MA, Hashimi MW: Obesity and the heart. Am J Med Sci 1993; 306:117–23.
48. Alexander JK: Obesity and cardiac performance. Am J Cardiol 1964; 14:860–5.

49. Stelfox HT, Ahmed SB, Ribeiro RA, et al.: Hemodynamic monitoring in obese patients: the impact of body mass index on cardiac output and stroke volume. Crit Care Med 2006; 34:1243–6.

50. Nakajima T, Fujioka S, Tokunaga K, et al.: Noninvasive study of left ventricular performance in obese patients: influence of duration of obesity. Circulation 1985; 71:481–6.

51. de Divitiis O, Fazio S, Petitto M, et al.: Obesity and cardiac function. Circulation 1981; 64:477–82.

52. Messerli FH: Cardiovascular effects of obesity and hypertension. Lancet 1982; 1:1165–8.

53. Hind D, Calvert N, McWilliams R, et al.: Ultrasonic locating devices for central venous cannulation: meta-analysis. BMJ 2003; 327:361.

54. Paul DR, Hoyt JL, Boutros AR: Cardiovascular and respiratory changes in response to change of posture in the very obese. Anesthesiology 1976; 45:73–8.

55. Vallejo MC, Sah N, Phelps AL, et al.: Desflurane versus sevoflurane for laparoscopic gastroplasty in morbidly obese patients. J Clin Anesth 2007; 19:3–8.

56. Arain SR, Barth CD, Shankar H, Ebert TJ: Choice of volatile anesthetic for the morbidly obese patient: sevoflurane or desflurane. J Clin Anesth 2005; 17:413–9.

57. Cork RC, Vaughan RW, Bentley JB: General anesthesia for morbidly obese patients—an examination of postoperative outcomes. Anesthesiology 1981; 54:310–3.

58. Schwartz AE, Matteo RS, Ornstein E, et al.: Pharmacokinetics of sufentanil in obese patients. Anesth Analg 1991; 73:790–3.

59. Leykin Y, Pellis T, Lucca M, et al.: The pharmacodynamic effects of rocuronium when dosed according to real body weight or ideal body weight in morbidly obese patients. Anesth Analg 2004; 99:1086–9.

60. Leykin Y, Pellis T, Lucca M, et al.: The effects of cisatracurium on morbidly obese women. Anesth Analg 2004; 99:1090–4.

61. Lemmens HJ, Brodsky JB: The dose of succinylcholine in morbid obesity. Anesth Analg 2006; 102:438–42.

62. Brodsky JB, Lemmens HJM, Brock-Utne JG, Saidman LJ: Anesthetic considerations for bariatric surgery: proper positioning is important for laryngoscopy. Anesth Analg 2003; 96:1841–2.

63. Adams JP, Murphy PG: Obesity in anaesthesia and intensive care. Br J Anaesth 2000; 85:91–108.

64. Gander S, Frascarolo P, Suter M, et al.: Positive end-expiratory pressure during induction of general anesthesia increases duration of nonhypoxic apnea in morbidly obese patients. Anesth Analg 2005; 100:580–4.

65. Dixon BJ, Dixon JB, Carden JR, et al.: Preoxygenation is more effective in the 25° head-up position than in the supine position in severely obese patients. Anesthesiology 2005; 102:1110–5.
66. Brodsky JB, Lemmens HJM, Brock-Utne JG, et al.: Morbid obesity and tracheal intubation. Anesth Analg 2002; 94:732–6.
67. Arbous MS, Meursing AE, van Kleef JW, et al.: Impact of anesthesia management characteristics on severe morbidity and mortality. Anesthesiology 2005; 102:257–68; quiz 491–2.
68. Frappier J, Guenoun T, Journois D, et al.: Airway management using the intubating laryngeal mask airway for the morbidly obese patient. Anesth Analg 2003; 96:1510–5.
69. Combes X, Sauvat S, Leroux B, et al.: Intubating laryngeal mask airway in morbidly obese and lean patients. Anesthesiology 2005; 102:1106–9.
70. Warner MA, Warner ME, Weber JG: Clinical significance of pulmonary aspiration during the perioperative period. Anesthesiology 1993; 78:56–62.
71. Vaughan RW, Bauer S, Wise L: Volume and pH of gastric juice in obese patients. Anesthesiology 1975; 43:686–9.
72. Harter RL, Kelly WB, Kramer MG, et al.: A comparison of the volume and pH of gastric contents of obese and lean surgical patients. Anesth Analg 1998; 86:147–52.
73. Maddox A, Horowitz M, Wishart J, Collins P: Gastric and oesophageal emptying in obesity. Scand J Gastroenterol 1989; 24:593–8.
74. Smith KJ, Dobranowski J, Yip G, et al.: Cricoid pressure displaces the esophagus: an observational study using magnetic resonance imaging. Anesthesiology 2003; 99:60–4.
75. Riess ML, Stowe DF, Warltier DC: Cardiac pharmacological preconditioning with volatile anesthetics: from bench to bedside? Am J Physiol Heart Circ Physiol 2004; 286:H1603–7.
76. Parlow JL, Ahn R, Milne B: Obesity is a risk factor for failure of "fast track" extubation following coronary artery bypass surgery. Can J Anaesth 2006; 53:288–94.
77. Cadi P, Guenoun T, Journois D, et al.: Pressure-controlled ventilation improves oxygenation during laparoscopic obesity surgery compared with volume-controlled ventilation. Br J Anaesth 2008; 100:709–16.
78. van den Berghe G, Wouters P, Weekers F, et al.: Intensive insulin therapy in the critically ill patients. N Engl J Med 2001; 345:1359–67.
79. Furnary AP, Gao G, Grunkemeier GL, et al.: Continuous insulin infusion reduces mortality in patients with diabetes undergoing coronary artery bypass grafting. J Thorac Cardiovasc Surg 2003; 125:1007–21.

80. Ouattara A, Lecomte P, Le Manach Y, et al.: Poor intraoperative blood glucose control is associated with a worsened hospital outcome after cardiac surgery in diabetic patients. Anesthesiology 2005; 103:687–94.
81. Kersten JR, Schmeling TJ, Orth KG, et al.: Acute hyperglycemia abolishes ischemic preconditioning in vivo. Am J Physiol 1998; 275:H721–5.
82. Fletcher EC, Shah A, Qian W, Miller CC, 3rd: "Near miss" death in obstructive sleep apnea: a critical care syndrome. Crit Care Med 1991; 19:1158–64.
83. Alpert MA: Obesity cardiomyopathy: pathophysiology and evolution of the clinical syndrome. Am J Med Sci 2001; 321:225–36.
84. Valencia-Flores M, Rebollar V, Santiago V, et al.: Prevalence of pulmonary hypertension and its association with respiratory disturbances in obese patients living at moderately high altitude. Int J Obes Relat Metab Disord 2004; 28:1174–80.
85. Bernstein AD, Parsonnet V: Bedside estimation of risk as an aid for decision-making in cardiac surgery. Ann Thorac Surg 2000; 69:823–8.
86. Downing SW, Edmunds LH, Jr.: Release of vasoactive substances during cardiopulmonary bypass. Ann Thorac Surg 1992; 54:1236–43.
87. Kirklin JK, Naftel DC, McGiffin DC, et al.: Analysis of morbid events and risk factors for death after cardiac transplantation. J Am Coll Cardiol 1988; 11:917–24.
88. Ruvolo G, Greco E, Speziale G, et al.: Nitric oxide formation during cardiopulmonary bypass. Ann Thorac Surg 1994; 57:1055–7.
89. Ruvolo G, Speziale G, Greco E, et al.: Nitric oxide release during hypothermic versus normothermic cardiopulmonary bypass. Eur J Cardiothorac Surg 1995; 9:651–4.
90. Speziale G, De Biase L, De Vincentis G, et al.: Inhaled nitric oxide in patients with severe heart failure: changes in lung perfusion and ventilation detected using scintigraphy. Thorac Cardiovasc Surg 1996; 44:35–9.
91. Speziale G, Ruvolo G, Marino B: A role for nitric oxide in the vasoplegic syndrome. J Cardiovasc Surg (Torino) 1996; 37:301–3.
92. Costard-Jackle A, Fowler MB: Influence of preoperative pulmonary artery pressure on mortality after heart transplantation: testing of potential reversibility of pulmonary hypertension with nitroprusside is useful in defining a high risk group. J Am Coll Cardiol 1992; 19:48–54.
93. Lesage AM, Tsuchioka H, Young WG, Jr., Sealy WC: Pathogenesis of pulmonary damage during extracorporeal perfusion. Arch Surg 1966; 93:1002–8.

94. Arain SR, Ruehlow RM, Uhrich TD, Ebert TJ: Efficacy of dexmedeto-midine versus morphine for post-operative analgesia following major inpatient surgery. Anesth Analg 2004; 98:153–8.
95. Herr DL: Phase IIIB, multi-center, open label, randomized study comparing the safety/efficacy of dexmedetomidine (Dex) to propo-fol, for ICU sedation after CABG surgery. Crit Care Med 2000:A124.

Peter Slinger, MD, FRCPC

Lung Isolation in a Patient with a
10 Difficult Airway

INTRODUCTION

Lung isolation is a standard part of anesthetic management for many patients scheduled to undergo thoracic surgical procedures. It improves surgical access during open thoracic procedures (particularly during minimally invasive procedures) and allows segregation of one lung from the other to prevent spillage during surgical manipulation. In addition, lung isolation is required for minimally invasive cardiac surgery and other intrathoracic procedures. The increasing clinical need is creating challenges for the anesthesiologist and requires that lung isolation techniques be mastered. With the increasing use of these techniques, anesthesiologists are being asked more frequently to provide lung isolation even in patients who have airways that are difficult to manage. Fortunately, a number of new devices and approaches are now available to optimize airway management and achieve lung isolation. At the same time, it is critical to emphasize that, for every patient, careful attention must be provided to understanding how to manage the patient with a difficult airway, as described in the American Society of Anesthesiologists algorithms (1), while also considering the goals of lung isolation and how best to fulfill them. This chapter provides an outline of how to develop an organized plan to provide lung isolation for patients with difficult airways and an overview of some of the newer techniques and equipment available to achieve lung isolation during thoracic surgery.

Medically Challenging Patients Undergoing Cardiothoracic Surgery, edited by Neal H. Cohen, MD, MPH, MS, Lippincott Williams & Wilkins, Baltimore © 2009.

LUNG ISOLATION TECHNIQUES

Lung isolation can be achieved by three different methods: double-lumen endobronchial tube (DLT), bronchial blocker, or single-lumen endobronchial tube (see Table 10–1). The most common technique for achieving lung isolation is with insertion of a DLT, which is a bifurcated tube with both a tracheal and a bronchial lumen. DLTs can be used to achieve isolation of either the right or left lung, using tubes with either a right or left bronchial lumen. The second method involves blockade of a right or left mainstem bronchus to facilitate collapse of the area of the lung distal to the occlusion (2). Recently, three new bronchial blockers have become available in North America: the Arndt® wire-guided bronchial blocker (Cook® Critical Care, Bloomington, IN) (3), the Cohen Flexitip® endobronchial blocker (Cook® Critical Care) (4), and the Fuji Uniblocker® (Fuji Systems, Tokyo, Japan) (5) (see Figure 10–1 and Table 10–2).These bronchial blockers can be inserted through a standard endo-tracheal tube (ETT) (see Figures 10–2 and 10–3).

The Univent bronchial blocker® (Fuji Systems) is a catheter contained within a separate channel inside a modified single-lumen ETT. The catheter is extended beyond the tip of the ETT into a mainstem bronchus and inflated to obstruct the bronchus. Although Univent tubes have been used for lung isolation in some patients with difficult airways (6), the tubes are made of silicon (vs. the common polyvinyl chloride ETTs), and many clinicians find the tubes to be somewhat stiffer and less easy to position in patients with more difficult airways.

Bronchial blockers can also be inserted intraluminally (coaxial) through a single-lumen ETT. They also can be placed independently through the glottis exterior to a single lumen tube, if necessary. This approach allows the use of a smaller size single-lumen tube; as a result, this technique is often preferred for use in pediatric patients. Another advantage of bronchial blockers can be seen when postoperative mechanical ventilation is planned after prolonged thoracic or esophageal surgery. In many instances, these patients have an edematous upper airway at the end of the procedure. If a bronchial blocker is used, there is no need to change the single-lumen ETT. The smallest internal diameter of ETT that will allow passage of both a bronchial blocker and a fiberoptic bronchoscope (FOB) depends on the diameters of the bronchoscope and blocker. For standard adult 9 French bronchial blockers, an ETT with an internal diameter >7.0 mm will allow passage of a bronchoscope <4 mm in diameter. Larger bronchoscopes will require an ETT with a size >7.5 mm in internal diameter. No matter what size bronchial blocker that is inserted, it must be well lubricated prior to insertion to facilitate manipulation within the ETT.

TABLE 10–1. Options for lung isolation

Options	Advantages	Disadvantages
Double Lumen Tube Direct laryngoscopy Via tube exchanger Fiberoptically	• Quickest to place successfully • Repositioning rarely required • Bronchoscopy to isolated lung • Suction to isolated lung • CPAP easily added • Can alternate OLV to either lung easily • Placement still possible if bronchoscopy not available	• Size selection more difficult • Difficult to place in patients with difficult airways or abnormal tracheas • Not optimal for postoperative ventilation • Potential laryngeal trauma • Potential bronchial trauma
Bronchial Blockers (BB) Arndt Cohen Fuji	• Size selection rarely an issue • Easily added to regular ETT • Allows ventilation during placement • Easier placement in patients with difficult airways and in children • Postoperative two-lung ventilation by withdrawing blocker • Selective lobar lung isolation possible • CPAP to isolated lung possible	• More time needed for positioning • Repositioning needed more often • Bronchoscope essential for positioning • Nonoptimal right-lung isolation due to right upper lobe anatomy • Bronchoscopy to isolated lung impossible • Minimal suction to isolated lung • Difficult to alternate OLV to either lung
Univent Tube	• Same as BBs • Less repositioning compared to BBs	• Same as BBs • ETT portion has higher air flow resistance than regular ETT • ETT portion has larger diameter than regular ETT
Endobronchial Tube	• Like regular ETTs, easier placement in patients with difficult airways • Longer than regular ETT • Short cuff designed for lung isolation	• Bronchoscopy necessary for placement • Does not allow for bronchoscopy, suctioning, or CPAP to isolated lung • Difficult right lung OLV
ETT advanced into bronchus	• Easier placement in patients with difficult airways	• Does not allow for bronchoscopy, suctioning, or CPAP to isolated lung • Cuff not designed for lung isolation • Difficult right OLV

CPAP = continuous positive airway pressure; OLV = one-lung ventilation.

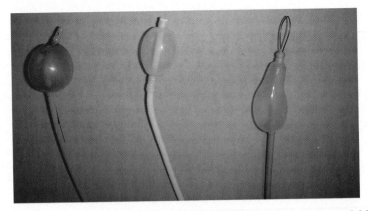

FIGURE 10–1. Three independent bronchial blockers currently available in North America (see Table 10–2 for details). Left: The Cohen® Tip-Deflecting Endobronchial Blocker 9F (Cook® Critical Care, Bloomington, IN), which allows anesthesiologists to establish single-lung ventilation by directing its flexible tip left or right into the desired bronchus using a control wheel device on the proximal end of the blocker in combination with fiberoptic bronchoscope (FOB) guidance. Middle: The Fuji Uniblocker®, 9F (Fuji Corp., Tokyo, Japan). It has a fixed distal curve that allows it to be rotated for manipulation into position with FOB guidance. Unlike its predecessor, the Univent, the Uniblocker is used with a standard endotracheal tube. Right: The wire-guided endobronchial blocker (Arndt® blocker; Cook® Critical Care) introduced in 1999. It contains a wire loop in the inner lumen; when used as a snare with a FOB, it allows directed placement. The snare is then removed, and the 1.4-mm lumen may be used as a suction channel or for oxygen insufflation.

TABLE 10–2. Characteristics of the Cohen, Arndt, and Fuji bronchial blockers

Characteristic	Cohen Blocker	Arndt Blocker	Fuji Uniblocker
Size	9F	5F, 7F, and 9F	5F, 9F
Balloon shape	Spherical	Spherical or elliptical	Spherical
Guidance mechanism	Wheel device to deflect the tip	Nylon wire loop that is coupled with the fiberoptic bronchoscope	None, preshaped tip
Smallest recommended ETT for coaxial use	9F (8.0 ETT)	5F (4.5 ETT), 7F (7.0 ETT), 9F (8.0 ETT)	9F (8.0 ETT)
Murphy eye	Present	Present in 9F	Not present
Center channel	1.6-mm internal diameter	1.4-mm internal diameter	2.0-mm internal diameter

ETT = single endotracheal tube.

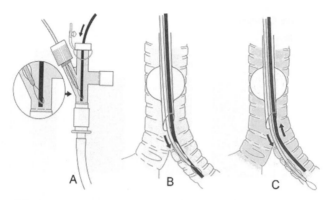

FIGURE 10–2. Placement of the Arndt wire-guided endobronchial blocker. A) Coupling of the nylon wire loop and the fiberoptic bronchoscope (FOB) through a single-lumen endotracheal tube. The multiorifice endotracheal tube connector pictured diagram is supplied with the blocker. B) Arndt blocker along with the FOB are advanced together into the desired mainstem bronchus. C) Disengagement of the blocker by withdrawing the fiberoptic bronchoscope. Diagram courtesy of Dr. J Campos.

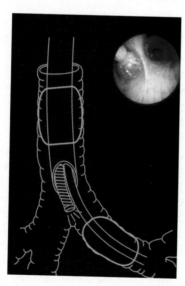

FIGURE 10–3. Diagram of a bronchial blocker placed into the left mainstem bronchus under direct visual guidance using a fiberoptic bronchoscope (FOB) in the endotracheal tube. Top right: FOB view. This technique of blocker placement in advance of the FOB is used with the Cohen and Fuji blockers and differs from the placement technique of the Arndt blocker (see Figure 10–2).

The recent introduction of new designs of bronchial blockers has led to a revival of interest in this technique, which previously had been used for lung isolation as long as 70 years ago. One of the reasons that the technique had been abandoned as the initial approach to lung isolation was the availability of a broader range of double-lumen ETTs. In addition, there is a common impression that the lung deflation is much

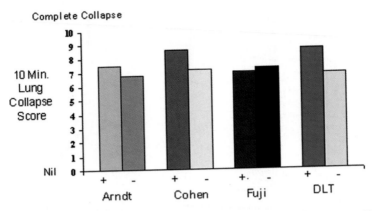

Complete Collapse

FIGURE 10–4. Comparison of the lung collapse scores after 10 minutes of lung isolation during left-sided thoracic surgery using an Arndt, Cohen, or Fuji bronchial blocker or a left-sided double-lumen endobronchial tube (DLT) with (+) or without (−) −20 cmH₂O suction to the lumen of the blocker or DLT. There were no differences between blockers and DLTs with respect to the degree of lung collapse (10 = complete collapse; 0 = no collapse). Suction was associated with an increase in lung collapse scores. (Based on data from [7].)

slower when accomplished through a bronchial blocker, thus risking persistent lung distension or delays in surgery, particularly for video-assisted thoracoscopic procedures. However, when the lung is carefully de-nitrogenated by ventilation with 100% oxygen prior to inflation of the blocker cuff (thus encouraging atelectasis of the nonventilated lung) and suction (−20 cmH₂O) is applied to the suction channel of the bronchial blocker, the time for lung collapse is equivalent to that seen with DLTs (see Figure 10–4). However, positioning of the bronchial blocker is less stable than is positioning of a DLT; therefore, the bronchial blocker often requires intraoperative repositioning (see Figure 10–5) (7). The Arndt blocker used in this study had the original ellipse-shaped cuff; newer blockers have a sphere-shaped cuff. It is not clear whether the change in cuff design will improve positioning (see Figure 10–6).

The final option for lung isolation is through the use of either a single-lumen ETT or endobronchial tube, which is advanced into the contralateral mainstem bronchus protecting this lung while allowing collapse of the lung on the opposite (surgical) side (see Figure 10–7). This technique is rarely used today in adult practice (except in some cases in which airway management is difficult, during emergencies such as in the event of an acute pulmonary bleed in an unstable patient, or after a pneumonectomy). The limitations of this approach are related to the limited access to the nonventilated lung and the difficulty of maintaining appropriate positioning of the standard single-lumen tube within the bronchus. This approach is more commonly used in infants and children, because of the lack of other appropriately sized options. In the pediatric population, an uncuffed, uncut pediatric ETT is advanced into the mainstem bronchus under direct guidance using a pediatric bronchoscope.

LUNG ISOLATION IN THE PATIENT WITH A DIFFICULT UPPER AIRWAY

A number of patients requiring one-lung ventilation (OLV) are identified during preoperative evaluation to have a potentially difficult upper (supraglottic) airway (see Figure 10–8); others present with unexpected difficulty to intubate after induction of anesthesia. The difficulty in managing the airway may be related to anatomic abnormalities or other associated lesions in the mouth, throat, or upper airway. For example,

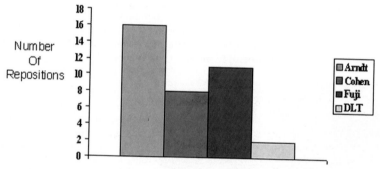

FIGURE 10–5. Comparison of the frequency of repositioning the airway device during left-sided thoracic surgery using an Arndt, Cohen, or Fuji bronchial blocker or a left-sided double-lumen endobronchial tube DLT (*n* = 26/group). Repositioning was required more often with the bronchial blockers than with DLTs. (Based on data from [8].)

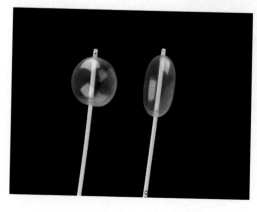

FIGURE 10–6. Left: Recently introduced spherical cuff. Right: original Arndt bronchial blocker cuff. Both designs are available. Some clinicians prefer to use the spherical cuff for right-sided surgery because of the short length of the right mainstem bronchus. (Photo courtesy of Dr. R. Purugganan.)

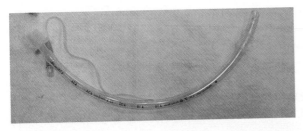
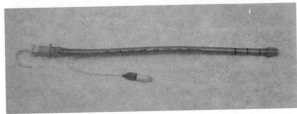
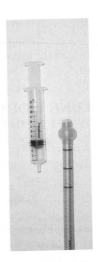

FIGURE 10–7. Standard single-lumen endotracheal tube (top left) and a specifically designed single-lumen endobronchial tube (bottom left and right) (Phycon, Fuji Systems Corp., Tokyo, Japan). The endobronchial tube is longer and has a shorter cuff without a Murphy eye. It can be used as an endotracheal tube and advanced into a mainstem bronchus with fiberoptic guidance when needed for lung isolation.

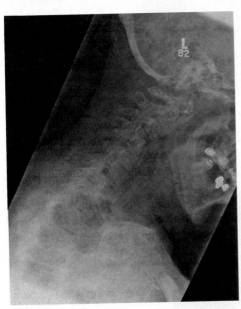

FIGURE 10–8. Lateral cervical spine x-ray of a patient with rheumatoid arthritis and anterior subluxation of C3 on C4. This patient required a thoracotomy for a lung tumor and was not felt to be a candidate for stabilization of the cervical spine. The anesthetic was managed with awake fiberoptic intubation with an endotracheal tube (ETT) and awake lateral decubitus positioning prior to induction of anesthesia. Lung isolation was provided by a bronchial blocker passed through the ETT.

between 5% and 8% of patients with primary lung carcinoma also have a carcinoma of the pharynx, usually located in the epiglottic area (8). In addition, many of the patients coming for thoracic surgery have had previous radiation therapy of the neck or previous airway surgery such as hemimandibulectomy or hemiglossectomy, making intubation and achievement of OLV difficult because of distorted upper airway anatomy. In patients who require OLV and present with a difficult upper airway, the primary goal of airway management is to establish a secure airway initially using a single-lumen ETT placed orally with the aid of a flexible FOB, after appropriate airway anesthesia is achieved. After the single-lumen ETT is in place, an independent bronchial blocker can be passed into the appropriate mainstem bronchus or the ETT can be exchanged for a DLT, if feasible. The decision about which option is best for an individual patient depends on the anatomy, difficulty with the initial intubation and passage of the single-lumen ETT, and the ability to manipulate the head and neck. In addition, the selection of the technique to isolate the lung will depend on an understanding of the risks, benefits, advantages, and disadvantages of each method of lung isolation for the individual patient and proposed surgical procedure (see Table 10–1). For example, if the patient requires OLV and cannot be intubated orally, an awake nasotracheal intubation can be performed with a single-lumen ETT; after the airway is established, then a bronchial blocker can be passed.

Another group of patients that may benefit from the use of bronchial blockers are those cancer patients who have undergone a previous contralateral pulmonary resection. In such cases, selective lobar blockade with a bronchial blocker in the ipsilateral side will improve oxygenation and facilitate surgical exposure.

An alternative technique to achieve OLV in the patient with a difficult upper airway is to intubate the patient's trachea with a single-lumen ETT, then utilize a tube exchanger to replace the existing single-lumen ETT with a DLT. When this technique is used, the tube-exchange catheter should have a hollow center channel, and universal adapters should be available to allow insufflation of oxygen or to facilitate jet ventilation, if necessary. The tube exchangers also should have numeric markings on the outer surface to allow careful control of the depth of insertion to minimize risks associated with manipulation of the exchanger. When placing a DLT over the exchange catheter, the catheter should be at least 83 cm long. A 14F exchange catheter can be used for placement of a 41F or 39F DLT; for placement of a 37F or 35F DLT, an 11F exchange catheter is needed. Specially designed tube-exchange catheters for DLTs are available with a softer distal tip to try to decrease the risk of distal airway trauma (Cook® exchange catheter, Cook Critical Care) (see Figure 10–9). The exchange catheter, single-lumen ETT, and the DLT combination should be tested in vitro before using them for tube placement in the patient.

The technique for placement of the tube exchanger is similar to the technique used to achieve tracheal intubation. A sniffing position facilitates the tube-exchange process. After the exchange catheter is lubri-

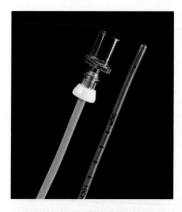

FIGURE 10–9. The recently introduced Cook airway catheter (Cook® Critical Care, Bloomington, IN) for exchanges between double-lumen endobronchial tubes and endotracheal tubes. This recent modification has a soft distal (purple) tip to attempt to decrease the risk of distal airway injury during tube exchange (right). The proximal stiffer green end (left) has detachable connectors for emergency ventilation. Shown is the standard 15-mm outside diameter breathing circuit connector. The exchange catheter also comes with a jet ventilation connector (not shown).

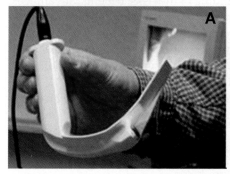
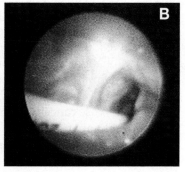

FIGURE 10–10. A: GlideScope® (Verathon Corp., Bothell, WA) video-laryngoscope. Note the acute flexion of the laryngoscope blade. (Photo courtesy of Dr. R. Cooper.) B: View of the glottis from a GlideScope® during a tube exchange. A tube-exchange catheter can be seen passing through the vocal cords. This clear view of the glottis facilitates manipulation of the airway device during replacement of an endotracheal tube with a double-lumen endobronchial tube.

cated, it is advanced through the single-lumen ETT. The catheter should not be inserted deeper than 24 cm measured at the lips to avoid accidental rupture or laceration of the trachea or bronchi (9). After insertion of the tube exchanger, the cuff of the ETT is deflated and the single-lumen ETT is withdrawn. Then the endobronchial lumen of the DLT is advanced over the exchange catheter. For this technique, a video-laryngoscope is helpful to facilitate the tube exchange and to guide the DLT through the glottis under direct vision (see Figure 10–10). If a video-laryngoscope is not available, having an assistant perform standard laryngoscopy during tube exchange partially straightens out the alignment of the oropharynx and glottis and facilitates the exchange. Proper final position of the DLT is then documented using clinical signs including auscultation as well as bronchoscopic confirmation of proper placement.

In selected patients for whom bag-mask ventilation is straightforward, oral intubation with a single-lumen ETT or DLT may be performed after induction of anesthesia using either an FOB or a video-laryngoscope (10). Although the GlideScope® (Verathon Corp., Bothell, WA) video-laryngoscope offers an excellent view of the glottis in the majority of the patients (see Figure 10–10), the acute angle of the laryngoscope blade may make it difficult to pass a DLT directly through the glottis in some cases. There are a variety of new video-laryngoscopes with more conventional styles of blades that some clinicians prefer in this situation such as the Video MACINTOSH System® (Karl Storz, Culver City, CA) (11) (see Figure 10–11) or the Airtraq® (Prodol Meditech S.A., San Jose, CA) (12), which has recently developed a blade specially designed to facilitate DLT placement (see Figure 10–12).

A final option for lung isolation in a patient who has a difficult upper airway is awake fiberoptic intubation using a DLT (13). This option is not commonly used because it requires excellent topical/regional anesthesia of the airway and a cooperative patient. Despite these limitations, this approach may be the best option for the patient with a bronchopleural fistula. Judicious use of dexmedetomidine or remifentanil infusions may be of some help as adjuncts for these cases. The standard pediatric FOB has a short working length beyond the bronchial lumen of a DLT. It is best to practice this technique on a mannequin and become comfortable with it before attempting this approach in a patient (see Figure 10–13).

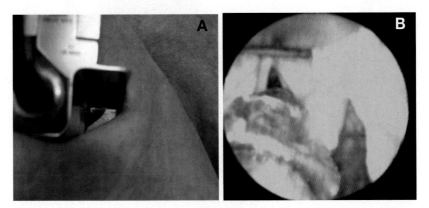

FIGURE 10–11.   A: Photograph of the Video MACINTOSH System® (Karl Storz, Culver City, CA) during intubation. Note the poor grade of view of the glottis seen with "line-of-sight." B: Photograph of the view on the video screen during placement of a double-lumen tube in the same patient. Note the improved view of the glottis compared to (A). (Photos courtesy of Dr. R. Purugganan.)

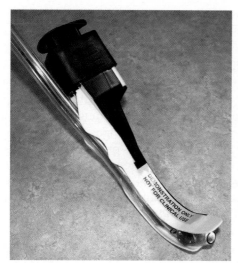

FIGURE 10–12. Recently introduced modification of the Airtraq® (12) (Prodol Meditech S.A., San Jose, CA) video-laryngoscope for intubation using a double-lumen tube. (Photo courtesy of Dr. R. Purugganan.)

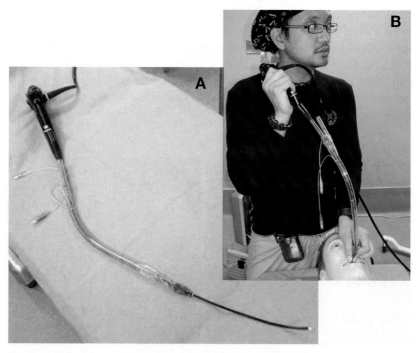

FIGURE 10–13. A: Pediatric fiberoptic bronchoscope passed through the bronchial lumen of a double-lumen endobronchial tube (DLT) for fiberoptic intubation. Note that the actual working length of the DLT beyond the distal bronchial orifice is only approximately 20–25 cm. B: Fiberoptic intubation of a mannequin with a DLT. (Photos courtesy of Dr. R. Purugganan.)

LUNG ISOLATION IN THE PATIENT WITH A DIFFICULT LOWER AIRWAY

A patient who requires OLV might have distorted anatomy below the glottis caused by a number of anatomic or pathologic abnormalities. For example, the patient with a descending thoracic aortic aneurysm may have compression of the left mainstem bronchus. Similarly, the presence of an intra- or extraluminal tumor near the tracheobronchial bifurcation may compromise the ability to insert a left-sided DLT. Such anomalies usually can be detected on preoperative chest radiographs or computed tomography (CT) scans, so these studies should be reviewed routinely prior to induction of anesthesia or attempted airway manipulation (see Figure 10–14). For some patients, flexible FOB examination is necessary to assess a distorted area of the airway prior to selection of a specific tube or blocker to achieve OLV (see Figure 10–15). The FOB can be passed through the bronchial lumen and used to guide the DLT under direct vision in cases in which lower airway anatomy is distorted (see Figure 10–16).

Another group of patients for whom airway management and lung isolation can be challenging are those patients who have previously undergone tracheostomy or laryngectomy. Placement of a DLT through a tracheostomy stoma can be difficult and often results in malpositioning because the upper airway has been shortened and the conventional DLT

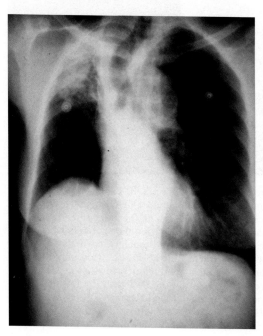

FIGURE 10–14.
Preoperative chest x-ray of a patient with a history of a previous right upper lobectomy and recent hemoptysis presenting for right thoracotomy possible completion pneumonectomy. The potential problems positioning a left-sided double-lumen tube (because of the tracheal deviation in this patient) are easily appreciated by viewing the x-ray but are not mentioned in the radiologist's report. The anesthesiologist must examine the chest imaging him/herself preoperatively to anticipate problems in lung isolation.

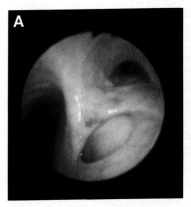
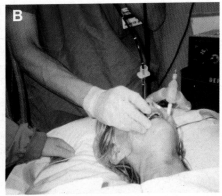

FIGURE 10–15. A: Fiberoptic bronchoscopic photograph of a tracheoesophageal fistula caused by esophageal cancer. The fistula is seen posteriorly at the level of carina at 5 o'clock. The left mainstem bronchus is at 9 o'clock, and the right mainstem bronchus is at 2 o'clock. B: Fiberoptic-guided placement of bilateral endobronchial tubes (5-mm internal diameter microlaryngoscopy tubes) for repair of tracheoesophageal fistula in the same patient. (Photos courtesy of Dr. R Grant.)

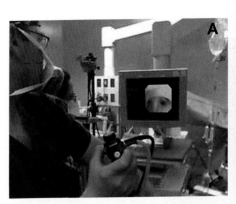
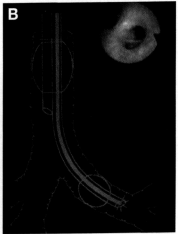

FIGURE 10–16. A: A fiberoptic bronchoscope (FOB) has been placed in the bronchial lumen of a double-lumen endobronchial tube DLT during intubation. The distal tip of the DLT is approaching the carina, seen on the video screen. The FOB is used to guide the DLT placement under direct vision. For patients who have a large angle between the trachea and left mainstem bronchus, having an assistant apply manual pressure displacing the trachea of the anesthetized patient to the right will often facilitate placing the DLT or blocker into the left mainstem bronchus. B: The FOB has been used to guide the DLT into the left mainstem bronchus. Top left: the left upper lobe bronchus can be seen at 10 o'clock and the left lower lobe bronchus just slightly toward 4 o'clock from center. This is the correct position of a left-sided DLT as seen from the bronchial lumen.

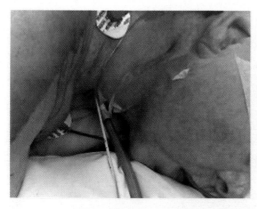

FIGURE 10–17. Patient with a tracheostomy in the left lateral decubitus position for right-sided thoracic surgery. An independent bronchial blocker has been placed through the small tracheostomy stoma, followed by a flexible 6-mm internal diameter endotracheal tube, for lung isolation.

may be too long. Before placing a device used for lung isolation through a tracheostomy stoma, it is important to determine whether it is a fresh stoma or has been in place for some time. For the patient with a relatively new tracheostomy, any manipulation of the stoma is fraught with significant risk and potential to lose control of the airway entirely. The alternative options for achieving OLV in a patient who has had a previous tracheostomy include 1) insertion of a single-lumen ETT either from above (if the upper airway is intact, as is often the case for a patient who underwent tracheostomy for long-term ventilatory management, but has no upper airway disease) or through the stoma and using an independent bronchial blocker, coaxial, or extralumenal (14) (see Figure 10–17); 2) insertion of an independent bronchial blocker through a disposable cuffed tracheostomy cannula; or 3) replacement of the tracheostomy cannula with a short DLT, specifically designed for use in a patient with a tracheostomy, such as the Naruke DLT (15).

CONCLUSION

The optimal method of lung isolation will depend on a number of factors, including the patient's airway anatomy, the indication for lung isolation, the available equipment, and the training and experience of the anesthesiologist. Whatever method of lung isolation is used, a general approach to airway management can be best defined using the "ABCs" of lung isolation:

Anatomy

Know the tracheobronchial anatomy. One of the major problems that many anesthesiologists have in achieving satisfactory lung isolation is caused by lack of familiarity with the distal airway anatomy and potential endobronchial or extrinsic abnormalities that deform the airway (16).

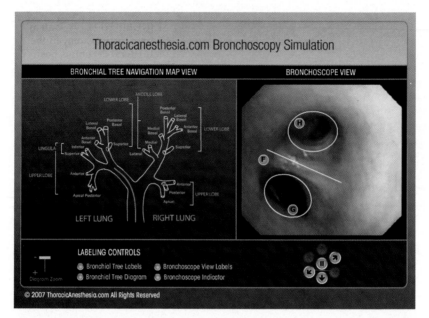

FIGURE 10–18.   Online bronchoscopy simulator. The user can navigate the tracheobronchial tree using real-time video by clicking on the lighted directional arrows under the "Bronchoscopic view" (right). Clicking on the labels on the "Bronchoscopic view" gives details of the anatomy seen. The process is aided by the "Bronchial Tree Navigational Map" (left), which shows the simultaneous location of the bronchoscope in the airway.

Bronchoscopy

Whenever possible, use a FOB to position endobronchial tubes and bronchial blockers. The ability to perform fiberoptic bronchoscopy is now a fundamental skill needed by all anesthesiologists providing anesthesia for thoracic surgery. An online bronchoscopy simulator has been developed to help train anesthesiologists in positioning double-lumen tubes and blockers (see Figure 10–18). This simulator, which uses real-time video, is available without cost at www.thoracicanesthesia.com.

Chest Imaging

The anesthesiologist should always review all chest images (CT, magnetic resonance imaging, etc.) prior to induction of anesthesia or placement of a double-lumen tube or bronchial blocker. Abnormalities of the lower airway often can be identified in advance. The information provided by the images will have an impact on the selection of the optimal method of lung isolation for a specific patient (see Figure 10–19). With

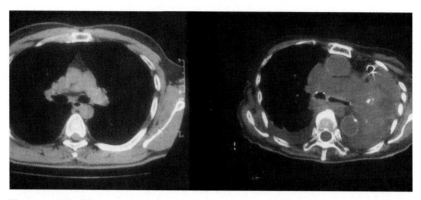

FIGURE 10–19. Computed tomography (CT) scans from just below the level of the carinal bifurcation. Left: CT from normal patient. Right: CT from patient scheduled for left lung biopsy. The patient has a left-sided lung tumor and effusion, which compresses the left mainstem bronchus. This bronchial compression was not evident on the chest x-ray. It may be difficult to place a left-sided double-lumen endobronchial tube (DLT) in this patient. A right-sided DLT or a bronchial blocker would be the preferred method of lung isolation if required for this patient.

these additional data, clinical management can be modified to address any structural changes that will influence tube placement and/or proper positioning of the endobronchial lumen or bronchial blocker or could potentially require an entirely different approach to lung isolation or surgical approach.

References

1. Practice guidelines for management of the difficult airway: a report by the American Society of Anesthesiologists Task Force on Management of the Difficult Airway. Anesthesiology 1993; 78:597–602
2. Campos JH: An update on bronchial blockers during lung separation techniques in adults. Anesth Analg 2005; 97:1266–74
3. Arndt GA, DeLessio ST, Kranner PW, Orzepowski W, Ceranski B, Valtysson B: One-lung ventilation when intubation is difficult—presentation of a new endobronchial blocker. Acta Anaesthesiol Scand 1999; 43: 356–8
4. Cohen E: The Cohen flexitip endobronchial blocker: an alternative to a double lumen tube. Anesth Analg 2005; 101:1877–9
5. Nishiumi N, Nakagawa T, Masuda R, Iwasaki M, Inokuchi S, Inoue H: Endobronchial bleeding associated with blunt chest trauma treated by bronchial occlusion with a Univent. Ann Thorac Surg 2008; 85:245–50

6. Baraka A: The Univent tube can facilitate difficult intubation in a patient undergoing thoracoscopy. J Cardiothorac Vasc Anesth 1996; 10:693–4

7. Narayanaswamy M, Lacroix M, Kanellakos G, et al.: A comparison of three designs of bronchial blockers with double-lumen tubes for lung isolation. Anesth Analg 2007: 104:SCA11

8. Hagihira S, Takashina M, Mori T, et al.: One-lung ventilation in patients with difficult airways. J Cardiothorac Vasc Anesth 1998; 12:186

9. DeLima L, Bishop M: Lung laceration after tracheal extubation over a plastic tube exchanger. Anesth Analg 1991; 73:350–1

10. Jones PM, Harle CC, Turkstra TP: The GlideScope® cobalt video-laryngoscope—a novel single-use device. Can J Anaesth 2007; 54: 677–8

11. Kaplan MB, Ward DS, Berci G: A new video laryngoscope—an aid to intubation and teaching. J Clin Anesth 2002; 14:620–6

12. Maharaj CH, O'Croinin D, Curley G, et al.: A comparison of tracheal intubation using the Airtraq® or the Macintosh laryngoscope in routine airway management: a randomised, controlled clinical trial. Anaesthesia 2006; 61:1093–9

13. Patane PA, Sell BA, Mahla ME: Awake fiberoptic endobronchial intubation. J Cardiothorac Vasc Anesth 1990; 4:229–31

14. Tobias JD: Variations on one-lung ventilation. J Clin Anesth 2001; 13:35–9

15. Saito T, Naruke T, Carney E, et al.: New double intrabronchial tube (Naruke tube) for tracheostomized patients. Anesthesiology 1998; 89:1038–9

16. Campos JH, Hallam E, Van Natta T, Kernstein KH: Devices for lung isolation used by anesthesiologists with limited thoracic experience: comparison of double-lumen endotracheal tube, Univent® torque control blocker, and Arndt wire-guided endobronchial blocker®. Anesthesiology 2006; 104:261–6

Javier H. Campos, MD

Managing the Patient with an Anterior Mediastinal Mass

11

INTRODUCTION

Anterior mediastinal masses are uncommon in the adult patient; however, they present significant challenges to the anesthesiologist because of their impact on the airway and cardiovascular system (1). The anatomic location and size of the mediastinal mass have significant implications related to compression of the airway, mainly in the lower third of the trachea and main bronchi; compression of major vessels, including superior vena cava and pulmonary vessels; as well as compression of adjacent organs (2–4). This review focuses on specific considerations, including 1) anatomy of the mediastinum; 2) preoperative assessment, with particular attention to radiological and diagnostic tests; 3) mechanism of an airway obstruction and adjacent structures by a mass effect; 4) intraoperative management, including the use of standby cardiopulmonary bypass (CPB); and 5) potential postoperative complications in the adult patient with an anterior mediastinal mass.

ANATOMY OF THE MEDIASTINUM

The mediastinum is situated between the two pleural cavities. It extends superiorly from the root of the neck and the thoracic inlet to the hemidiaphragm inferiorly. It is divided into the superior and inferior mediastinum by the transverse thoracic plane, which is an imaginary plane extending horizontally from the sternal angle anteriorly to the border of

Medically Challenging Patients Undergoing Cardiothoracic Surgery, edited by Neal H. Cohen, MD, MPH, MS, Lippincott Williams & Wilkins, Baltimore © 2009.

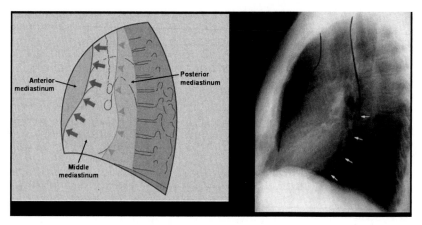

FIGURE 11–1. A. Schematic representation of mediastinal anatomy. B. Lateral radiograph of the chest.

the fourth thoracic vertebra posteriorly. The inferior mediastinum is sub-divided into anterior, middle, and posterior compartments. The anterior mediastinum contains the thymus, trachea, esophagus, vessels and arter-ies, as well as lymph nodes. Any abnormal growth in this region will affect the adjacent area. The impact includes potential compression of the tracheobronchial tree and occlusion of major vessels (superior vena cava and pulmonary vessels). The middle mediastinum is the space occupied by the heart and pericardium (5, 6). Figure 11–1 shows a) schematic representation of mediastinal anatomy and b) lateral radi-ograph of the chest.

A variety of neoplasms and other lesions present with anterior mediastinal involvement. Thymoma is the most common primary neo-plasm of the anterior mediastinum. Other tumors include germ cell tumors, Hodgkin or non-Hodgkin lymphomas, bronchiogenic carci-noma, and thyroid tumors. Thymomas are classified as invasive or non-invasive. Approximately 30% of thymomas are invasive and may cause pleural, pericardial, and great vessel invasion although rarely will they invade the superior vena cava.

AIRWAY AND CARDIOVASCULAR COMPLICATIONS ASSOCIATED WITH ANTERIOR MEDIASTINAL MASS

Tracheal obstruction and compression may result from extrinsic com-pression by a tumor of the mediastinum, thyroid gland, or metastatic hilum or by mediastinal lymphadenopathy in adult patients. The liter-ature is filled with case reports involving compromise of the airway in adult patients with anterior mediastinal masses when the patient was placed in the supine position (7), at the induction of anesthesia (8), during the intraoperative period, at extubation (9), or in the postoperative period (1). The complete collapse and loss of the airway in the adult patient in the intraoperative period is considered a rare event based upon two retrospective reports (1, 10).

The mechanism of airway compression by a mediastinal mass is multifactorial. For example, during administration of general anesthesia, the tumor that was previously supported by muscle tone in an awake patient now collapses because of its weight onto the larger airways rendered compressible by relaxation of the smooth muscle. In addition, the airway loses the distinctive transpleural gradient—the tethering effect of expanded lungs by a reduction of inspiratory muscle tone and an increase in abdominal muscle tone. Tracheal narrowing by more than 35% increases the risk of airway obstruction during general anesthesia.

With a patient in the supine position, the effects of anesthetics and muscle relaxants lead to a decrease in the dimensions of the rib cage, a cephalad displacement of the dome of the diaphragm, and a reduction in thoracic gas volume. The reduction in the dimension of the chest wall may limit the available space for the trachea relative to the tumor, and the decrease in tracheal distending pressure at low lung volumes promotes collapse, particularly in the presence of tracheomalacia.

Another area of concern with an anterior mediastinal mass is the extension of the compression or obstruction of the airway into the bronchi. As a result of the extensive nature of the airway obstruction, in some selected patients it may be necessary to advance the endotracheal tube into a bronchus or to place a stent into the distal airway to maintain expansion of the lung distal to the obstruction (11). Many of these tumors can compress the superior vena cava, compress the lower part of the trachea, and potentially involve the right and left mainstem bronchi as well. In addition, patients with an anterior mediastinal mass can have progressive hypoxemia caused in part by compression of pulmonary vessels or the presence of a large pleural effusion creating intrapulmonary shunting and compromising gas exchange.

Compression of the larger airways also can cause significant changes in gas exchange and patient morbidity. For example, some patients with an anterior mediastinal mass develop severe hypoxemia caused by a total obstruction of the left mainstem bronchus and compression of the pulmonary artery. Takeda and colleagues (12) reported the case of a 19-year-old male with a large anterior mediastinal mass seen on chest computed tomography (CT) scan as compressing the trachea, left main bronchus, and right pulmonary artery. Approximately 60 minutes after induction of anesthesia, the patient developed progressive hypoxemia and desaturation (<80%). Intraoperative bronchoscopy showed total occlusion of the left main bronchus. Because of progressive hypoxemia, percutaneous cardiopulmonary support was used with extracorporeal membrane oxygenation. As part of a median sternotomy, the tumor was lifted and removed, improving arterial oxygenation. Therefore, lifting the tumor or immediate surgical suspension should be considered when all conventional approaches fail to restore arterial oxygenation.

Another potential complication related to airway obstruction is the development of noncardiogenic pulmonary edema, particularly in patients with severe airway obstruction either before or after surgical intervention. In a case report by Price and Hecker (13), a 27-year-old patient with a large anterior mediastinal mass received general anesthesia with endotracheal intubation without problems in the intraoperative period. The mediastinal mass was not resected. After extubation, the patient developed respiratory insufficiency with cyanosis and copious pink frothy secretions, with a diagnosis of noncardiogenic pulmonary edema. The potential explanation of this event included the transmission to the interstitial space of negative intrapleural pressure, generated by inspiratory efforts against an obstructed airway leading to pulmonary edema.

PREOPERATIVE ASSESSMENT

Patients with anterior mediastinal masses may present with a variety of symptoms. Moderate symptoms include persistent cough, dyspnea, chest pain, fatigue, diaphoresis, and vocal cord paralysis caused by compression from mass effect. Severe symptoms may include orthopnea, stridor, cyanosis, dysphagia, syncope, and superior vena cava syndrome (jugular vein distension and facial edema). The symptoms can be exacerbated depending upon the size of the mass (i.e., >15 cm^3), compression of adjacent structures, or changes in patient position from upright, seated, supine, prone, or lateral decubitus position (14). As a result of the varying symptomatic presentation of the patient with an anterior mediastinal mass and the impact of changes in position and venous return on the hemodynamics and the airway, a comprehensive preoperative evaluation is critical. The evaluation should define the anatomic relationship between the mass and the airway and great vessels, and, to the extent possible, identify the dynamic nature of the mass and its effects to define the most appropriate approach to induction and maintenance of anesthesia.

Radiological Studies in Patients with an Anterior Mediastinal Mass

The initial study in patients with a suspected anterior mediastinal mass generally is a standard biplane chest radiography, which will identify

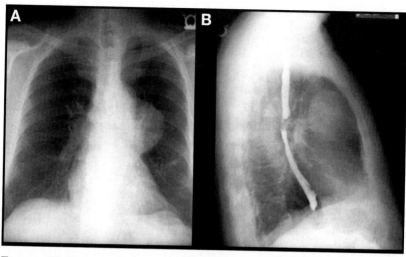

FIGURE 11–2. A: Anterior mediastinal mass in the left hemithorax of a posterior–anterior chest radiograph. B: Mediastinal mass without compromise to the tracheobronchial tree shown in a lateral radiograph with esophageal contrast.

up to 97% of mediastinal tumors. The chest x-ray also provides important information regarding the size and location of the mass (15). In addition, in this patient group in particular, special attention must be paid to the lateral radiograph of the chest to determine the overall extent of the mass and potential involvement of adjacent structures. A barium contrast esophagogram also will be useful to determine whether there is tracheobronchial tree involvement, although other dynamic studies may be more useful in defining the characteristics of the mass. An anterior mediastinal mass can be seen clearly in the left hemithorax of the posterior–anterior chest radiograph of Figure 11–2A. A lateral radiograph with esophageal contrast shows a mediastinal mass without compromise to the tracheobronchial tree in Figure 11–2B.

Most patients subsequently will have a CT scan of the chest to confirm the presence of a mediastinal mass and clarify the anatomy (16, 17). The CT scan of the chest will define the precise size and location of the mediastinal mass, any involvement with adjacent structures, as well as the degree of compression of the airway (trachea and/or bronchi). It is important during the assessment of the CT scan to identify the location of the mass, define its relationship to adjacent structures, assess the extent and degree of tracheal and/or vascular compression, and assess the patency of the airway at the tracheal and bronchial level. The CT scan also will permit accurate measurement of the airway diameter and will determine the precise level and extent of compression of the trachea. The average cross-sectional diameter of the trachea in a 70-kg, 170-cm-

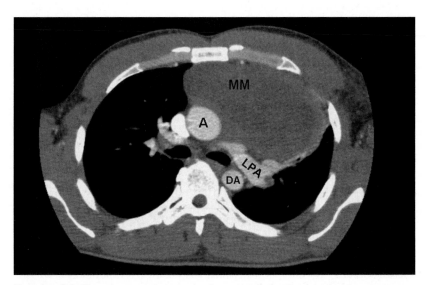

FIGURE 11–3.   Computed tomography scan of the chest with a large anterior mediastinal mass. MM = mediastinal mass; LPA = left pulmonary artery; A = ascending aorta; DA = descending aorta.

tall person is 18–23 mm (18). A tracheal diameter narrowing of 10 mm on CT corresponds to a 50% reduction in the tracheal cross-sectional area at that level. Figure 11q–3 shows a CT scan of the chest with a large anterior mediastinal mass.

Magnetic resonance imaging (MRI) is an adjunct to CT scan evaluation reserved for patients in whom CT scans did not resolve the anatomic issues or for whom additional information about the mass and its relationship to other vital organs is required (19). Because approximately 30% of thymomas are invasive, cardiac MRI allows the identification of soft tissue location, morphology, and degree of intracardiac vessel invasiveness of the tumor. Therefore, cardiac MRI should be ordered if an invasion of the mediastinal mass into the vessels or the heart is suspected.

Pulmonary Function Studies

Pulmonary function tests (PFTs) should be obtained in the patient with an anterior mediastinal mass to clarify the impact on the airway. The PFTs provide a dynamic assessment of airway obstruction throughout the respiratory cycle. The flow volume loop (FVL) is probably the most helpful in identifying the presence of an upper airway obstruction. Interpretation of the FVL is critical to define the extent of airway obstruction caused by the mass and to determine if the obstruction is inspiratory, expiratory, or both. A plateau on inspiratory flow of the FVL is consistent with a variable extrathoracic upper airway obstruction. A plateau of the expiratory flow with a normal inspiratory flow suggests an intrathoracic upper airway obstruction. In contrast, patients who have flattening of both the inspiratory and expiratory flows have a pattern indicative of a fixed obstruction.

Historically, based upon one anecdotal case report (20), anesthesiologists have requested upright and supine spirometry as a part of the preoperative assessment in patients with an anterior mediastinal mass. A recent retrospective cohort study of adults with known mediastinal masses identified 37 patients who had spirometry ordered as a part of their preoperative assessment (10). The overall mean values reported in a seated position include forced vital capacity (FVC) and forced expiratory volume in 1 second (FEV$_1$) of 4.02 ± 0.75 L (90.7 ± 13.3% predicted volume) and 3.22 ± 0.56 L (89.6 ± 14.2% predicted volume), respectively. Only ten patients had both upright and supine spirometry ordered, including four who had abnormal results suggestive of upper airway obstruction. Of the patients who had upright and supine spirometry performed, the test was ordered more commonly in the younger and symptomatic patients. Perioperative complications did not significantly occur more frequently in the patients who had upright and supine spirometry ordered than in those who did not have these tests performed. Although the results of spirometry were abnormal in four patients, suggesting upper airway obstruction, all received general anesthesia; no airway collapse, obstruction, or other perioperative complications occurred while receiving general anesthesia. The perioperative complications rate was 5.4%. The study did not demonstrate any correlation between abnormal upright and supine spirometry results and symptoms, with abnormal chest CT scan findings, or with the anesthetic technique or the development of intra- and/or postoperative complications. Therefore, upright and supine spirometry may not be any better in predicting complications than are symptoms and chest CT scan and should not be routinely obtained in patients with anterior mediastinal masses.

In another retrospective study (21), this one involving 36 adults with intrathoracic Hodgkin's disease, the incidence of upper airway obstruction was examined to correlate FVL pattern with changes in the CT scan of the chest before and after chemotherapy and radiation therapy. Of the 36 patients included in the study, 25 had baseline and follow-up PFTs. The results showed that 14 of 25 patients (56%) had an abnormal FVL pattern prior to chemotherapy; seven of these patients had a flattening pattern during inspiratory and expiratory loop compatible with a fixed obstruction pattern. Seven patients had only a flattening pattern during inspiratory loop, and eleven had a normal FVL. In contrast, 4 months after chemotherapy with reduction in the size of the tumor, only 6 of 25 patients (25%) had an abnormal FVL. One patient had a fixed pattern on FVL, and five had flattening on inspiratory loop compatible with extrathoracic obstruction.

The abnormal patterns seen were either fixed obstruction or variable extrathoracic obstruction. To correlate the FVL with abnormal findings on the chest CT scan, the tracheal configuration from the CT scan was graded accordingly: grade I, minimal tracheal distortion and being round and symmetrical in shape; grade II, moderate distortion and oval in shape; and grade III, severe distortion and narrowing of the trachea lumen >50%. On chest CT scan, 16 patients were identified as having a grade I tracheal deformity, 6 had grade II deformity, and 3 had grade III deformity. All patients with grade III deformity had a fixed obstruction pattern. The study also showed that patients with a fixed pattern on FVL had significant decreases in inspiratory and expiratory flow rates. This study clearly demonstrated that a fixed pattern of obstruction was associated with lower flow rates and severe tracheal distortion on CT; this finding suggests that *asymptomatic* patients with an abnormal FVL but a normal tracheal size on CT scan do not require a more extensive preoperative evaluation.

Another interesting study evaluated 32 patients who had orthopnea associated with a nontoxic goiter. The study was designed to assess the extent of postural changes in respiratory function (22). Pulmonary function assessment was performed in a seated and supine position. Expiratory flows were assessed. In addition, the goiter–trachea radiologic relationships were subdivided into 3 groups: grade I, no evidence of tracheal deviation; grade II, tracheal deviation present in lateral and/or anteroposterior plane with tracheal compression <20%; and grade III, tracheal compression >20%. Overall in the three groups studied, the average maximal expiratory flow at 50% of FVC/maximal inspiratory flow at 50% was >1.1, suggesting the presence of upper airway obstruction. The patients who had grade II tracheal deviation/compression had a lower expiratory reserve volume and maximal expiratory flow at 25% of FVC and higher airway resistance. The prevalence of orthopnea was highest in patients whose goiter–trachea relationships were classified as a grade III, where 75% presented with orthopnea as compared to 18% with orthopnea in the grade I group. Also in patients with orthopnea, the prevalence of patients who had intrathoracic goiters was higher (78% vs. 21% in patients without orthopnea). In addition, obesity (body mass index > 30) was associated with orthopnea in this group of patients.

These studies clearly showed a consistent pattern on pulmonary dynamics and association with severe tracheal deviation or compression. Therefore, any patient with an anterior mediastinal mass who has a fixed pattern on FVL and severe tracheal distortion or compression (i.e., >50%) on chest CT scan requires a more extensive evaluation. Although the specific additional studies that are required have not been systematically evaluated, the assessment now often includes awake flexible fiberoptic bronchoscopy to assess the specific area(s) of potential distortion or compression through an endoscopic view.

Transthoracic and transesophageal echocardiography are also useful in evaluating the patient with an anterior mediastinal mass. It can not only define the extent of cardiac involvement, if any, but also the presence of pericardial effusion, impact of the mass on cardiac filling, and any other associated abnormalities that might impact anesthetic or surgical management (23). In addition, during the anesthetic management as part of the intraoperative care, if an extension of the tumor invades the great vessels or the heart, an evaluation with intraoperative transesophageal echocardiography is necessary to rule out the presence of thrombus. Transesophageal echocardiography will also be helpful in determining if there is any compression to right ventricular outflow tract (24, 25). Transesophageal echocardiography is also useful in determining if there is a pericardial effusion associated with the anterior mediastinal mass (26, 27).

SURGICAL CONSIDERATIONS

Patients with an anterior mediastinal mass require a number of procedures both for diagnosis and treatment. The specific approach to the patient depends on the size of the tumor and the extent of compression of the airway or major vessels. Anesthetic management will depend on an understanding of the anatomy and physiology and the goals of the surgical procedure. Needle aspiration biopsy of a solid mass using local anesthesia may provide tissue diagnosis, allowing radiation or chemotherapy to reduce the size of the mass. If a mediastinal mass appears to have a cystic component, needle aspiration of the mass under local anesthesia may relieve the airway compression (28). Transsternal core biopsy has been used as an alternative to mediastinoscopy in patients with an anterior mediastinal mass using local anesthesia under CT guidance as an outpatient procedure (29). CT-guided biopsy is done under local anesthesia by introducing a cannula with a stylet through the sternal bone. A drill with an eccentric tip is inserted in the cannula, and a hole is manually drilled. The inner cannula contains an automatic cutting needle allowing the retrieval of a tissue sample with CT guidance; the biopsy can be performed from the desired area of the tumor. An alternative for the diagnosis of an anterior mediastinal mass is a biopsy through mini-mediastinoscopy under local anesthesia through a

3-cm parasternal incision at the 2nd or 3rd intercostal space according to the location of the mass. This procedure is carried out under local anesthesia, sedation, and ultrasonography guidance in the operating room (30). In addition, parasternal anterior mediastinotomy under local anesthesia has been used with percutaneous needle biopsy for malignant anterior mediastinal masses with success (31). Another alternative for the diagnosis of mediastinal masses is transcervical mediastinoscopy under general anesthesia (6).

Different surgical and therapeutic interventions for an anterior mediastinal mass resection include median sternotomy and resection, conventional thoracoscopic approach, or thoracoscopic thymectomy using the da Vinci® robot-assisted system (Intuitive Surgical, Inc., Sunnyvale, CA) (32). The advantage of using the da Vinci robotic system is that it is considered a minimally invasive surgery (33). Bodner and colleagues (34) reported good results in ten patients undergoing thymectomies and five patients who had removal of other mediastinal masses. Other studies involving only mediastinal mass resection with the da Vinci robotic system have reported similar good results (35, 36). In one study (36), the intraoperative management of patients with mediastinal masses included selective single-lung ventilation and CO_2 insufflation to a pressure of 10–15 mmHg to facilitate surgical exposure. Another advantage of the robotic approach is reduced hospital length of stay. A nonrandomized study comparing median sternotomy with robotically assisted surgery for thymectomy demonstrated that the hospital length of stay was an average of 5 days with the robotic surgery versus 10 days with median sternotomy (37).

ANESTHETIC CONSIDERATIONS

Anesthetic management must be determined based on an understanding of the extent of involvement of the mass into adjacent structures such as an airway or great vessel, the physiologic consequences, and the proposed surgical procedure. Airway obstruction can occur at any stage of anesthesia. The potential causes of airway obstruction include change in position to the supine position, which allows the weight of the mass to be distributed directly over the trachea or bronchi; the effects of anesthetics in decreasing smooth muscle tone within the trachea and decreasing the tethering effect on airway diameter; and the change from spontaneous to positive pressure ventilation, potentially decreasing the airway patency or diameter and paradoxically worsening the obstruction by creating increased postobstructive turbulent flow (38).

Patients with a large anterior mediastinal mass who require general anesthesia have the potential for an unexpected airway obstruction or car-

TABLE 11–1. Basic components for managing the airway in patients with a large anterior mediastinal mass

- Rigid bronchoscope
- Flexible fiberoptic bronchoscope (different sizes)
- Laryngeal mask airways
- Laryngoscopes
- Armored single-lumen endotracheal tubes
- Double-lumen endotracheal tubes (DLTs)
- Suction devices connected to bronchoscopes
- Surgical team ready to intervene
- Transesophageal echocardiogram (cases involving heart and great vessels)

diovascular collapse. Therefore, if the preoperative evaluation documents a major compromise to the airway, an awake intubation should be attempted with minimal sedation while maintaining spontaneous ventilation. A rigid bronchoscope and an experienced bronchoscopist must be available in the operating room prior to manipulation of the airway. The advantage of a rigid bronchoscopy is that it can bypass the obstruction and provide a ventilation pathway if complete obstruction occurs. After the airway is secured by an endotracheal tube (armored single-lumen endotracheal tube, a double-lumen endobronchial tube [DLT], or a regular endotracheal tube), positive pressure ventilation can be attempted, followed by the administration of muscle relaxants if necessary. An alternative is to use an inhalational induction by a face mask with sevoflurane, most appropriate for the asymptomatic patients without documented airway compression. In these patients spontaneous ventilation should be maintained until the airway is secured.

Intraoperative life-threatening airway compression can be managed first by making the diagnosis with a flexible fiberoptic bronchoscope and second by changing the patient position to lateral decubitus, head up, semisitting position or a lateral side where ventilation can be managed (9, 39). The use of a rigid bronchoscope should be considered to reestablish air patency of the airway. Table 11–1 describes the basic preparation for managing patients with a large anterior mediastinal mass.

In a retrospective study (1) involving 98 patients with an anterior mediastinal mass, the use of general anesthesia was selected for 97 of 105 anesthetic cases. In the study, 79 of 97 patients received neuromuscular blockade as part of the anesthetic management. In 15 patients, spontaneous ventilation was kept followed by neuromuscular blockade and controlled ventilation. Another three patients received general anesthesia with spontaneous ventilation throughout the case because they were considered at very high risk for airway obstruction because of the presence of the mass. There were eight cases that received local anesthesia and sedation. These patients were considered a higher-risk group based on symptomatology and radiological evaluation; also, they had larger anterior mediastinal masses (734 ± 643 cm³) and more tracheal compression on the chest CT scan. Of note, in this report none of the patients experienced occlusion of the airway despite the fact that some patients had severe compression (i.e., >50%) of the tracheobronchial tree as determined by a chest CT scan and bronchoscopic examination.

Another therapeutic option that can be helpful in selected patients with an anterior mediastinal mass and major airway obstruction is the use of a helium/oxygen mixture (40). It can be useful during perioperative management or in emergency situations of either inoperable airway obstruction or to overcome the increases in airway resistance associated with chemotherapy- or radiation therapy–induced edema. In one report, the use of helium/oxygen 80%:20% delivered by a mask during chemotherapy and radiation therapy reduced the tumor size and has been used as a potentially lifesaving therapy in an emergency situation (41). The advantage of using helium is its very low density, which is useful in overcoming airway resistance and obstruction. The administration of a helium/oxygen mixture improves laminar flow and reduces airway resistance and breathing work. Although it is only a temporary intervention, it can be lifesaving for selected patients. The higher the helium concentration, the better the effect on gas flow, i.e., fixed helium/oxygen mixtures of 60% helium, 40% oxygen or 80% helium, 20% oxygen. As a result, this approach is useful in only those patients who do not require high inspired oxygen concentrations.

AIRWAY MANAGEMENT FOR THE PATIENT WITH ANTERIOR MEDIASTINAL MASS

Although most patients scheduled for surgery for an anterior mediastinal mass do not have total airway obstruction at the time of presentation, they can deteriorate rapidly as either a result of edema or hemorrhage or after loss of normal airway tone during induction of anesthesia. Total occlusion of the airway can lead to respiratory and cardiovascular collapse. Maintaining airway patency represents a challenge, specifically if the obstruction is located at the middle or lower third of the trachea or at the entrance of a mainstem bronchus because patients who require general anesthesia will have the potential for unexpected airway obstruction. If during the preoperative assessment a major compromise to the airway is already present (i.e., tracheal deviation with >50% compression at the level of trachea, or lesions close to the tracheal carina), an awake intubation with flexible fiberoptic bronchoscopy must be performed with minimal sedation and spontaneous ventilation (4, 42).

At the time of manipulation of the airway, and (in the most tenuous patients) at the induction of anesthesia, an experienced bronchoscopist must be available immediately in the operating room to intervene if necessary (43). For some patients, rigid bronchoscopy is necessary to bypass the obstruction and provide a pathway for ventilation if complete obstruction occurs. After the airway is secured and the patient intubated, subsequent management of the patient must be individualized based on the location and size of the mass, the intended surgical procedure, and the hemodynamic changes associated with position changes, manipulation of the mass, and effects of positive pressure ventilation. The selection of endotracheal tube also requires careful consideration of the size and location of the mass, the anticipated surgical procedure, and the plans for postoperative airway management. In many cases an armored single-lumen endotracheal tube is useful to prevent compression of the endotracheal tube from compromising the ability to ventilate the patient. For the patient with a distal extrathoracic lesion that is causing compression of a bronchus, a left- or right-sided DLT may be more appropriate. The DLT has a number of advantages in this situation, including the increased tube length, which allows bypassing the point of obstruction, and the ability to independently ventilate each lung, if necessary, to optimize the surgical field and ensure gas exchange (44).

CPB FOR THE PATIENT WITH AN ANTERIOR MEDIASTINAL MASS

CPB with cannulation of femoral vessels has been used in patients with progressive hypoxemia and very narrow airways, specifically in patients with tracheal tumors obstructing the tracheal carina and bronchi (45). Also, standby CPB via femorofemoral access has been reported as a prophylactic measure if severe hypoxemia occurs because of major airway obstruction (46). The evidence does not strongly support the need for standby CPB; however, the use of CPB can be justified for the patient with an anterior mediastinal mass who has compression of the tracheal carina with imminent total occlusion of the bronchi and associated severe hypoxemia that has not responded to conventional maneuvers.

POSTOPERATIVE COMPLICATIONS IN PATIENTS WITH ANTERIOR MEDIASTINAL MASS

Patients with an anterior mediastinal mass are at risk for developing postoperative complications for a number of reasons. For those patients who undergo a biopsy procedure without resection of the mass, the risk of airway compromise is high. For those who have the mass excised surgically, there is risk of tracheomalacia after the procedure. (47, 48). A

TABLE 11–2.   Perioperative complications

Author	N	Intra-operative complications	Post-operative complications	Airway collapse	Life-threatening complications in the post-operative period
Béchard et al. (1)	97	4/97	11/97	0	7/97
Hnatiuk et al. (10)	37	1	0	0	0

number of other respiratory complications can occur. A study by Béchard and colleagues (1), involving 98 patients with mediastinal masses who underwent 105 anesthetic procedures, showed that the incidence of early respiratory complications in the postoperative period (>48 hours) was 6.7% (11/98 patients). These complications included airway edema, development of pneumonia, and atelectasis. In these patients, only 7 of the 105 anesthetic procedures had life-threatening respiratory complications including reintubations. The complications were associated more commonly with patients who had tracheal compression of >50% on the preoperative chest CT scan and a mixed pulmonary syndrome on PFTs. Also of interest in this report is the fact that no airway collapses occurred in the intra- or postoperative period, nor were any deaths reported. Table 11–2 shows the perioperative complications in patients undergoing mediastinal mass resection from two recent retrospective studies.

CONCLUSION

Airway collapse caused by an anterior mediastinal mass is a rare event in the adult patient. However, the adult patient with an anterior mediastinal mass requires careful preoperative assessment and anesthetic management, particularly when there is evidence of airway compression of >50% and/or major vessel obstruction. Preoperative assessment should include chest radiograph and CT scan of the chest to estimate the degree of involvement. Intravascular and intracardiac involvement of the mass should be evaluated with transthoracic or transesophageal echocardiography. Spirometry in the upright and supine position is not better at predicting perioperative complications than is a CT scan alone. FVL testing with confirmation of tracheal deviation by CT scan can predict intraoperative complications. Anterior mediastinal mass cases in which the airway is compressed require standby rigid bronchoscopy and an experienced bronchoscopist as part of the anesthetic management. The incidence of postoperative complications remains low and is most evident within the first 48 hours after surgery.

References

1. Béchard P, Létourneau L, Lacasse Y, et al.: Perioperative cardiorespiratory complications in adults with mediastinal mass: incidence and risk factors. Anesthesiology 2004; 100:826–34.
2. Capdeville M: The management of a patient with tracheal compression undergoing combined resection of an anterior mediastinal mass and aortic valve replacement with coronary artery bypass graft surgery: utility of the laryngeal mask airway and Aintree intubation catheter. J Cardiothorac Vasc Anesth 2007; 21:259–61.
3. Harte BH, Jaklitsch MT, McKenna SS, et al.: Use of a modified single-lumen endobronchial tube in severe tracheobronchial compression. Anesthesiology 2002; 96:510–11.
4. Goh MH, Liu XY, Goh YS: Anterior mediastinal masses: an anaesthetic challenge. Anaesthesia 1999; 54:670–74.
5. Datt V, Tempe DK: Airway management in patients with mediastinal masses. Indian J Anaesth 2005; 49:344–52.
6. Ahmed-Nusrath A, Swanevelder J: Anaesthesia for mediastinoscopy. Contin Educ Anaesth Crit Care Pain 2007; 7:6–9.
7. Cho Y, Suzuki S, Yokoi M, et al.: Lateral position prevents respiratory occlusion during surgical procedure under general anesthesia in the patient of huge anterior mediastinal lymphoblastic lymphoma. Jpn J Thorac Cardiovasc Surg 2004; 52:476–9.
8. Bitter D: Respiratory obstruction associated with induction of general anesthesia in a patient with mediastinal Hodgkin's disease. Anesth Analg 1975; 59:399–402.
9. Prakash UBS, Abel MD, Hubmayr RD: Mediastinal mass and tracheal obstruction during general anesthesia. Mayo Clin Proc 1988; 63:1004–11.
10. Hnatiuk OW, Corcoran PC, Sierra A: Spirometry in surgery for anterior mediastinal masses. Chest 2001; 120:1152–6.
11. Narang S, Harte BH, Body SC: Anesthesia for patients with a mediastinal mass. Anesthesiol Clin North Am 2001; 19:559–79.
12. Takeda S, Miyoshi S, Omori K, et al.: Surgical rescue for life threatening hypoxemia caused by a mediastinal tumor. Ann Thorac Surg 1999; 68:2324–6.
13. Price SL, Hecker BR: Pulmonary oedema following airway obstruction in a patient with Hodgkin's disease. Br J Anaesth 1987; 59:518–21.

14. Slinger P, Karsli C: Management of the patient with a large anterior mediastinal mass: recurring myths. Curr Opin Anaesthesiol 2007; 20:1–3.
15. Harris GJ, Harman PK, Trinkle JK, et al.: Standard biplane roentgenography is highly sensitive in documenting mediastinal masses. Ann Thorac Surg 1987; 44:238–41.
16. Mendelson DS: Imagining of the thymus. Chest Surg Clin North Am 2001; 11:269–93.
17. Sorgho-Lougue LC, Luciani A, Kobeiter H, et al.: Adenocarcinomas of unknown primary (ACUP) of the mediastinum mimicking lymphoma: CT findings at diagnosis and follow-up. Eur J Radiol 2006; 59:42–8.
18. Campos JH: An update on tracheobronchial anatomy and fiberoptic bronchoscopy on thoracic anesthesia. Curr Opin Anaesthesiol 2009; 22:4–10.
19. Chiles C, Woodard PK, Gutierrez FR, et al.: Metastatic involvement of the heart and pericardium: CT and MR imaging. Radiographics 2001; 21:439–49.
20. Neuman GG, Weingarten AE, Abramowitz RM, et al.: The anesthetic management of the patient with an anterior mediastinal mass. Anesthesiology 1984; 60:144–7.
21. Vander Els NJ, Sorhage F, Bach AM, et al.: Abnormal flow volume loops in patients with intrathoracic Hodgkin's disease. Chest 2000; 117:1256–61.
22. Torchio R, Gulotta C, Perboni A, et al.: Orthopnea and tidal expiratory flow limitation in patients with euthyroid goiter. Chest 2003; 124:133–40.
23. Dursun M, Sarvar S, Cekrezi B, et al.: Cardiac metastasis from invasive thymoma via the superior vena cava: cardiac MRI findings. Cardiovasc Intervent Radiol 2008; 31:S209–S212.
24. Redford DT, Kim AS, Barber BJ, et al.: Transesophageal echocardiography for the intraoperative evaluation of a large anterior mediastinal mass. Anesth Analg 2006; 103:578–9.
25. D'Cruz IA, Feghali N, Gross CM: Echocardiographic manifestations of mediastinal masses compressing or encroaching on the heart. Echocardiography 1994; 11:523–33.
26. Webster JA, Self DD: Anesthesia for pericardial window in a pregnant patient with cardiac tamponade and mediastinal mass. Can J Anaesth 2003; 50:815–8.
27. Allen GC, Byford LJ, Shamji FM: Anterior mediastinal mass in a patient susceptible to malignant hyperthermia. Can J Anaesth 1993; 40:46–9.

28. Flaherty S, Grishkin BA: Airway obstruction by anterior mediastinal mass. Successful management by percutaneous aspiration. Chest 1994; 106:947–8.

29. Hagberg H, Ahlström HK, Magnusson A, et al.: Value of transsternal core biopsy in patients with a newly diagnosed mediastinal mass. Acta Oncol 2000; 39:195–8.

30. Fang WT, Xu MY, Chen G, et al.: Minimally invasive approaches for histological diagnosis of anterior mediastinal masses. Chin Med J 2007; 120:675–9.

31. Watanabe M, Takagi K, Aoki T, et al.: A comparison of biopsy through a parasternal anterior mediastinotomy under local anesthesia and percutaneous needle biopsy for malignant anterior mediastinal tumors. Surg Today 1998; 28:1022–6.

32. Yoshino I, Hashizume M, Shimada M, et al.: Thoracoscopic thymomectomy with the da Vinci computer-enhanced surgical system. J Thorac Cardiovasc Surg 2001; 122:783–5.

33. DeRose JJ, Jr., Swistel DG, Safavi A, et al.: Mediastinal mass evaluation using advanced robotic techniques. Ann Thorac Surg 2003; 75:571–3.

34. Bodner J, Wykypiel H, Wetscher G, et al.: First experiences with the da Vinci operating robot in thoracic surgery. Eur J Cardiothorac Surg 2004; 25:844–51.

35. Bodner J, Wykypiel H, Greiner A, et al.: Early experience with robot-assisted surgery for mediastinal masses. Ann Thorac Surg 2004; 78:259–65.

36. Savitt MA, Gao G, Furnary AP, et al.: Application of robotic-assisted techniques to the surgical evaluation and treatment of the anterior mediastinum. Ann Thorac Surg 2005; 79:450–5.

37. Cakar F, Werner P, Augustin F, et al.: A comparison of outcomes after robotic open extended thymectomy for myasthenia gravis. Eur J Cardiothorac Surg 2007; 31:501–5.

38. Silbert KS, Biondi JW, Hirsch NP: Spontaneous respiration during thoracotomy in a patient with a mediastinal mass. Anesth Analg 1987; 66:904–7.

39. Pullerits J, Holzman R: Anaesthesia for patients with mediastinal masses. Can J Anaesth 1989; 36:681–8.

40. Mizrahi S, Laari Y, Lugassy G, et al.: Major airway obstruction relieved by helium/oxygen breathing. Crit Care Med 1986; 14:986–7.

41. Curtis JL, Mahlmeister M, Fink JB, et al.: Helium-oxygen gas therapy. Use and availability for the emergency treatment of inoperable airway obstruction. Chest 1986; 90:455–7.

42. Younker D, Clark R, Coveler L: Fiberoptic endobronchial intubation for resection of an anterior mediastinal mass. Anesthesiology 1989; 70:144–6.

43. Petruzzelli GJ, deVries EJ, Johnson J, et al.: Extrinsic tracheal compression from an anterior mediastinal mass in an adult: the multidisciplinary management of the airway emergency. Otolaryngol Head Neck Surg 1990; 103:484–6.
44. Narula N, Katyal S, Tewari A, et al.: Intraoperative life threatening airway obstruction in a patient with mediastinal mass. Indian J Anaesth 2006; 50:214–7.
45. Jensen V, Milne B, Salerno T: Femoral-femoral cardiopulmonary bypass prior to induction of anaesthesia in the management of upper airway obstruction. Can Anaesth Soc J 1983; 30:270–2.
46. Tempe DK, Arya R, Dubey S, et al.: Mediastinal mass resection: femorofemoral cardiopulmonary bypass before induction of anesthesia in the management of airway obstruction. J Cardiothorac Vasc Anesth 2001; 15:233–6.
47. Sinha PK, Dubey PK, Singh S: Identifying tracheomalacia. Br J Anaesth 2000; 84:127–8.
48. Geelhoed GW: Tracheomalacia from compression goiter: management after thyroidectomy. Surgery 1988; 104:1100–8.

Jeremy L. Bricker, MD, MS
Jerry V. Young, PharmD, MD
John Butterworth, MD

The Patient with a Tumor Invading the Vena Cava

12

INTRODUCTION

Tumors that invade the vena cava present a number of challenges to the anesthesiologist and surgeon when the time comes for surgical resection. This chapter will review the characteristics of the various tumors known to invade the vena cava. It will provide a discussion of the typical clinical presentation and the differential diagnosis, and recommended work-up of the patient with an invasive vena cava tumors. The chapter will include a description of the suggested approach to preoperative anesthetic evaluation and intraoperative management and monitoring of these complex patients. The overall goal of the management is to decrease the perioperative risks associated with resection of vena caval tumor thrombi, while ensuring intraoperative stability. Finally, the surgical techniques for tumor resection will be discussed with particular emphasis on the anesthetic implications of the surgical options. Much of the content of this chapter will relate to renal cell carcinoma (RCC) because of the frequency with which this cell type invades the vena cava as well as the abundance of literature on the subject (1–4). One of the most critical factors for optimizing perioperative care of these complex cases is to ensure a thoughtful dialog between the anesthesiologist and surgeon(s).

Medically Challenging Patients Undergoing Cardiothoracic Surgery, edited by Neal H. Cohen, MD, MPH, MS, Lippincott Williams & Wilkins, Baltimore © 2009.

TUMOR CELL TYPES

Renal Cell Carcinoma (RCC)

RCC is probably the most-studied and most frequently encountered of all the tumors that invade the vena cava. RCC accounts for 2%–3% of adult cancers and 85% of all primary malignant renal tumors (5–9). RCC originates from proximal renal tubular epithelium and is classified histologically as converted clear cell, papillary (chromophilic), chromophobe, collecting duct, neuroendocrine, or unclassified. The most common form of RCC is the converted clear cell carcinoma type (5, 6, 10, 11). Worldwide, there are 210,000 new cases of RCC diagnosed annually (6). The peak incidence occurs in the fifth and sixth decades of life. No matter the age of presentation, RRC has a 2:1 male/female predominance (5).

Patients with RCC typically present with hematuria, flank pain, palpable flank mass, weight loss, anemia, and/or fever. Over the past few years, an increasing number of cases have been detected in asymptomatic patients who have undergone routine screening or imaging for an unrelated problem (5, 7, 10, 12, 13). In 4%–10% of patients with RCC, the tumor invades the lumen of the inferior vena cava (IVC), and in up to one quarter of these patients the tumor extends cephalad to the level of the hepatic veins (9, 12–16). IVC invasion may lead to bilateral pedal edema with or without deep vein thrombosis (DVT) [and its associated risk of pulmonary embolism (PE)], Budd–Chiari syndrome (with associated liver dysfunction or failure), and/or varicosities (secondary to IVC obstruction) (12, 13, 17–20). In 1% of RCC cases, the most cephalad portion of the tumor will extend into the right atrium or ventricle, often leading to syncope, arrhythmias, dyspnea on exertion, palpitations, and/or other signs and symptoms of tricuspid regurgitation or obstruction (3, 9, 12, 15, 21–23). Because of the risk of sudden death from thrombosis or embolism, patients presenting with cardiac involvement require prompt evaluation and surgical resection (3, 23, 24). Curiously, direct extension of RCC into the venous system can occur in the absence of metastatic disease, even though roughly one quarter of all newly diagnosed patients with RCC present with metastases (5, 6, 8, 12, 25). Metastases are most commonly found in the lungs, but can also be found in bone (osteolytic), regional lymph nodes, the liver, the brain, and the adrenal glands (5).

Risk factors for RCC include cigarette smoking, exposure to asbestos/petroleum products/heavy metals, and cystic disease associated with end-stage renal disease (5). Only a small fraction of RCC cases are familial, occurring in the forms of hereditary clear cell carcinoma, hereditary papillary renal carcinoma, and RCC associated with von Hippel–Lindau syndrome (5).

Staging using the diagnostic modalities discussed later in this chapter provides an important basis for formulating an appropriate treatment plan and determining the prognosis for an individual patient (5). The American Joint Committee on Cancer's 2002 Tumor–Node–etastasis (TNM) Staging System for RCC is generally recommended for clinical and scientific use (Table 12–1) (7, 26).

RCC is poorly responsive to either cytotoxic agents or immunotherapy (interferon-α and interleukin-2); therefore, the primary treatment remains radical nephrectomy, with removal of the kidney, surrounding fascia, ipsilateral adrenal gland, and upper portion of the ureter (5, 6, 10, 13, 14, 17, 27–29). Patients with metastatic disease formerly were not regarded as surgical candidates because of the low survival rate. The 5-year survival for the patient with metastatic RCC is <10%. In the past surgery was performed to provide palliative relief of pain or hemorrhage from the primary tumor (1, 5, 14). However, recent data suggest that surgical resection followed by immunotherapy improves survival in some patients with metastatic disease (5, 6, 10, 30). As a result, more patients with metastatic RCC are being referred for surgical resection.

Survival following tumor resection is directly related to the initial tumor stage (including the presence or absence of lymph node or visceral metastasis or perinephric fat invasion) and the completeness of tumor resection (complete vs. incomplete) (5, 10, 13, 28, 31–33). Interestingly, there are many reports that involvement of the IVC by RCC tumor thrombus does not affect the prognosis of patients following complete surgical resection, but does increase the surgical morbidity and mortality of tumor resection (6, 9, 13, 16, 28, 31, 33, 34). Recent 5-year survival rates for stages I, II, III, and IV are 96%, 82%, 64%, and 23%, respectively (26).

Testicular Carcinoma

Testis cancers may sometimes invade the lumen of the IVC, either by intravascular extension or IVC wall erosion. The incidence of testicular tumors in the United States is 9 per 100,000 males, and testicular tumors are the most common malignancy in men 18–35 years old (35–37). Ninety-five percent of testicular cancers are germ cell tumors (GCTs), which can be highly aggressive; the remaining 5% of testicular tumors are typically benign (35). Twenty to thirty percent of patients with GCTs present with metastatic disease; nevertheless, even with widespread disease, the prognosis remains favorable, with 80%–90% of newly diagnosed patients obtaining a cure (35, 36). When present, metastases are most often found in the retroperitoneal lymph nodes, the lungs, the liver, the brain, or bone (35, 37).

TABLE 12-1. The American Joint Committee on Cancer's 2002 Tumor–Node–Metastasis (TNM) Staging System for RCC

Primary Tumor (T)

TX: Primary tumor cannot be assessed

T0: No evidence of primary tumor

T1: Tumor 7 cm or less in greatest dimension, limited to the kidney

T1a: Tumor 4 cm or less in greatest dimension, limited to the kidney

T1b: Tumor .4 cm but not .7 cm in greatest dimension, limited to the kidney

T2: Tumor .7 cm in greatest dimension, limited to the kidney

T3: Tumor extends into major veins or invades adrenal gland or perinephric tissues but not beyond Gerota's fascia

T3a: Tumor directly invades the adrenal gland or perirenal and/or renal sinus fat but not beyond Gerota's fascia

T3b: Tumor grossly extends into the renal vein or its segmental (muscle-containing) branches, or vena cava below the diaphragm

T3c: Tumor grossly extends into vena cava above diaphragm or invades the wall of the vena cava

T4: Tumor invades beyond Gerota's fascia

Regional Lymph Nodes (N)

NX: Regional lymph nodes cannot be assessed

N0: No regional lymph node metastases

N1: Metastases in a single regional lymph node

N2: Metastases in more than one regional lymph node

Distant Metastasis (M)

MX: Distant metastasis cannot be assessed

M0: No distant metastasis

M1: Distant metastasis

Stage Grouping

Stage I	T1, N0, M0
Stage II	T2, N0, M0
Stage III	T1, N1, M0
	T2, N1, M0
	T3, N0, M0
	T3, N1, M0
Stage IV	T4, N0, M0
	T4, N1, M0
	Any T, N2, M0
	Any T, Any N, M1

Risk factors for GCTs include cryptorchidism, exogenous estrogen administration to the mother during pregnancy, trauma, and infection-related testicular atrophy (35). For patients with cryptorchidism, orchiopexy early in life, although not altering malignant potential, does facilitate examination and tumor detection (35). The classic presentation of a testicular tumor is painless enlargement of the testis. Any such masses should be considered cancerous until proven otherwise (19, 35). Other presenting signs and symptoms may include testicular pain, anorexia, lymphadenopathy, gynecomastia, bone pain (if bone metastasis is present), back pain (if retroperitoneal lymph nodes are involved), and/or dyspnea (if pulmonary metastasis is present) (35, 36). Lower extremity edema with or without DVT and the associated risk of PE can be seen in cases of IVC involvement (35, 36, 38).

Treatment plans for testicular cancer begin with radical orchiectomy using an inguinal approach and definitive, histological diagnosis (20, 35), assuming there is no evidence of IVC extension. Following orchiectomy, treatment depends on staging and the tumor cell type and may include any one or combination of observation, radiation, platinum-based chemotherapy, and surgery (19, 35).

Between 3% and 11% of testis tumors will invade the IVC and only rarely will there be right-heart involvement (19, 37–39). As with any caval tumor, it is important to determine the proximal extent of IVC invasion preoperatively to plan for the appropriate surgical technique and anesthetic management (14, 15, 17). Whereas RCC spreads intravascularly to the IVC via the renal vein, testicular cancer spreads to the IVC via the gonadal vein (36). Unlike RCC, testicular cancer can also invade the IVC by eroding into the cava when tumor spreads to the retroperitoneal lymph nodes (36, 38). Both forms of IVC involvement occur more often with right-sided than left-sided tumors (36). Surgical techniques for resection of testicular tumors that have spread intravascularly to the IVC are similar to those used for RCC (see "Surgical Techniques" section).

Intravenous Leiomyomatosis

Intravenous leiomyomatosis (IVL) is a condition in which a benign, smooth muscle tumor grows into venous channels and/or lymphatics (3, 40). IVL typically arises from uterine leiomyomas (fibroids) or the smooth muscle portion of uterine venous walls (3, 18, 22). IVL occurs most commonly in middle aged, white women, 90% of whom will be parous (3, 22, 40). Signs and symptoms of IVL include menstrual irregularity, dysmenorrhea, pelvic or abdominal pain, and/or palpable masses (18, 22). Some patients remain asymptomatic until IVC or right-heart involvement occurs (22, 24). Patients may undergo treatment with a gonadotropin-releasing hormone agonist to decrease tumor size prior to having a total abdominal hysterectomy (TAH) with bilateral salpingo-oophorectomy (BSO) and surgical resection of intravenous tumor thrombus (21, 40, 41).

In 10% of IVL cases the intravenous tumor thrombus can extend to the IVC and/or right heart (3, 18). The tumor typically gains access to the venous system via the uterine or ovarian vein, then grows through the common iliac vein to the IVC (18, 22). IVC or right heart/tricuspid valve involvement produces the expected signs and symptoms, including lower extremity or abdominal wall edema, Budd–Chiari syndrome, ascites, syncope, dyspnea on exertion, palpitations, orthopnea, pleuritic chest pain, paroxysmal nocturnal dyspnea, and/or sudden death (3, 18, 22). Patients with IVC and/or right-heart involvement should undergo prompt preoperative evaluation and complete surgical resection of the tumor thrombus, in much the same way as is done for patients with RCC, with simultaneous TAH/BSO (3, 21, 24).

Additional Tumors

Other tumors that will occasionally invade the vena cava include hepatocellular, thyroid, and adrenal carcinoma; pheochromocytoma; and leiomyosarcoma. The management of the primary tumor will vary, but the surgical and anesthetic issues related to the IVC extension are similar to the management of the other IVC tumors.

DIAGNOSTIC EVALUATION

Standard diagnostic evaluation of a patient with a suspected abdominal or pelvic tumor typically includes a medical history, physical examination, computed tomography (CT) or magnetic resonance imaging (MRI) of the abdomen and pelvis, and a chest radiograph (5). Laboratory testing often includes a basic metabolic panel (BMP, which includes measurement of electrolytes, blood urea nitrogen, and creatinine), liver function tests, and a complete blood count (CBC) (5). Tumor markers (such as human chorionic gonadotropin and alpha-fetoprotein) and urine analysis/cytology should be obtained when indicated based on the presumed type of tumor (5, 20, 35, 37). Some tumor forms may be initially diagnosed using pelvic, abdominal, or testicular ultrasonography (17, 35, 40). If metastatic disease is suspected, CT or MRI of the chest and head and a radionuclide bone scan may be indicated (5, 13, 28).

Invasion of the renal vein, IVC, or right atrium can be determined using a number of techniques, including MRI or CT, inferior venacavography, or echocardiography (12). Preoperative transesophageal echocardiography (TEE) should be considered if tumor thrombus extends to the level of the diaphragmatic IVC or when other modalities are inconclusive (17). MRI has been shown to be superior to CT when vascular extension is present (6, 12, 42). Currently, venacavography is used only when venous anatomy is poorly visualized with other types of imaging (5, 16, 43).

Tumor extension to these intravascular locations will greatly affect the surgical technique employed to resect the tumor as well as the anesthetic management of the patient (14, 15, 17).

PREOPERATIVE ANESTHETIC EVALUATION

For patients scheduled to undergo primary tumor excision, and for whom IVC invasion is not present, preoperative evaluation includes a comprehensive medical history and physical examination. It will usually include a chest radiograph and an electrocardiogram, although multiple studies have shown that these studies have a low diagnostic yield in the absence of symptoms. Laboratory studies should include a measurement of hemoglobin, to which many clinicians will add a CBC and BMP. Additional testing may be indicated by the patient's concomitant disease(s), functional status, and physiologic stress associated with the particular type of tumor resection being undertaken. For example, additional assessment of pulmonary function might be indicated in a patient with severe chronic lung disease who will undergo a thoracoabdominal incision.

Tumor extension to intravascular locations may greatly change the surgical and anesthetic approach to the patient (14, 15, 17) and mandates a more comprehensive preoperative evaluation. As noted earlier for RCC, patients with tumors that invade the vena cava have an increased risk of surgical morbidity and mortality: Invasion of the IVC increases surgical risk fourfold, largely because of increases in the rates of perioperative stroke and myocardial infarction (16, 44, 45). Additionally, the risk of surgical complications is twofold greater when tumor thrombi extend to the level of the hepatic veins (or more proximal) compared to thrombi that have a less proximal extension (28).

To develop an anesthetic plan that will address the clinical needs of the patient and clarify the surgical approach, the anesthesiologist should review all imaging studies to document the cephalad extension of the tumor thrombus, to determine whether the thrombus adheres to, or invades, the wall of the IVC, and to evaluate the degree of IVC obstruction (11–13). Ideally, these studies should be completed within a short period of time before surgery, because tumor thrombus may extend "further" during the interval between evaluation and surgery if there is a prolonged delay between imaging and induction of anesthesia (12, 17).

Paraneoplastic syndromes secondary to abnormal production of hormones often occur in patients with malignant disease and may lead to a required alteration in anesthetic management. For example, frequent paraneoplastic syndromes associated with RCC include erythrocytosis, hypercalcemia, nonmetastatic hepatic dysfunction (Stauffer syndrome), hypertension, feminization or masculinization, and Cushing syndrome

TABLE 12–2. Commonly used chemotherapeutic agents for
testicular cancer and their associated side effects

Cisplatin: Renal impairment, myelosuppression, peripheral neuropathy
Bleomycin: Pulmonary fibrosis, fevers, chills
Vinblastine: Peripheral and autonomic neuropathy, myelosuppression
Ifosfamide: Central nervous system toxicity, myelosuppression
Cyclophosphamide: Myelosuppression
Dactinomycin: Myelosuppression
Etoposide: Myelosuppression

(5). The preoperative evaluation should include an assessment of the
physiologic sequelae associated with these paraneoplastic syndromes.

Direct and indirect actions of chemotherapeutic agents also must be
considered during the preoperative anesthetic evaluation for those
patients who have received preoperative chemotherapy. As previously
noted, RCCs are rarely treated with cytotoxic agents because of their usual
lack of response; in contrast, testicular cancers are often treated with
chemotherapy. Common chemotherapeutic agents used in the treatment
of testicular cancer, and their side effects, are outlined in Table 12–2 (46).

Postoperative respiratory failure or acute respiratory distress syndrome has been reported following retroperitoneal lymph node dissection
and other major surgeries in patients treated with bleomycin. Respiratory
complications associated with bleomycin toxicity typically occur 3–10
days after the operation (47, 48). A long list of risk factors, many still controversial, have been identified, including overly generous perioperative
fluid administration (which we believe to be the most important factor),
intraoperative hyperoxia (still controversial since it was first proposed in
the early 1980s), preexisting pulmonary injury (including prior irradia-
tion of the chest), significant smoking history, age >70 years, renal failure,
concomitant administration of other chemotherapeutic agents, and total
bleomycin dose >450–500 mg (as opposed to a lower total dose) (47, 48).
Based on these observations, our recommendation is to maintain FiO_2 at
a level <0.3 (provided arterial oxygen saturation can be maintained) and
to minimize fluid administration using a 1:2 ratio of colloid to crystalloid
consistent with hemodynamic stability and adequate urine output (38,
47, 48). Some authors recommend that nitrous oxide not be used because
of a perceived risk for worsening bone marrow suppression; however,
we can find no data that confirm that there is a bone-marrow–related benefit to avoiding nitrous oxide in these patients. We recommend postoperative neuraxial analgesia both for the better quality of analgesia and in

TABLE 12–3.   System of classification for cephalad extent of IVC tumor thrombus

Level I: <2 cm above the ostium of the renal vein in the IVC

Level II: Below the origin of the hepatic veins

Level III: Above the level of the hepatic veins but below the diaphragm

Level IV: Above the level of the diaphragm

the hope of preventing postoperative splinting and atelectasis through reducing the pain from upper abdominal and flank incisions.

Many surgical techniques are feasible for resection of tumors invading the IVC, and different techniques have different intraoperative anesthetic requirements (see "Surgical Techniques" section).

ASSESSING THE EXTENT OF IVC INVOLVEMENT

The level of invasion of the IVC by tumor thrombus dictates the surgical technique (14, 15, 17, 42). There are many systems available to classify the level of IVC involvement by tumor thrombus. One such system commonly used for classifying the extent of cephalad spread of tumor thrombus in the IVC is provided in Table 13–3 (11).

Levels I and II are treated similarly in terms of surgical technique and anesthetic management (13, 14). Moreover, the associated risk is also similar (28). Tumors that extend beyond the level of the hepatic veins (Levels III and IV) are more troublesome and dangerous to resect (14, 28, 45).

INTRAOPERATIVE MONITORING

The need for monitoring beyond the "standard" devices (continuous electrocardiography, noninvasive blood pressure, pulse oximetry, temperature, capnography, and inspired/expired gas analysis) depends on the patient's physical status, extent of disease and level of tumor extension proximally in the IVC or heart, and the surgical technique to be employed. For resection of vena caval invasive tumors, invasive blood pressure and central venous pressure (CVP) monitoring are often used. The placement of central catheters has greater potential risk in these patients. Care must be exercised not to dislodge intracardiac tumor thrombus with guide wires when placing subclavian or internal jugular catheters with the Seldinger technique (18). TEE guidance may be of value in this clinical situation (18). When there is complete occlusion of the IVC by tumor thrombus or when there is tumor extension to the tricuspid valve, we recommend that invasive blood pressure monitoring

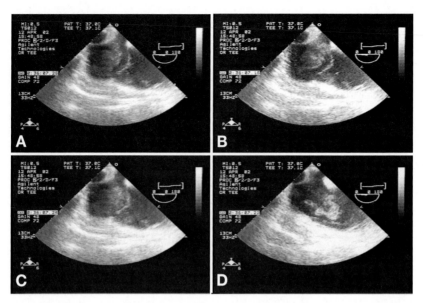

FIGURE 12–1. Transesophageal images of a patient undergoing resection of renal cell carcinoma. The echocardiographer was called emergently by a colleague to diagnose the cause of sudden hemodynamic collapse in a patient undergoing resection of a Level II, Stage III renal cell carcinoma. All images were obtained with the probe in the midesophageal position at 0°. In ventricular systole, a 2 × 3 cm mass is seen to spin freely in the right atrium (A and B). With the approach of ventricular diastole, the mass approaches the tricuspid valve (C). During diastole filling of the right ventricle, the tumor fills but is unable to cross the tricuspid valve (D), then returns to a right atrial position (not shown).

be initiated prior to induction of anesthesia, given the risk for sudden and profound hypotension (Figure 12–1). CVP monitoring may not be possible.

The indications for pulmonary artery catheterization remain controversial for nearly all surgical patients, and the use of the catheter for these patients has the same potential risks and benefits. However, we do not place pulmonary artery catheters when there is an intraatrial tumor thrombus because of our concern about the potential for the catheter to dislodge and propagate tumor emboli (9, 49). We strongly recommend TEE as a safer and more useful monitoring option.

TRANESOPHAGEAL ECHOCARDIOGRAPHY (TEE)

In cases with IVC or atrial involvement, we find TEE exceptionally useful for multiple reasons, perhaps most importantly because we can use TEE to define the most cephalad extent of tumor thrombus accurately

TABLE 12–4.   Advantages of intraoperative TEE during resection of vena caval invasive tumors

Minimally invasive, accurate measurement of cephalic spread of intracaval tumor

Differentiation of free floating tumor thrombus and adherent tumor thrombus

Determination of degree of IVC occlusion

Assessment of the completeness of tumor thrombus resection

Diagnosis of tumor embolization

Evaluation of cause of hemodynamic instability

Assessment of right- and left-heart function

Guidance for placement of clamps, guide wires, and catheters

Evaluation of cardiac anatomy

and safely at the time of operation (13, 17, 44, 50). A long-axis view of the IVC will define the cephalic extent of tumor, the degree of caval occlusion, and the characteristics of the tumor "head" (51). In case reports and in our personal experiences, some patients have a more cranial extension of tumor thrombus on intraoperative TEE then had been reported in preoperative imaging studies (12, 17, 44, 50). The tumor extension will sometimes be great enough to necessitate significant changes in the surgical plan (12, 17, 27).

After defining the extent of tumor invasion, continuing use of TEE can provide valuable information during the surgical resection (see Table 12–4). A properly performed and interpreted TEE examination is of value in assessing right- and left-heart function, evaluating cardiac valves and other features of cardiac anatomy, and determining the adequacy of ventricular end-diastolic volume (42, 51, 52). When there are sudden and unexplained changes in vital signs, TEE can identify intracardiac obstructing lesions in real time (52). An echocardiographer faced by sudden, severe hypotension associated with tumor thrombus near the tricuspid valve, right atrial dilation, failure of tricuspid leaflets to coapt, and an underfilled right ventricle can recommend immediate surgical removal of a tumor thrombus obstructing the tricuspid valve using cardiopulmonary bypass (CPB) as a life-saving maneuver (9, 49). Specific diagnosis of intraoperative PE can be challenging: The signs and clinical symptoms are often nonspecific (53). In this setting, continuous TEE examination aids in safe resection of IVC tumor thrombus by allowing rapid diagnosis of tumor embolization (42, 44, 50–54) (Figure 12–1).

Whenever tumor thrombus is present in the IVC and whenever major vessels will be opened to air there will be a risk of embolism; however, fewer than 0.4% of all RCCs and no more than 5% of those with IVC involvement will embolize during surgery (50, 52). The risk of intraoperative PE *may* be lower in cases of IVL because of the less friable, firm consistency of the tumor (18). Nevertheless, we (and others) recommend TEE whenever a vena caval tumor thrombus is present.

When tumor emboli are detected in the right heart by TEE, manipulation of the embolic source should stop and the IVC may need clamping to prevent additional emboli from entering the heart (53, 54). TEE will often fail to identify pulmonary emboli that have migrated to the periphery of the pulmonary circulation or that are located in the left pulmonary artery (visualization is impaired by the left main bronchus) (52, 53). If other causes of severe hypotension, including acute hemorrhage, IVC compression, anaphylaxis, pericardial tamponade, or myocardial ischemia, have been ruled out and no cause can be found, one can presumptively diagnose PE using indirect evidence obtained by TEE examination (53). Signs of right ventricular outflow obstruction, including right atrial, right ventricular, or pulmonary artery dilation, interatrial septal bulging into the left atrium, or right-to-left shunting through a patent foramen ovale, support a diagnosis of PE (9, 53). Other signs consistent with PE include increased pulmonary artery pressure or CVP, hepatic engorgement, decreased end-tidal CO_2 tension, and an increased ratio of arterial CO_2 tension to end-tidal CO_2 tension (50, 52, 53). If hemodynamic instability continues, CPB and pulmonary artery embolectomy may be required to optimize perfusion and cardiac function and facilitate safe tumor removal (9, 42, 50, 52, 53, 55).

Finally, although continuous monitoring has some value, particularly for diagnosing tumor emboli, it is important to use TEE to confirm tumor and/or thrombus removal after the surgical excision is completed (12, 13, 42, 50, 52, 53).

INDUCTION AND MAINTENANCE OF ANESTHESIA

In most patients with IVC tumors, induction and maintenance of anesthesia can be guided by the preferences of the individual clinician although they must be modified based on the clinical manifestations of the tumor and associated medical conditions. For example, in some cases as a result of renal or hepatic dysfunction, drug doses may require adjustments although typically no specific changes in selection of induction agents are required. A more significant concern is the effect of tumor occlusion of the IVC on venous return, particularly after administration of drugs that compromise venous return or after initiation of positive pressure ventilation. Patients with complete occlusion of the IVC by tumor thrombus are often assumed to present special concerns with regard to hypotension during anesthesia. In these cases, have vasopressor solutions mixed and ready for use before induction. As discussed previously, this is a setting in which TEE would likely be of value in differentiating the cause of hypotension.

Patients with Level IV IVC involvement may have tricuspid regurgitation or obstruction secondary to tumor thrombus. If so, the manifestations of these complications must be considered during induction of anesthesia. Tricuspid regurgitation, even when associated with moderate-to-severe degrees of right atrial volume overload, is usually well-tolerated provided that adequate ventricular filling is maintained. Conversely, acute tricuspid obstruction can lead to cardiac arrest and may require initiation of CPB to facilitate immediate thrombectomy (49).

Our preference is to titrate ketamine for induction of anesthesia in patients with Level IV IVC tumors, although other induction agents can be used safely as well. One of the primary goals during induction is to ensure maintenance of CVP and intravascular volume (as assessed by TEE) in the "high normal range," and to avoid potential triggers of increased pulmonary vascular resistance (e.g., hypercarbia) during maintenance of anesthesia in these patients.

ADDITIONAL ANESTHETIC CONSIDERATIONS

Many patients with RCC will present with anemia, and an occasional patient may require preoperative blood transfusion (27). The "trigger" for transfusion before, during, and after surgery is poorly defined and represents the point where a clinician's best estimate is that the risks of transfusion are fewer than the risks of avoiding transfusion. In most cases, we transfuse patients with cerebrovascular and/or coronary artery disease (both of which are common in patients with RCC) to hematocrits of 25% or greater. Whether preoperative transfusion is provided or not, every patient who undergoes surgical excision of an IVC tumor must have secure venous access including one or more large-bore intravenous catheters (14 or 16 g).

One of the most challenging aspects of the surgical and anesthetic management of the patient with IVC tumor occurs at the time of cross-clamping of the vena cava. The degree to which blood pressure and heart rate respond to IVC cross-clamping will vary widely from patient to patient and depend on the level at which the IVC is clamped (42). Patients who present to the operating room with nearly complete occlusion of the IVC by tumor thrombus often have little hemodynamic instability, probably because they have well-established collateral venous channels (4, 11, 14, 38, 56). These channels also will tend to increase the risk of intraoperative blood loss (11, 36). For other patients, the hemodynamic changes can be significant. As will be discussed in greater detail later in this chapter, severe cardiovascular instability may be associated with IVC cross-clamping above the level of the hepatic veins and may require creation of a venovenous shunt or initiation of CPB (28, 42). Additionally, many patients will have abrupt declines in blood pressure following release of the IVC clamp.

The other potential risk related to manipulation of the tumor within and around the IVC is embolization of tumor. The tumor can dislodge during palpation of the IVC or cross-clamping. In addition, the risk of tumor or clot embolization does not necessarily end after completion of the surgical procedure, but may also occur in some patients postoperatively (50). Therefore, embolism should remain in the differential diagnosis of unexplained postoperative hypotension.

SURGICAL TECHNIQUES

The surgical approach will be dictated by the extent of the tumor thrombus into the proximal vena cava, the degree of vena caval wall involvement, the tumor size, and surgeon preference, in large part based on past clinical experience and an understanding of the anatomy. In addition, as part of the assessment of the patient, the surgeon should discuss with the anesthesiologist whether the procedure can be most successfully completed with or without CPB (12–15, 17, 42). We and others recommend that these complex operations be undertaken only in specialized facilities where TEE and CPB are readily available (13, 42, 56). As is usually the case in surgical oncology, a complete resection of the tumor and any associated tumor thrombus will increase the chances for prolonged survival, so the surgical approach and experience of the surgeon in complete resection become critical factors in the postoperative course of the patient (3, 14, 22).

The likelihood that segmental cavectomy will be needed varies depending on the tumor type. RCCs with vena caval extension usually will not adhere to or invade the IVC wall or right atrium, obviating the need for caval resection (5, 13, 56, 57). In most of these cases, the tumor can be removed from the IVC without compromising the integrity of the vena cava itself. Testicular cancers, in contrast, have a greater tendency to invade the wall of the retroperitoneal IVC, often requiring that a portion of the IVC be resected (36, 38, 58). The reported incidence of IVC involvement by metastatic testicular cancer necessitating IVC resection is 7%–11% (58). IVC resection for testicular cancer normally presents few intraoperative hemodynamic problems because the involved vena cava is typically inferior to the renal veins (19, 38). Because extensive collateral venous channels usually have developed, most surgeons perform cavectomy with ligation, without reconstruction (38, 58). A patch or graft can be placed if deemed necessary (59). When larger and/or more cephalad portions of the cava must be removed, replacement of the resected vena cava with prosthetic or autologous (vein or pericardium) grafts is usually required (13, 56, 57). Renal vein involvement may require nephrectomy for complete tumor resection (38). Some surgeons will resect testicular IVC tumor thrombus or place an IVC filter prior to initiating chemotherapy to reduce the risk of tumor embolization during chemotherapy and radiotherapy (19).

Tumor thrombi located below the insertion of the hepatic veins (Levels I and II) are typically removed following IVC isolation (33, 45). IVC isolation includes clamping of the infrarenal IVC, contralateral renal vein, and IVC between the most cephalad extent of tumor thrombus and the hepatic veins (13, 14, 56, 60). Many Level I tumor thrombi can be removed without IVC isolation or cross-clamping simply by reducing the tumor thrombus into the renal vein and placing a distal renal vein clamp (11, 61). These maneuvers are done in an attempt to prevent migration of tumor emboli to the heart or pulmonary vasculature where they could result in pulmonary metastatic disease or hemodynamic instability (4, 13, 25, 42, 45). The tumor thrombus then can be removed via inferior venacavotomy or a circumferential cut around the insertion of the affected renal vein (13, 45, 60). Depending on the location of the tumor, limited liver mobilization or retraction may be needed (50). Only occasionally will an infrahepatic tumor thrombus require extracorporeal circulation (11, 61).

Tumor thrombi extending above the level of the hepatic veins (Levels III and IV) create a greater challenge by increasing the risk for bleeding, tumor embolization, and postoperative hepatic and/or renal dysfunction (14, 45). There is only limited consensus as to the optimal operative treatment for these patients (14, 32, 33, 45). Extensive liver mobilization and dissection often will be required to achieve adequate IVC exposure for segmental isolation (11, 62). It is sometimes possible to convert a Level III or Level IV thrombus to a Level II thrombus by "milking" the IVC to reduce the cephalad extension of the tumor thrombus (14, 50, 61). When successful, this approach allows the surgical team to clamp the IVC below the hepatic veins, allowing better blood return to the heart for greater hemodynamic stability, and leading to less engorgement of the liver and associated postoperative liver dysfunction (14, 44). At this time, the tumor thrombus can be removed by venacavotomy as described earlier in this chapter.

If the proximal extent of a Level III tumor thrombus cannot be moved caudad to the hepatic veins, an IVC clamp or an endoluminal occluder must be placed in a suprahepatic location cephalad to the furthest extent of the tumor thrombus (13, 28, 61). After cross-clamping, if the patient develops hemodynamic instability, extensive bleeding from collateral veins, or hepatic engorgement, venovenous shunting, hepatic vascular occlusion (Pringle maneuver), or initiation of cardiopulmonary bypass may be required (11, 28, 61).

As mentioned previously, some patients with supradiaphragmatic tumor thrombus (Level IV) will demonstrate free-floating tumor thrombi on TEE (11). In these cases it may be possible to reduce the tumor thrombus to a location below the diaphragm and, if successful, treat it as a Level III tumor thrombus (11, 45, 56, 63). CPB with or without deep hypothermic circulatory arrest (DHCA), as described later in this chapter, is used by many surgeons to resect nonreducible Level IV tumor thrombi (32, 45, 62).

Venovenous Bypass

For patients with tumor thrombi extending to a level between the hepatic veins and the diaphragm in which the IVC must be cross-clamped at a "high" location, venovenous bypass may be required to prevent hemodynamic instability and decrease perioperative morbidity (6, 11). Venovenous bypass is performed by inserting one venous cannula into the IVC distal to the most caudad extent of tumor thrombus and inserting another venous cannula into the right atrium (11, 61). The cannulae are then connected with heparin-bonded shunt tubing and attached to a centrifugal pump (11, 61). Alternative sites for cannulation include the femoral, internal jugular, or axillary vein (4, 11, 34, 42, 61, 64). The specific sites for cannulation will be determined by the location of the tumor thrombus and other anatomic considerations for each patient.

As noted previously, patients presenting with complete or near-complete occlusion of the IVC often tolerate "high" IVC cross-clamping without hemodynamic compromise because of the established collateral venous channels that have developed (4, 11, 14, 38, 56). Venovenous bypass is most often used in patients with tumor thrombi extending to a level between the hepatic veins and the diaphragm, although some surgeons will also use this technique for patients with supradiaphragmatic tumor thrombi and only partial occlusion of the IVC (11, 60). In those situations, venovenous bypass serves not only to prevent hemodynamic instability, but also to increase the chances for complete tumor resection by allowing for an unhurried, thorough inspection of the IVC (11, 34, 61). Additional advantages of venovenous bypass versus CPB with DHCA include decreased operating time, avoidance of hypothermia and systemic anticoagulation (and the associated risk of coagulopathy), decreased blood loss, and decreased rate of postoperative complications (11, 34, 60, 61, 65). Disadvantages of venovenous bypass versus CPB with DHCA include increased risks of PE, warm ischemic injury to the kidneys and liver, and incomplete tumor thrombus resection

(60, 62). When compared to a "clamp and run" technique without extracorporeal perfusion or shunt devices, disadvantages of venovenous bypass include increased blood loss, operating time, and length of hospital stay, as well as increases in the risk of air embolism, thromboembolic complications, and vessel injury (11, 14, 34).

CPB

CPB with or without DHCA has long been a useful technique for resection of IVC invasive tumors. With advances in surgical techniques such as liver mobilization and venovenous bypass, its use has diminished (11, 14, 42, 56, 66, 67). Many surgeons advocate the use of CPB for Level IV tumor thrombi that cannot be reduced to a level below the diaphragm and for cases of intraatrial thrombus, whereas others restrict use of CPB to extensive intraatrial tumor or tumor thrombus adherent to the wall of the IVC or right atrium (11, 13, 14, 45, 56, 68). When utilizing CPB with or without DHCA for resection of tumors invading the right heart or with high level IVC involvement, some surgeons recommend that the abdominal procedure be performed first so that retroperitoneal hemostasis can be obtained prior to anticoagulation (39). Others recommend a two-stage procedure in which resection of the intrathoracic/intracardiac portion of the tumor thrombus is performed first and abdominal resection is performed at a later date to decrease intraoperative blood loss and decrease operating time (43).

Use of CPB during resection of tumor thrombi decreases the risk of tumor embolization, improves surgical field conditions and visualization, and circumvents the issue of hemodynamic stability discussed previously (69, 70). Traditionally, CPB with the addition of DHCA has been used to provide a bloodless surgical field allowing for complete resection of IVC/atrial tumor thrombi (55, 56, 60, 64, 71). Additional advantages of DHCA include a further decrease in the risk of PE, as well as decreases in the risk of massive hemorrhage, incomplete tumor resection, and warm ischemic injury to organs (60, 62, 71, 72). Although many surgeons continue to use CPB with DHCA, a few restrict its use to resection of tumors adherent to the supradiaphragmatic IVC/atrium or when visualization is not adequate with CPB alone (56, 63). DHCA increases bypass and operating time and increases the risks of coagulopathy (likely secondary to platelet dysfunction), perioperative bleeding, and neurologic sequelae above those posed by CPB alone (14, 29, 61, 62, 70, 71, 73).

CPB, in the setting of IVC/atrial tumor thrombus resection, is typically initiated after systemic anticoagulation and the placement of one or two venous cannula(s) in the SVC and/or right atrium (taking care to not dislodge any tumor thrombus) for venous drainage and one arterial can-

320 Bricker, Young, and Butterworth

nula in the ascending aorta for arterial return (4, 23, 62, 64, 70, 72). Some surgeons will cannulate a femoral vein to assure adequate venous drainage of the lower body although, for most patients, this is not necessary in the setting of extensive IVC obstruction and development of collateral venous channels (71). Following cooling of the patient's core temperature to 15–20°C, CPB can be discontinued for the duration of the surgical excisions and is deemed safe for 20–25 minutes (45, 49, 62, 65, 70, 74). Addition of anterograde cerebral perfusion via cannulae placed in the right subclavian artery and left common carotid artery increases safe DHCA time to 60–80 minutes (23, 70, 74). Packing the head in ice likely reduces the rate at which the brain warms during DHCA (75).

Prior to initiating DHCA, and following the onset of ventricular fibrillation, the aorta is cross-clamped and cold cardioplegia is administered for myocardial protection (62, 64, 70, 73). Following the initiation of DHCA, the IVC is entered near the renal vein of tumor thrombus origin, and the heart is entered through a right atriotomy (60, 62). Following complete removal of the tumor thrombus, atriotomies and venacavotomies are closed with suture and, if needed, patch placement (60, 70). Following resumption of CPB, the patient is gradually rewarmed (70, 72). Weaning from CPB is typically well tolerated in patients with good preoperative ventricular function, although positive inotropic drug support (20–40 ng/kg/min epinephrine or 2–5 µg/kg/min dobutamine) may be required for a few hours.

Neuroprotection is of utmost importance during DHCA and is almost exclusively provided by the profound hypothermia. Many clinicians administer methylprednisolone, mannitol, thiopental, lidocaine, and/or magnesium sulfate in the hope of providing additional protection, although convincing evidence for the efficacy of any of these agents is lacking (62, 65, 70–72, 74). We and others feel that the important features of anesthetic management in cases where DHCA is employed include maintaining brain hypothermia during arrest and keeping blood glucose in the normal range through use of an insulin infusion protocol (65, 70, 76).

CONCLUSION

The management of the patient with an IVC tumor represents a challenging clinical situation that requires special knowledge, skills, and coordination. For the patient scheduled for surgical removal of a vena caval tumor or thrombus, the anesthesiologist must have a more comprehensive understanding of the anatomy, the extent of the tumor involvement, and the hemodynamic consequences associated with it than often is required for other surgical procedures. In addition, the anesthetic management must take into account the potential impact of induction agents, and intraoperative management on hemodynamics. Intraoperative TEE can provide important information about the status of the tumor or thrombus and the hemodynamic sequelae associated with surgical manipulation. The most critical aspect of the perioperative care of these patients—and perhaps more important in this situation than most other procedures—is the careful coordination and ongoing communication between the anesthesiologist and surgeon prior to and during the surgical procedure.

References

1. Montie JE, el Ammar R, Pontes JE, et al.: Renal cell carcinoma with inferior vena cava tumor thrombi. Surg Gynecol Obstet 1991; 173(2):107–15
2. Katsumata T, Shinfeld A, Houel R, et al.: Pelvic leiomyoma in the right atrium. Ann Thorac Surg 1998; 66:2095–6
3. Stolf NA, Santos GG, Haddad VL, et al.: Successful one-stage resection of intravenous leiomyomatosis of the uterus with extension into the heart. Cardiovasc Surg 1999; 7(6):661–4
4. Jibiki M, Iwai T, Inoue Y, et al.: Surgical strategy for treating renal cell carcinoma with thrombus extending into the inferior vena cava. J Vasc Surg 2004; 39(4):829–35
5. Konety BR, Williams RD: Chapter 21: Renal parenchymal neoplasms. In: Smith's general urology, 17th Edition. New York, NY, McGraw-Hill, 2008
6. Keane T, Gillatt D, Evans CP, et al.: Current and future trends in the treatment of renal cancer. Eur Urol Suppl 2007; 6:374–84
7. Ljungberg B, Hanbury DC, Kuczyk MA, et al.: Renal cell carcinoma guideline. Eur Urol 2007; 51:1502–10
8. Lam JS, Shvarts O, Leppert JT, et al.: Renal cell carcinoma 2005: new frontiers in staging, prognostication and targeted molecular therapy. J Urol 2005; 173:1853–62
9. Windokun A, Duncan AI, Koch CG: Occult tumor embolization detected by intraoperative transesophageal echocardiography. J Cardiothorac Vasc Anesth DOI: 10.1053/j.jvca.2007.12.011
10. Parekh DJ, Cookson MS, Chapman W, et al.: Renal cell carcinoma with renal vein and inferior vena caval involvement: clinicopathological features, surgical techniques and outcomes. J Urol 2005; 173(6):1897–902
11. Blute ML, Leibovich BC, Lohse CM, et al.: The Mayo Clinic experience with surgical management, complications and outcomes for

patients with renal cell carcinoma and venous tumour thrombus. Br J Urol Int 2004; 94:33–41

12. Singh I, Jacobs LE, Kotler MN, et al.: The utility of transesophageal echocardiography in the management of renal cell carcinoma with intracardiac extension. J Am Soc Echocardiogr 1995; 8:245–250

13. Zini L, Haulon S, Decoene C, et al.: Renal cell carcinoma associated with tumor thrombus in the inferior vena cava: surgical strategies. Ann Vasc Surg 2005; 19:522–8

14. Ciancio G, Soloway MS: Renal cell carcinoma with tumor thrombus extending above diaphragm: avoiding cardiopulmonary bypass. Urology 2005; 66:266–70

15. Gindea AJ, Gentin B, Naidich DP, et al.: Unusual cardiac metastasis in hypernephroma: the complementary role of echocardiography and magnetic resonance imaging. Am Heart J 1988; 116(5):1359–61

16. Sigman DB, Hasnain JU, Del Pizzo JJ, et al.: Real-time transesophageal echocardiography for intraoperative surveillance of patients with renal cell carcinoma and vena caval extension undergoing radical nephrectomy. J Urol 1999; 161:36–8

17. Harkin CP, Roberts PF, Nelson RS, et al.: Re-evaluation of renal cell carcinoma tumor thrombus extension by intraoperative transesophageal echocardiography. J Cardiothorac Vasc Anesth 2000; 14(2):182–5

18. Subramaniam B, Pawlowski J, Gross BA, et al.: TEE-guided one-stage excision of intravenous leiomyomatosis with cardiac extension through an abdominal approach. J Cardiothorac Vasc Anesth 2006; 20(1):94–5

19. Masui S, Onishi T, Arima K, et al.: Successful management of inferior vena cava thrombus complicating advanced germ cell testicular tumor with temporary inferior vena cava filter. Int J Urol 2005; 12:513–5

20. Sharifi R, Ray P, Schade SG, et al.: Inferior vena cava thrombosis: unusual presentation of testicular cancer. Urology 1988; 32(2):146–50

21. Ricci MA, Cloutier LM, Mount S, et al.: Intravenous leiomyomatosis with intracardiac extension. Cardiovasc Surg 1995; 3(6):693–6

22. Nam MS, Jeon MJ, Kim YT, et al.: Pelvic leiomyomatosis with intracaval and intracardiac extension: a case report and review of the literature. Gynecol Oncol 2003; 89:175–80

23. Wu C-C, Hseih S, Ho W-M, et al.: Surgical treatment for recurrent hepatocellular carcinoma with tumor thrombi in right atrium: using cardiopulmonary bypass and deep hypothermic circulatory arrest. J Surg Oncol 2000; 74:227–31

24. Topcuoglu MS, Yaliniz H, Poyrazoglu H, et al.: Intravenous leiomyomatosis extending into the right ventricle after subtotal hysterectomy. Ann Thorac Surg 2004; 78:330–2

25. Swenson JD, Hullander RM, Nolan JF, et al.: Renal cell carcinoma in the inferior vena cava demonstrated by transesophageal echocardiography. J Cardiothorac Vasc Anesth 1993; 7(3):335–6

26. American Cancer Society. "How is kidney cancer (renal cell carcinoma) staged?" Retrieved from http://www.cancer.org/docroot/home/index.asp. Accessed on 6 March 2009.

27. Plowman AN, Bolsin SN, Patrick AJ: Unusual cause of intraoperative hypotension diagnosed with transesophageal echocardiography in a patient with renal cell carcinoma. Anaesth Intensive Care 1999; 27:63–5

28. Lubahn JG, Sagalowsky AI, Rosenbaum DH, et al.: Contemporary techniques and safety of cardiovascular procedures in the surgical management of renal cell carcinoma with tumor thrombus. J Thorac Cardiovasc Surg 2006; 131(6):1289–95

29. Ruel M, Bedard P, Morash CG, et al.: Resection of right atrial tumor thrombi without circulatory arrest. Ann Thorac Surg 2001; 71:733–4

30. Mosharafa A, Koch M, Shalhav A, et al.: Nephrectomy for metastatic renal cell carcinoma: Indiana University experience. Urology 2003; 62(4):636–40

31. Tsuji Y, Goto A, Hara I, et al.: Renal cell carcinoma with extension of tumor thrombus into the vena cava: surgical strategy and prognosis. J Vasc Surg 2001; 33(4): 789–96

32. Nesbitt JC, Soltero ER, Dinney CP, et al.: Surgical management of renal cell carcinoma with inferior vena cava tumor thrombus. Ann Thorac Surg 1997; 63:1592–9

33. Kaplan S, Ekici S, Dogan R, et al.: Surgical management of renal cell carcinoma with inferior vena cava tumor thrombus. Am J Surg 2002; 183(3):292–9

34. Browning AJ, Eardley I, Joyce AJ, et al.: Percutaneous veno-venous bypass in surgery for renal cell carcinoma with associated vena caval tumour thrombus. Br J Urol Int 1999; 83:850–2

35. Presti JC. Chapter 23: Genital tumors. In: Smith's general urology, 17th Edition. New York, NY, McGraw-Hill, 2008

36. Hassan B, Tung K, Weeks R, et al.: The management of inferior vena cava obstruction complicating metastatic germ cell tumors. Cancer 1999; 85:912–8

37. Fishman AD, Hoffman A, Volterra F, et al.: Intracaval and intracardiac metastatic nonseminomatous germ cell tumor: a rare cause of hemolytic anemia and thrombocytopenia. Cancer Invest 2002; 20(7–8):996–1001

38. Spitz A, Wilson TG, Kawachi MH, et al.: Vena caval resection for bulky metastatic germ cell tumors: an 18-year experience. J Urol 1997; 158:1813–8

39. Moon TD, Fox LS, Varma DG: Testicular teratocarcinoma with intracaval metastases to the heart. Urology 1992; 40(4):368–70

40. Khayata GM, Thwaini S, Aswad SG: Intravenous leiomyomatosis extending to the heart. Int J Gynecol Obstet 2003; 80:59–60

41. Podolsky LA, Jacobs LE, Ioli A, et al.: TEE in the diagnosis of intravenous leiomyomatosis extending into the right atrium. Am Heart J 1993; 125(5):1462–4

42. Chan F, Ngan Kee WD, Low JM: Anesthetic management of renal cell carcinoma with inferior vena cava extension. J Clin Anesth 2001; 13:585–7

43. Castelli P, Caronno R, Piffaretti G, et al.: Surgical treatment of malignant involvement of the inferior vena cava. Int Semin Surg Oncol 2006; 3:19

44. Mizoguchi T, Koide Y, Ohara M, et al.: Multiplane echocardiographic guidance during resection of renal cell carcinoma extending into the inferior vena cava. Anesth Analg 1995; 81:1102–5

45. Vaidya A, Ciancio G, Soloway M: Surgical techniques for treating a renal neoplasm invading the inferior vena cava. J Urol 2003; 169: 435–44

46. Small EJ. Chapter 19: Chemotherapy of urologic tumors. In: Smith's general urology, 17th Edition. New York, NY, McGraw-Hill, 2008

47. Donat SM, Levy DA: Bleomycin associated pulmonary toxicity: is perioperative oxygen restriction necessary? J Urol 1998; 160:1347–52

48. Waid-Jones MI, Coursin DB: Perioperative considerations for patients treated with bleomycin. Chest 1991; 99:993–9

49. Takeda K, Sawamura S, Tamai H, et al.: Reversible tricuspid valve obstruction during removal of renal cell carcinoma with intracardiac tumor extension. Anesth Analg 2000; 91:1137–8

50. Chen H, Ng V, Kane CJ: The role of transesophageal echocardiography in rapid diagnosis and treatment of migratory tumor thrombus. Anesth Analg 2004; 99(2):357–9

51. Koide Y, Mizoguchi T, Ischii K, et al.: Intraoperative management for removal of tumor thrombus in the inferior vena cava or the right atrium with multiplane transesophageal echocardiography. J Cardiovasc Surg 1998; 39(5):641–7

52. Larney V, Charles R, Brown AS, et al.: Value of transesophageal echocardiography for diagnosis of intraoperative tumour embolization. Anaesth Intensive Care 2006; 34(6):797–800

53. O'Hara JF, Sprung J, Whalley D, et al.: Transesophageal echocardiography in monitoring of intrapulmonary embolism during inferior

vena cava tumor resection. J Cardiothorac Vasc Anesth 1999; 13(1):69–71

54. Fayad A: Echocardiography images of inferior vena cava tumor thrombus in patient with renal cell carcinoma. Can J Anaesth 2008; 55(8):557–8

55. Belis JA, Levinson ME, Pae WE: Complete radical nephrectomy and vena caval thrombectomy during circulatory arrest. J Urol 2000; 163(2):434–6

56. Ciancio G, Hawke C, Soloway M: The use of liver transplant techniques to aid in the surgical management of urological tumors. J Urol 2000; 164:665–72

57. Ciancio G, Soloway M: Resection of the abdominal inferior vena cava for complicated renal cell carcinoma with tumour thrombus. Br J Urol Int 2005; 96:815–8

58. Albers P, Melchior D, Muller SC: Surgery in metastatic testicular cancer. Eur Urol 2003; 44:233–44

59. Yoshidome H, Takeuchi D, Ito H, et al.: Should the inferior vena cava be reconstructed after resection for malignant tumors? Am J Surg 2005; 189:419–24

60. Chowdhury UK, Mishra AK, Seth A, et al.: Novel techniques for tumor thrombectomy for renal cell carcinoma with intraatrial tumor thrombus. Ann Thorac Surg 2007; 83:1731–6

61. Boorjian SA, Sengupta S, Blute ML: Renal cell carcinoma: vena caval involvement. Br J Urol Int 2007; 99:1239–44

62. Chiappini B, Savini C, Marinelli G, et al.: Cavoatrial tumor thrombus: single-stage surgical approach with profound hypothermia and circulatory arrest, including a review of the literature. J Thorac Cardiovasc Surg 2002; 124(4):684–8

63. Ciancio G, Soloway M: Renal cell carcinoma invading the hepatic veins. Cancer 2001; 92(7):1836–42

64. Kleisli T, Raissi SS, Nissen NN, et al.: Cavo-atrial tumor resection under total circulatory arrest without a sternotomy. Ann Thorac Surg 2006; 81:1887–8

65. Babayan E, Zelman V, Berger JM, et al.: Brain protection: pathophysiology and clinical application. Semin Anesth Perioperative Med Pain 2004; 23(3):160–73

66. Taweemonkongsap T, Nualyong C, Leewansangtong S, et al.: Surgical treatment of renal cell carcinoma with inferior vena cava thrombus: using liver mobilization technique to avoid cardiopulmonary bypass. Asian J Surg 2008; 31(2):75–82

67. Hogue CW, Palin CA, Arrowsmith JE: Cardiopulmonary bypass management and neurologic outcomes: an evidence-based appraisal of current practices. Anesth Analg 2006; 103:21–37

68. Blanloeil Y, Le Roux C, Rigal JC, et al.: Transesophageal echocardiography diagnosis of tricuspid obstruction by a vena cava tumour. Can J Anaesth 2001; 48:401–4
69. Kawahito S, Kitahata H, Kitagawa T, et al.: Non-cardiac surgery applications of extracorporeal circulation. J Med Invest 2007; 54:200–10
70. Welch M, Bazaral M, Schmidt R, et al.: Anesthetic management for surgical removal of renal carcinoma with caval or atrial tumor thrombus using deep hypothermic circulatory arrest. J Cardiothorac Anesth 1989; 3(5):580–6
71. Wotkowicz C, Libertino JA, Sorcini A, et al.: Management of renal cell carcinoma with vena cava and atrial thrombus: minimal access vs median sternotomy with circulatory arrest. Br J Urol Int 2006; 98:289–97
72. Moskowitz DM, Perelman SI, Cousineau KM, et al.: Multidisciplinary management of a Jehovah's Witness patient for the removal of a renal cell carcinoma extending into the right atrium. Can J Anaesth 2002; 49:402–8
73. Pochettino A, Cheung AT: Pro: Retrograde cerebral perfusion is useful for deep hypothermic circulatory arrest. J Cardiothorac Vasc Anesth 2003; 17(6):764–7
74. Apostolakis E, Akinosoglou K: The methodologies of hypothermic circulatory arrest and of antegrade and retrograde cerebral perfusion for aortic arch surgery. Ann Thorac Cardiovasc Surg 2008; 14:138–48
75. Brooker RF, Zvara DA, Velvis H, et al.: Topical ice slurry prevents brain rewarming during deep hypothermic circulatory arrest in newborn sheep. J Cardiothorac Vasc Anesth 1997; 11(5):591–4
76. Bellinger DC, Wypij D, du Plessis AJ, et al.: Developmental and neurologic effects of alpha-stat versus Ph-stat strategies for deep hypothermic cardiopulmonary bypass in infants. J Thorac Cardiovasc Surg 2001; 121:374–83

Steven E. Hill, MD

Care of the Cardiothoracic Surgical Patient Refusing
13 Transfusion

INTRODUCTION

Some patients seeking medical care refuse to accept allogeneic blood or blood products. When they do so, the health care provider is presented with a challenge in determining how best to treat the patient, optimize clinical care, and at the same time respect the patient's wishes. The dilemma is probably best defined in the modern version of the Hippocratic Oath that states, "I will apply, for the benefits of the sick, all measures that are required, avoiding those twin traps of overtreatment and therapeutic nihilism" (1). A literal interpretation of this statement supports transfusion therapy as a 'required measure' in the face of life-threatening hemorrhage while also acknowledging the duty to the patient of avoiding 'overtreatment'. Although most physicians abhor the prospect of allowing a patient to exsanguinate because of a treatable anemia or coagulopathy, most physicians recognize the right of the patient or surrogate to make the decision to withhold blood products. The paternalistic practices of the past are no longer acceptable; patient autonomy is accepted as a right.

As early as 1914, the basis for patient autonomy as the guiding principle for decisions regarding medical management including transfusion therapy was established in a U.S. Supreme Court ruling on the case of *Schloendorff v. Society of New York Hospitals*. Based upon the constitutional right to liberty, the Court ruled that, "Every human being of adult years and sound mind has a right to determine what shall be done with

Medically Challenging Patients Undergoing Cardiothoracic Surgery, edited by Neal H. Cohen, MD, MPH, MS, Lippincott Williams & Wilkins, Baltimore © 2009.

his own body; and a surgeon who performs an operation without his patient's consent commits an assault for which he is liable in damages" (2). Although transfusion is not a surgical procedure, the intent of the ruling is clear and can be extrapolated to all medical interventions. It is conflict between the desire to provide all required measures for the benefit of the patient and the wish to honor patient autonomy in decision making that creates a conundrum for physicians caring for patients refusing transfusion. In this chapter, a clinical case will be used as the basis for a discussion of the issues involved in caring for the patient who refuses transfusion for a high-blood-loss emergent procedure with emphasis on preparation, consent, medico-legal guidelines, alternatives to transfusion therapy and formulation of an anesthetic plan.

CLINICAL SCENARIO

An 18-year-old unmarried male with a known history of bicuspid aortic valve and a minor factor VII deficiency presents to a local emergency department with dyspnea following an episode of ripping/tearing chest pain radiating to the back while lifting weights in the gym. Examination is notable for a blowing diastolic murmur, tachycardia, and poor peripheral perfusion. Auscultation of the chest reveals diffuse rales. Urine output is minimal. Chest x-ray demonstrates a prominent aorta and bilateral pulmonary edema. Computerized tomography reveals a Type A aortic dissection and moderate pericardial effusion.

Because of the patient's deteriorating clinical condition and severe dyspnea, he undergoes tracheal intubation, and he is sedated and transferred to your facility for definitive care. The patient's driver's license from the neighboring state reveals a birth date of January 23, 1990. A laminated wallet card entitled "Durable Power of Attorney for Health Care" that is witnessed but not notarized is found. The document includes a statement that the patient refuses transfusion of whole blood and its primary components, but accepts all blood fractions as well as procedures for which the patient's blood remains within a circuit which is never detached from the patient. The health care power of attorney was signed on July 30, 2007. The patient's health care agents are listed as (1) an adult sibling, and (2) the patient's mother.

At the time of admission, the patient's vital signs include a blood pressure of 96/35 mmHg, heart rate of 120 beats per minute, temperature of 36.8°C, and respiratory rate of 10 while the patient is receiving controlled ventilation with a ventilatory rate of 10 breaths per minute. His peak inspiratory pressure is 20 cm H_2O, positive end-expiratory pressure is 5 cm H_2O, and FiO_2 is 0.4. Arterial blood gases reveal a pH of 7.32, $PaCO_2$ of 32 mmHg, PaO_2 of 137 mmHg, and base excess of –6 mEq/L.

The patient's hemoglobin is 14.0 g/dL, platelet count is 171,000, and white blood cell count is 10,600. His basic chemistry panel is normal except for serum bicarbonate of 20 mEq/L. Coagulation parameters include a prothrombin time of 17.1 minutes with an *international normalized ratio* (INR) of 1.4, partial thromboplastin time of 31 minutes, and fibrinogen level of 472 mg/dL. Previous factor VII activity based on outside hospital records is 33% predicted with no other significant abnormalities noted according to a consultation by a hematologist. The patient is 180 cm tall with a weight of 90 kg.

Optimal Management Versus Patient Autonomy

Although the clinical diagnosis for this patient is obvious, the optimal management of the patient is complicated by his refusal to accept transfusion of blood products. Given the clinical presentation of ascending aortic dissection with aortic insufficiency, pulmonary edema, and pericardial effusion with evidence of impaired cardiac output, the preferred surgical intervention includes emergency repair of the aortic dissection while optimizing oxygen-carrying capacity with transfusion of packed red blood cells and correction of coagulation parameters with targeted blood component transfusion as indicated by the patient's course. In most clinical situations like this one (in which the procedure is emergent and the patient lacks capacity to consent), surgery with administration of blood products would be considered standard of care. If neither the patient nor an appropriate surrogate were available to consent to the procedure, it would be performed emergently and so documented in the medical record. However, for this patient the previously expressed and documented wishes are clearly defined and include refusal to accept blood products. As a result, the management decisions must take into account his wishes. The options are significantly affected by his determination not to accept blood products. Given the risk of exsanguination weighed against the benefit of the procedure, the surgeon's options are limited. Although medical management carries the lowest risk of exsanguination, the likelihood of this patient surviving without surgical intervention is very low in the presence of significant aortic insufficiency and an acute pericardial effusion that is likely enlarging. The possible surgical interventions include 1) aortic valve replacement with ascending aortic tube graft, 2) Bentall procedure, 3) homograft or xenograft of the aortic valve and ascending aorta, 4) aortic valve replacement or resuspension with hemiarch ascending aortic repair using deep hypothermic circulatory arrest, or 5) aortic valve replacement or resuspension with total arch replacement and "elephant trunk" descending aortic graft with deep hypothermic circulatory arrest. All of these interventions carry significant risk, further complicated by the transfusion limitations. Although the extent of the surgical intervention may be dictated by findings at the time of surgery, the higher risk of bleeding with more extensive surgery and deep hypothermic circulatory arrest limits the planned intervention to the less extensive procedures. This limitation likely compromises long-term success of the repair in a young patient and again places the providers in conflict with the desire to help the patient; some of the options may be considered below standard of care for this clinical problem and raise further concerns for the patient, the providers, and the hospital.

BELIEFS OF THE JEHOVAH'S WITNESS CHURCH

Although not all patients refusing transfusion therapy do so for religious reasons, the majority of the patients who refuse blood and blood products are members of the Jehovah's Witness Church. Therefore, an understanding of some of the beliefs of the Church relating to allogeneic blood is helpful in understanding the basis for their request and in caring for these patients. Based upon Scripture, Jehovah's Witness Church members believe that allogeneic whole blood and its primary components defile the body and are therefore forbidden. The primary components of blood include red blood cells, white blood cells, platelets, and unfractionated plasma. These products are absolutely forbidden based on their religious beliefs. Baptized Church members would rather die than receive these products. Most church members also do not accept stored autologous blood, as it has been separated from the patient and stored for a prolonged period.

Although prolonged storage of autologous blood is strictly forbidden by the Jehovah's Witness Church, procedures that maintain the patient's blood within a *continuous* circuit (such as hemodialysis, cardiopulmonary bypass [CPB], cell salvage, and intraoperative normovolemic hemodilution) are considered "matters of conscience" by the Church, allowing the individual Church members to make their own judgment as to whether they will consent to these procedures. Acceptance of "minor fractions" of blood is also considered a matter of conscience. Minor fractions include concentrated albumin solutions, purified plasma protein fraction, recombinant human protein medications, and clotting factor concentrates. Because plasma proteins are capable of crossing the placental barrier, protein fractions derived from whole plasma are considered acceptable therapeutic options for a large proportion of, but not all, Church members.

Cryoprecipitate, because it is the protein precipitate that is expressed from a bag of thawed whole plasma, is also considered a minor fraction and accepted by most Church members. In the past few years, the

Church Council also has determined that the residual "cryosupernatant" remaining after the cryoprecipitate is expressed from whole plasma is a minor fraction and acceptable as a matter of conscience. This product, referred to as *cryo-poor plasma* in most blood banks, has markedly improved the outcome for Church members suffering from disease states treated most effectively by plasmapheresis, especially thrombotic thrombocytopenic purpura (TTP). Although it makes patient management easier with improved outcomes, administration of minor fractions as well as procedures involving the recirculation of the patient's blood may be rejected by some Church members. As a result, specific discussions must be initiated with each patient regarding personal beliefs and wishes related to administration of blood products, minor fractions, and procedures such as CPB. If the patient does not have a clear understanding of matters of conscience within the Church, help is readily available from the Jehovah's Witness Hospital Liaison Committee in explaining and determining the Church's position on these issues for the patient. This resource is frequently underutilized, but can save time and frequently enhance therapeutic options for the physician and patient. Because many decisions are left to the personal judgment of the individual patient, it is critical for the anesthesiologist and surgeon to have a personal and private discussion with the patient to discuss the patient's beliefs and wishes regarding blood or blood products, and to provide an explanation of the management implications of the decision. If the patient decides to reject fractions or specific procedures, the risk to the patient may increase and outweigh benefits, even in urgent or emergent procedures. The patient should be given information about these risks and alternatives and be aware of the consequences of the decision. Documentation of the discussion should be recorded in the medical record.

MEDICO-LEGAL IMPLICATIONS OF TRANSFUSION REFUSAL

Before caring for patients refusing transfusion, an understanding of the legal precedents guiding patient autonomy is recommended. It is interesting that the landmark legal case that set much of the precedent for current legal support of patients refusing transfusion does not involve transfusion at all. The case of *Angela Carder v. George Washington University Hospital* (1990) (3) involved a pregnant patient at 26.5 weeks gestation who was terminally ill with metastatic osteogenic sarcoma. After discussion with her physicians in the presence of her family, Mrs. Carder agreed to palliative treatment designed to extend her life to 28 weeks to improve potential fetal outcome if the need to "intervene" and deliver the fetus developed. Mrs. Carder acutely deteriorated prior to 28 weeks, losing capacity to decide. The family, particularly the patient's mother, opposed Caesarean section as contrary to Mrs. Carder's wishes. Under the impression that the fetus was viable, the medical team obtained a court order for Caesarean section in the interest of the fetus. The decision to proceed with the Caesarean delivery was upheld by a three-judge motions division. The Caesarean section was performed, with death of both the mother and baby. Citing substituted judgment, the ruling was overturned on appeal, leaving the medical team and the hospital liable for damages. The hospital settled for an undisclosed amount and agreed to rewrite hospital policy to respect the autonomy of the pregnant patient. Since this ruling, autonomy of the adult patient with capacity to decide has been consistently upheld by the courts.

More recent cases have addressed the issue of refusal of transfusion in pregnancy. In the case of Vega versus Stamford Hospital (4), a pregnant woman was transfused against her wishes. The Connecticut Supreme Court ruled in favor of the patient and directed damages to be paid. Also in 1996, in the case of St. Mary's Hospital (FL) versus Harrell (5), transfusion of a pregnant woman was ordered by the court against her wishes. This ruling was overturned on appeal prior to transfusion. In the case of Fetus Brown versus D. Brown (6), a woman of 34.5 weeks gestation underwent resection of a urethral mass with subsequent postoperative anemia (hemoglobin 8.4 g/dL). A court-ordered transfusion was administered against patient wishes on behalf of the fetus. The pregnancy was successful with a healthy baby and mother, but the court-ordered transfusion decision was reversed later on appeal. With existing legal precedents such as these, the rights of the competent pregnant adult patient are clear. Until the child takes his or her first breath, the mother has the right to refuse transfusion therapy.

Less clear are the rights of the pregnant minor to refuse transfusion. In North Carolina, although able to make medical decisions regarding her prenatal care, a minor not emancipated by marriage or court order cannot refuse transfusion therapy if, in the opinion of her attending physician and one other person, her life would be threatened. The legal rights of the minor vary from state to state and should be clearly understood prior to proceeding with surgery when the parents or guardians refuse to allow the minor to receive blood products.

Any adult patient is competent unless determined otherwise by a court of law. Physicians do not determine competency. However, patients may lack capacity to decide because of medical conditions, and in that circumstance the physician is obligated to act on his or her behalf. The ability to provide or withhold consent to a medical intervention follows ethical guidelines established for capacity to decide. The patient must understand 1) the nature of the illness, 2) the natural history of the illness if untreated, 3) the treatment options available, and 4) the ramification of the decision. Without capacity to decide, informed consent is not possible, nor is refusal of potentially life-saving therapy. Therefore, it is the responsibility of the care providers to verify the patient's capacity to decide and the patient's uncoerced wishes prior to withholding transfusion in the face of life-threatening hemorrhage or anemia.

In this particular case, the patient lacks capacity to decide because of sedative medications and the underlying condition; discontinuation of sedation would be potentially life-threatening in the face of an unstable ascending aortic dissection. However, evidence of his prior wishes is present in the form of a Health Care Power of Attorney found in his wallet. If a valid Health Care Power of Attorney is produced and the attending physician has no reason to suspect that the patient's wishes are other than those listed for a patient lacking capacity to decide, then the physician must follow the preferences for refusal of transfusion as documented.

In the case presented, the Health Care Power of Attorney was signed and witnessed before the patient's 18th birthday, rendering the document invalid. As a result, further evidence of the patient's wishes since becoming an adult must be sought. Table 13–1 lists the current medical decision hierarchy in North Carolina (those in other states may vary). In this case, although an adult sibling was listed as the patient's first health care agent, his parents are, in fact, the next of kin because the document was signed while the patient was a minor. Advice of the parents should be sought, if time permits.

An additional problem with the wallet card involves differences between state laws. In Virginia, a Health Care Power of Attorney requires two witnesses but does not need to be notarized. In North Carolina, a valid Health Care Power of Attorney requires notarization, rendering the wallet card from the neighboring state technically invalid. If the patient had signed the power of attorney after becoming an adult and this document were otherwise valid in the patient's state of residence, reliance upon the document could be defended on the basis that it represents the

TABLE 13–1. Medical decision hierarchy in North Carolina

1. Adult or emancipated minor with capacity to decide
2. Court-appointed guardian for incompetent patient
3. Surrogate decision-maker identified by valid Health Care Power of Attorney
4. Spouse
5. Adult children
6. Parents of adult
7. Siblings
8. Other competent adult sufficiently related to patient to reliably express patient's prior wishes

best evidence available. However, in this case the treating physician could be criticized for actions based on an invalid legal document. In our program for managing patients who refuse transfusion, we have decided to err on the side of honoring valid Health Care Powers of Attorney from other states in an emergency. If the patient possesses capacity to decide and the clinical situation permits, we request that an out-of-state patient complete and notarize a North Carolina Health Care Power of Attorney. Once again, both state law and institutional policies may dictate alternative approaches to patient consent and decision making.

Although the wallet card in this case cannot be relied upon as a legally binding document because of the age of the patient at signing and possibly because of differing state laws, it remains helpful as evidence of the patient's wishes as he approached adulthood. It may also provide information about next of kin, allowing contact with the patient's parent. The overriding principle involved in this process is to obtain the best information available as to the adult patient's prior wishes. If, in the opinion of the treating physician, the wishes of the patient when possessing capacity to decide are sufficiently clear, then refusal of transfusion may be honored; it will likely be upheld by a court of law. However, if the treating physician has any doubts as to the validity of reported preferences given on behalf of the adult patient lacking capacity to decide, then treatment such as transfusion must be administered by the physician in the best interest of the patient with appropriate documentation of the process for determining the patient's wishes and the decision making clearly outlined in the medical record.

Each institution has its own policies and procedures for determining how to obtain consent, ensure patient competence to refuse treatment(s), and ensure that the patient decisions are made knowledgeably and without coercion. Some institutions have formalized the process and created specific teams of professionals to address these challenging issues. A multidisciplinary team with a program manager dedicated to care of patients refusing transfusion can provide the necessary infrastructure to determine how to deliver optimal medical care while honoring patient autonomy. Because clinical situations requiring allogeneic blood transfusion are frequently emotionally charged and often urgent or emergent, careful preparation and documentation of patient wishes is essential. In anticipation of elective surgical intervention, completion of an institution-specific refusal of treatment form as well as a state-specific Health Care Power of Attorney should be obtained outlining choices made by the patient in a nonurgent setting. In our institution, all patients refusing transfusion are referred to the Center for Blood Conservation for counseling and completion of documentation. The patient is counseled both in the presence as well as the absence of family members and must state that he or she would rather die than receive an allogeneic transfusion. Refusal of transfusion as well as specific preferences for minor fractions of whole blood and acceptable medical procedures involving the patient's blood are documented. Upon completion of documentation, an electronic block is placed on the patient's medical record number at the blood bank, assuring that a provider unaware of the patient's wishes is unable to have blood released for the patient. The encounter is entered into the electronic medical record by a midlevel provider and cosigned after review by the Medical Director. For each hospitalization, the patient's wishes are confirmed and a refusal of treatment form completed. In the event of an emergency, the patient is counseled by the accepting physician with phone consultation from Center for Blood Conservation personnel, and a refusal of treatment form is completed and signed by the patient possessing capacity to decide and by the counseling physician.

Pediatric patients present a different challenge for the care provider. Although they are able to sign all other consent forms for their child, parents of an unemancipated minor cannot refuse transfusion therapy on behalf of the minor. The process for addressing the need for transfusion and obtaining approval to transfuse varies from one state to another, however. At this time, no state in the United States allows a minor to die for lack of transfusion. If parents demand no transfusion be given their child under any circumstances and time permits, a court order is usually required to comply with state law and protect the institution from potential litigation. In our institution, parents are forbidden from marking out portions of procedural consent forms relating to transfusion for their children. Without a signature on the procedural consent form, the procedure will not be done unless emergent. If emergent and necessary to protect the child, the procedure will be performed and transfusion administered if needed. We have developed separate acknowledgment forms for these cases that recognize the parents' wishes and agree to attempt avoidance of transfusion for their child. However, these forms also state that we must comply with North Carolina state law, and the parents are counseled that state law forbids withholding medically necessary transfusion from a minor. Each provider should be aware of the legal requirements of the state in addressing transfusion or other therapies for minor patients.

In this particular case, although the Health Care Power of Attorney itself was not valid, the wishes outlined in the wallet card were confirmed by the mother (next of kin) as well as by the patient's sister. Transfusion of whole blood or component therapy is not an option.

One final point warrants discussion. A physician is not obligated to provide care to a patient who refuses transfusion, but he or she cannot abandon the patient. If the physician is not willing to follow the patient's wishes, care must be immediately transferred to another physician capable of providing care within the limits documented by the patient.

CLINICAL DECISION MAKING

Balancing the risk of exsanguination with the need for definitive repair of the dissection in this case limits the surgical options. Although the optimal procedure likely would be an aortic valve resuspension with ascending aortic replacement and hemiarch repair, the need for prolonged CPB, multiple suture lines, and deep hypothermic circulatory arrest produce an unacceptable risk of hemorrhage for most surgeons. A simpler aortic valve replacement with an ascending aortic tube graft reinstating normal flow through the true lumen and closing off the false lumen would be the quickest procedure with the least likelihood of severe bleeding and a reasonable chance of long-term success. Focused attention on hemostasis and effective blood conservation is also obviously critical. According to guidelines for blood conservation in cardiac surgical procedures described by Moskowitz and Shander (7), the mainstays of effective blood management include 1) preoperative optimization of hemoglobin, 2) intraoperative normovolemic hemodilution, 3) tolerance of anemia, 4) meticulous surgical technique, 5) on-site coagulation monitoring, and 6) targeted pharmacotherapy with antifibrinolytics. One of the most common causes of anemia in critically ill patients is phlebotomy (8). Although blood sampling is necessary for optimal patient care, phlebotomy can be minimized through judicious testing, small sample tubes, and "zero-waste" blood-drawing sets that allow return of blood drawn through the line prior to sampling to the patient. Preoperative administration of vitamin K, 10 mg subcutaneously, would be beneficial to assure substrate for hepatic generation of vitamin K–dependent factors in the perioperative period.

BLOOD CONSERVATION MODALITIES

Treatment alternatives for patients wishing to avoid allogeneic blood transfusion are limited. No artificial agents capable of supporting oxygen delivery in lieu of red blood cell hemoglobin are available currently. The poor safety profile of these agents limits their benefit and may worsen clinical outcome (9, 10). Because no oxygen therapeutic agents are in late-phase clinical trials, they are not available for release on a compassionate use basis at the present time.

Erythropoietin has been proposed for management of anemia and to reduce the need for transfusion. Although previously U.S. Food and Drug Administration (FDA)-approved as a method for reducing the need for allogeneic blood transfusion in patients with anemia of chronic disease (Hgb ≥10.0 and ≤13.0 g/dL) (11), recombinant erythropoietin therapy is undergoing progressive restriction by Medicare because of safety concerns. Although it does increase hemoglobin and decrease allogeneic transfusion in the perioperative period when given prior to major orthopedic surgery in randomized, controlled trials (12–14), it's use has been associated with increased risk for death and serious cardiovascular events when administered to achieve a target Hgb > 12 g/dL in cancer, renal failure, and surgical patients (15). Erythropoietin is approved for prophylactic use in anticipated high-blood-loss surgery with lower target hemoglobin of 12.0 g/dL. In this case, starting hemoglobin is normal and erythropoietin use would not meet labelled indications. However, for a patient refusing transfusion, recovery from surgically induced anemia could be aided by preoperative erythropoietin therapy and intravenous iron supplementation, although neither would have an immediate effect on hemoglobin.

Cell salvage is a widely used technique for preservation of intraoperative hemoglobin mass. Although the quality of blood returned to the patient is dependent on the skill of the operator and the hemoglobin of the shed blood, cell salvage has effectively minimized the need for transfusion when used as part of a blood management plan (16–18). Cell salvage returns only red blood cells in saline with removal of platelets and plasma proteins. Compared with fresh whole blood, this product has no hemostatic activity, and processing of large volumes of shed blood from the surgical field may produce a dilutional coagulopathy in major surgery (19–20). Whether perioperative cell salvage is superior to, or synergistic with, intraoperative normovolemic hemodilution has yet to be determined (21). Before initiating cell salvage, it is essential to determine if the patient is willing to accept shed blood returned from the surgical field.

Some patients who refuse to receive banked blood products will accept their own conserved blood. Cell conservation in such cases can be helpful in both optimizing clinical care and improving outcome. Conservation of red blood cell mass via intraoperative normovolemic hemodilution is a technique that has been studied in orthopedic, cardiac, and urologic surgery patients with varying results (22). The concept of hemodilution involves harvest of a predetermined volume of autologous whole blood into anticoagulant-containing blood donation bags identical to those used in blood banks. The harvested blood may be removed via a central venous catheter, an arterial catheter, or a large-bore peripheral intravenous catheter, but flow must be reliable and at an adequate flow rate to prevent clot formation prior to reaching the anticoagulant in the donor bag. The autologous blood is then kept at room temperature with gentle mixing for up to 8 hours prior to reinfusion (23). Harvested volume is replaced with colloid or crystalloid via a separate peripheral intravenous line to maintain normovolemia. After hemodilution, subsequent blood lost in the surgical field has a reduced red cell mass, and fluid replacement at the end of the case consists of fresh whole blood instead of intravenous fluid. Small volume hemodilution is ineffective (24). To conserve a significant volume of hemoglobin mass, the patient's starting hemoglobin and blood volume need to be high enough to allow harvest of a large volume of whole blood; surgical loss of diluted blood needs to be extensive enough to make the procedure worthwhile. For example, normovolemic harvest of 2000 mL of whole blood from a theoretical patient with starting hemoglobin of 15 g/dL and an estimated blood volume of 6000 mL followed by a 2000 mL intraoperative blood loss results in nadir intraoperative hemoglobin of 6.7 g/dL. Overall, 1.23 units of whole blood with the same hemoglobin content as the average hemoglobin content of the harvested blood would be preserved (25). Although this extent of blood conservation may enhance avoidance of allogeneic transfusion, the procedure involves significant alteration of intravascular oxygen-carrying capacity that could prove problematic for patients with limited physiologic reserve (26).

A meta-analysis of randomized normovolemic hemodilution trials, including 24 prospective, randomized, controlled trials with 1218 patients undergoing major surgery such as cardiac and orthopedic procedures, reported the overall likelihood of exposure to allogeneic blood to be reduced (odds ratio 0.31, 95% confidence interval, 0.15–0.62) However, caution was recommended in the interpreatation of these results due to heterogeneity of study design (22). Whereas the efficacy of hemodilution in reducing the number of allogeneic units transfused per patient undergoing high-blood-loss surgical procedures is supported by recent literature reviews, the literature is equivocal regarding the ability of hemodilution to significantly increase transfusion avoidance altogether (26, 27). When compared with perioperative cell salvage in a mathematical model of hemoglobin mass preservation, cell salvage shows a theoretical advantage over hemodilution (21). Whether hemodilution provides added benefit to cell salvage alone is untested. However, in a patient who refuses transfusion therapy and undergoes a high-blood-loss surgical procedure, intraoperative normovolemic hemodilution has an added benefit of sequestering 30%–50% of the patient's circulating blood volume from the surgical field with the ability to reinfuse whole blood in the event of a catastrophic hemorrhage after the bleeding is controlled, thus providing a safety net in these difficult cases. Table 13–2 outlines one method for calculation of hemodi-

TABLE 13–2.   Calculation of hemodilution harvest volume

- Weight = IBW + 0.33(actual weight − IBW)
- Volume = [weight × 70 (Hgb – target Hgb)] ÷ Hgb,
  where Volume = harvest volume in mL,
          IBW = ideal body weight from MetLife table, and
          Hgb = postinduction hemoglobin.
          Use weight × 65 for females and children.
          Target Hgb is usually around 8.0 g/dL, but may be lower in an otherwise
          healthy Jehovah's Witness patient undergoing noncardiac surgery.

lution harvest volume (25). Although relatively accurate in a normovolemic patient, alteration of circulating blood volume will create error in the calculation. Assuming an ideal body weight of 75 kg and a drop in hemoglobin to 13.5 g/dL with the fluids administered with induction of anesthesia, the calculated harvest volume for this patient to reach a normovolemic prebypass hemoglobin of 8.0 would be 2281 mL (five 450 mL units of whole blood).

Antifibrinolytic therapy has been used to address the bleeding diathesis often accompanying cardiac surgery performed with CPB. Tranexamic acid and aminocaproic acid are widely used lysine analogues, but are not FDA approved for this indication and serve as specific antifibrinolytic agents. In randomized, controlled trials, administration of either lysine analogue decreases postoperative bleeding, but neither has been proven to decrease reoperation rate for cardiac surgery (26). Aprotinin previously carried FDA approval as a prophylactic agent for reduction of bleeding in coronary artery bypass grafting surgery. In randomized, controlled trials, aprotinin decreased blood loss, allogeneic blood exposure, and rate of reoperation for bleeding following cardiac surgery (28–33). However, observational database studies questioned the safety profile of aprotinin in 2006 (34, 35). Further reports of safety concerns (36, 37), as well as results from a randomized, controlled comparison of aprotinin with tranexamic acid and aminocaproic acid showing a increased mortality in the aprotinin group (38)have resulted in withdrawal of this agent from the market (39). Aprotinin is no longer commercially available for clinical use. In this case either lysine analogue would be an acceptable option and should be used.

MANAGEMENT OF SEVERE BLEEDING

Despite surgical attention to hemostasis and use of topical agents to assist clot formation in the surgical field, the proposed procedure has a high risk for hemorrhage. For a patient refusing blood and its primary components but accepting minor blood fractions, there are several therapeutic options for treating coagulopathy. Unfortunately, platelet transfusion is not an option for this patient. Thrombocytopenia and thrombasthenia associated with CPB may be a fatal development for this patient. Without the ability to transfuse platelets, postbypass thrombocytopenia may be treated only by return of the sequestered whole blood harvested during intraoperative normovolemic hemodilution.

Platelet Dysfunction

In the clinical situation described, options for treatment of bypass-induced thrombasthenia are limited. DDAVP (1-deamino-8-d-argininevasopressin) administration in a dose of 0.3 mcg/kg briefly increases glycoprotein-1b expression, increases von Willebrand factor-to-antigen levels, and increases ristocetin cofactor activity for up to 4 hours following administration (40, 41). Because an acquired von Willebrand factor deficiency has been associated with aortic stenosis (42), some surgeons advocate use of this agent for treatment of thrombasthenia following CPB. Meta-analysis of the use of DDAVP as an adjunctive agent for hemostasis following coronary revascularization has failed to show benefit from DDAVP (43, 44). In fact, when used for patients undergoing coronary artery bypass graft surgery, DDAVP was associated with a 2.4-fold increase in the risk of perioperative myocardial infarction (44). However, when thromboelastography or other studies document that platelet dysfunction and platelet transfusion are not options, one-time administration of this agent may be indicated.

Fibrinogen Deficiency and von Willebrand Disease

Another treatable cause of coagulopathy in this patient is absolute fibrinogen deficiency. Although blood sampling should be limited in a patient refusing transfusion, measurement of serum fibrinogen and a point-of-care coagulation test such as thromboelastography prior to discontinuation from CPB is indicated to identify treatable causes of coagulopathy. If the fibrinogen level is <80 mg/dL and there is evidence of significant nonsurgical bleeding after heparin reversal and return of harvested blood from hemodilution, administration of cryoprecipitate, which contains primarily fibrinogen, factor VIII, von Willebrand factor, and fibronectin, should be considered before severe thrombocytopenia or anemia develop (45). Even if the fibrinogen level is not < 80 mg/dL, the possibility of undiagnosed von Willebrand disease exists and cryoprecipitate may be beneficial in the context of life-threatening nonsurgical bleeding without an identifiable cause.

Factor VII Deficiency

Recombinant factor concentrates have been developed for factors VIII, IX, and recently VII. These agents are considered minor fractions by the Jehovah's Witness Church and are widely accepted, even by patients refusing other fractions such as cryoprecipitate. For this patient with a known factor VII deficiency, the administration of recombinant factor VII should be considered. Because activated factor VII stimulates clot formation via the extrinsic pathway and represents one of the factors with the shortest half-life that tends to be depressed following prolonged CPB, it represents an attractive adjunct for treatment of coagulopathic bleeding in the postbypass cardiac surgical patient. Unfortunately, case reports of excessive thrombosis and poor outcome associated with its use raise concern about its safety (46). Factor VII stimulates clot formation in response to tissue factor expression. Because tissue factor levels are elevated by passage of blood through the CPB machine as well as by the surgical procedure itself, administration of this agent on bypass is contraindicated. According to a case–control study of the use of activated factor VII guided by protocol, Karkouti and colleagues (46) found a risk-adjusted decrease in mortality for cardiac surgical patients with excessive bleeding when factor VII was administered at least 2 hours following cardiac surgery. In this study, all surgical sources of bleeding had been ruled out and all other means to correct coagulopathy and severe anemia, including transfusion of red blood cells and blood components, had been exhausted (46). For the case described, the benefit of administration of 30–45 mcg/kg of activated factor VII in the presence of clinically significant nonsurgical postbypass bleeding would likely outweigh the risk. Delay of factor VII administration until after full heparin reversal, return of all harvested whole blood, and 2 hours of elapsed time since separation from CPB would be recommended. However, exsanguination in a patient refusing transfusion would alter the risk/benefit ratio toward earlier administration following separation from bypass and heparin reversal. Because the desired endpoint of factor VII administration is cross-linked fibrin, cryoprecipitate should be administered prior to factor VII to ensure that fibrinogen levels are adequate.

Unidentified Factor Deficiency

When significant bleeding continues after administration of DDAVP, cryoprecipitate, and activated factor VII, the presence of unidentified factor deficiency should be considered. Assuming that the patient would accept "cryosupernatant," administration of cryoprecipitate-poor plasma is indicated if bleeding continues. Although the volume of cryo-poor plasma required for replacement of vitamin K–dependent factors (8–10 mL/kg of plasma) (45) may dilute already low platelet levels, continued hemorrhage would also contribute to thrombocytopenia. Administration of cryo-poor plasma might also be superior to volume resuscitation with colloid or crystalloid alone. Administration of factor concentrates prepared from pooled plasma also might be effective. However, these agents are not extensively tested for safety, may cause undesirable thrombosis, and should be used only if the patient will not accept cryo-poor plasma or will not tolerate intravascular volume administration.

Postoperative Management

According to studies in healthy volunteers, acute normovolemic anemia is well compensated and does not result in a metabolic acidosis until the hemoglobin level falls to < 5.0 g/dL (47). However, without supplemental oxygen, short-term memory becomes affected below a hemoglobin level of 6.0 g/dL (48). When hemoglobin level drops to < 3.0 g/dL, compensatory mechanisms to increase oxygen delivery begin to fail and mortality rises abruptly (49) . In the event of severe postoperative anemia in a patient refusing transfusion therapy, balancing oxygen demand with available supply becomes essential to preventing tissue ischemia. Bone marrow stimulation with erythropoietin accompanied by supplemental intravenous iron therapy will encourage recovery of hemoglobin mass over time. However, hemoglobin levels rise over days to weeks. In the immediate postoperative period without additional hemoglobin, administration of supplemental oxygen may be the only means of increasing supply. In the presence of severe anemia, dissolved oxygen levels become increasingly important. The PaO_2 should be maintained at as high a level as possible, initially by administering 100% oxygen. The administration of hyperbaric oxygen, although theoretically beneficial, is not likely to be readily available and cannot be maintained while also addressing other clinical needs of the patient. In addition to optimizing the oxygen tension, oxygen demand should be minimized as much as possible. The patient should remain sedated and should receive ventilatory support to minimize work of breathing. Although there is little evidence to document its benefit, core cooling will reduce metabolic rate. When core cooling is used, the patient should also receive muscle relaxants and other agents to minimize shivering. This therapy would have to be maintained until recovery of sufficient hemoglobin to meet higher levels of oxygen demand.

TABLE 13–3. Recommended anesthetic plan

In this particular case, a rational anesthetic plan might include:
- Administer preoperative dose of 40,000 units of erythropoietin alfa subcutaneously with 125 mg of elemental iron in the form of ferric gluconate intravenously
- Minimize perioperative blood sampling and sampling waste
- Perform intraoperative normovolemic hemodilution with a target prebypass hemoglobin of 8.0 g/dL and a calculated harvest volume of 5 units of whole blood
- Perform cell salvage outside the pericardium with use of cardiotomy suction for cell salvage inside the pericardium
- Administer aminocaproic acid, 10 g intravenously following induction followed by 1 g/h by continuous infusion for the duration of surgery
- Minimize CPB circuit volume
- Perform rapid autologous priming upon initiation of CPB to eliminate unnecessary crystalloid from the pump prime solution
- Accept hemoglobin of 6.0 g/dL on bypass before returning harvested whole blood
- Recycle salvaged red blood cells to the bypass reservoir to maintain hemoglobin while on bypass
- Fully reverse heparin with protamine and monitor for heparin rebound with serial Activated clotting time measurements each hour for the first 2 hours in the intensive care unit; administer additional protamine if necessary
- Monitor point-of-care coagulation testing such as the thromboelastogram.
- If coagulation testing indicates thrombasthenia and the patient is bleeding postbypass, administer DDAVP
- If the patient is bleeding excessively and coagulation testing indicates deficiency, measure fibrinogen and prothrombin time. If fibrinogen level is <80,000 and bleeding continues postbypass, administer cryoprecipitate
- If the fibrinogen level is acceptable, the prothrombin time is prolonged, harvested whole blood has been returned, and bleeding continues in this patient with a known factor VII deficiency, administer activated factor VII in a dose of 30–45 mcg/kg and repeat if necessary
- If bleeding persists despite factor VII, consider administration of cryo-poor plasma
- Early reexploration is recommended for excessive chest tube output in the early postoperative period
- Postoperative erythropoietin and intravenous iron should be administered to stimulate recovery of hemoglobin mass if postoperative anemia is significant
- If severely anemic, maximize oxygen and limit metabolic demand
- Clearly document plan and rationale for decisions

CONCLUSION

Adult patients refusing transfusion are protected under the law; physicians are also protected when the patient's wishes, as known, are honored. At the same time, in cases such as the one presented in this chapter, refusal of transfusion complicates care but does not necessarily contraindicate a surgical intervention. When considering therapeutic alternatives, it is essential to develop a comprehensive, multidisciplinary approach to understand the patient's specific wishes and to ensure that appropriate blood products and other therapeutic options are available. Table 13–3 outlines some of the recommended approaches to the perioperative management of the patient who refuses transfusion. Patients who refuse blood and blood products have taught us a great deal about effective blood management strategies and have fostered continued research in search of an acceptable replacement for allogeneic human blood transfusion. The therapeutic options are limited, but can result in a satisfactory outcome for many patients presenting for complex surgical procedures, including those requiring CPB.

References

1. Definition of Hippocratic oath. (2002). Available at: http://www.medterms.com/script/main/art.asp?articlekey=20909. Accessed March 11, 2009
2. Schloendorff v. Society of New York Hospitals: NY, 1914, 211, pp 125
3. In re a.C.: A 2d, 1990, 573, pp 1235
4. Stamford Hospital v. Vega: A 2d, 1996, 674, pp 821
5. Harrell v. St. Mary's Hospital, Inc.: So 2d, 1996, 678, pp 455
6. In re Fetus Brown: NE 2nd, 1997, 689, pp 397
7. Moskowitz DM, Klein JJ, Shander A, et al.: Predictors of transfusion requirements for cardiac surgical procedures at a blood conservation center. Ann Thorac Surg 2004; 77:626–634
8. Vincent JL, Baron JF, Reinhart K, et al.: Anemia and blood transfusion in critically ill patients. JAMA 2002; 288:1499–1507
9. Natanson C, Kern SJ, Lurie P, et al.: Cell-free hemoglobin-based blood substitutes and risk of myocardial infarction and death: a meta-analysis. JAMA 2008; 299:2304–2312
10. Hill SE, Grocott HP, Leone BJ, et al.: Cerebral physiology of cardiac surgical patients treated with the perfluorocarbon emulsion, af0144. Ann Thorac Surg 2005; 80:1401–1407
11. Procrit prescribing information, 2007. Ortho Biotech Products, LP, Raritan, NJ
12. Goldberg MA, McCutchen JW, Jove M, et al.: A safety and efficacy comparison study of two dosing regimens of epoetin alfa in patients undergoing major orthopedic surgery. Am J Orthop 1996; 25:544–552
13. de Andrade JR, Jove M, Landon G, et al.: Baseline hemoglobin as a predictor of risk of transfusion and response to epoetin alfa in orthopedic surgery patients. Am J Orthop 1996; 25:533–542
14. Faris P: Use of recombinant human erythropoietin in the perioperative period of orthopedic surgery. Am J Med 1996; 101:28S–32S
15. FDA. (2008). Questions and answers on medication guidelines for erythropoiesis-stimulating agents (ESAS). Available at: http://www.fda.gov/cder/drug/infopage/RHE/qa2008.htm. Accessed March 12, 2009

16. Carless P, Moxey A, O'Connell D, et al.: Autologous transfusion techniques: a systematic review of their efficacy. Transfus Med 2004; 14:123–144
17. Murphy GJ, Allen SM, Unsworth-White J, et al.: Safety and efficacy of perioperative cell salvage and autotransfusion after coronary artery bypass grafting: a randomized trial. Ann Thorac Surg 2004; 77:1553–1559
18. Huet C, Salmi LR, Fergusson D, et al.: A meta-analysis of the effectiveness of cell salvage to minimize perioperative allogeneic blood transfusion in cardiac and orthopedic surgery. International Study of Perioperative Transfusion (ISPOT) Investigators. Anesth Analg 1999; 89:861–869
19. Vanderlinde ES, Heal JM, Blumberg N: Autologous transfusion. BMJ 2002; 324:772–775
20. Laub GW, Riebman JB: Autotransfusion: methods and complications. In Lake CL, Moore RA, eds.: Blood: hemostasis, transfusion, and alternatives in the perioperative period. Baltimore, MD, Lippincott Williams & Wilkins, 1995:382–394
21. Waters JH, Lee JS, Karafa MT: A mathematical model of cell salvage compared and combined with normovolemic hemodilution. Transfusion 2004; 44:1412–1416
22. Bryson GL, Laupacis A, Wells GA: Does acute normovolemic hemodilution reduce perioperative allogeneic transfusion? A meta-analysis. The International Study of Perioperative Transfusion. Anesth Analg 1998; 86:9–15
23. Ilstrup S, ed.: Handling, storage, and expiration of perioperative autologous red blood cell products. Standards for perioperative autologous blood collection and administration, 4th Edition. Bethesda, MD, AABB, 2009
24. Casati V, Speziali G, D'Alessandro C, et al.: Intraoperative low-volume acute normovolemic hemodilution in adult open-heart surgery. Anesthesiology 2002; 97:367–373
25. Hill SE, D'Alonzo RC: Perioperative management of bleeding and transfusion. In Newman MF, Fleischer L, Longnecker DE, eds.: Perioperative medicine: managing for outcome. Philadelphia, PA, Elsevier, 2007, Chapter 27
26. Ferraris VA, Ferraris SP, Saha SP, et al.: Perioperative blood transfusion and blood conservation in cardiac surgery: The Society of Thoracic Surgeons and the Society of Cardiovascular Anesthesiologists Clinical Practice Guideline. Ann Thorac Surg 2007; 83:S27–86
27. Helm RE, Klemperer JD, Rosengart TK, et al.: Intraoperative autologous blood donation preserves red cell mass but does not decrease postoperative bleeding. Ann Thorac Surg 1996; 62:1431–1441

28. Cosgrove DM, 3rd, Heric B, Lytle BW, et al.: Aprotinin therapy for reoperative myocardial revascularization: a placebo-controlled study. Ann Thorac Surg 1992; 54:1031–1036; discussion 1036–1038

29. Lemmer JH, Jr., Stanford W, Bonney SL, et al.: Aprotinin for coronary bypass operations: efficacy, safety, and influence on early saphenous vein graft patency. A multicenter, randomized, double-blind, placebo-controlled study. J Thorac Cardiovasc Surg 1994; 107:543–551; discussion 551–543

30. Levy JH, Pifarre R, Schaff HV, et al.: A multicenter, double-blind, placebo-controlled trial of aprotinin for reducing blood loss and the requirement for donor-blood transfusion in patients undergoing repeat coronary artery bypass grafting. Circulation 1995; 92: 2236–2244

31. Lemmer JH, Jr., Dilling EW, Morton JR, et al.: Aprotinin for primary coronary artery bypass grafting: a multicenter trial of three dose regimens. Ann Thorac Surg 1996; 62:1659–1667; discussion 1667–1658

32. Alderman EL, Levy JH, Rich JB, et al.: Analyses of coronary graft patency after aprotinin use: results from the International Multicenter Aprotinin Graft Patency Experience (IMAGE) Trial. J Thorac Cardiovasc Surg 1998; 116:716–730

33. Sedrakyan A, Treasure T, Elefteriades JA: Effect of aprotinin on clinical outcomes in coronary artery bypass graft surgery: a systematic review and meta-analysis of randomized clinical trials. J Thorac Cardiovasc Surg 2004; 128:442–448

34. Mangano DT, Tudor IC, Dietzel C: The risk associated with aprotinin in cardiac surgery. N Engl J Med 2006; 354:353–365

35. Karkouti K, Beattie WS, Dattilo KM, et al.: A propensity score case-control comparison of aprotinin and tranexamic acid in high-transfusion-risk cardiac surgery. Transfusion 2006; 46:327–338

36. Mangano DT, Miao Y, Vuylsteke A, et al.: Mortality associated with aprotinin during 5 years following coronary artery bypass graft surgery. JAMA 2007; 297:471–479

37. Shaw AD, Stafford-Smith M, White WD, et al.: The effect of aprotinin on outcome after coronary-artery bypass grafting. N Engl J Med 2008; 358:784–793

38. Fergusson DA, Hebert PC, Mazer CD, et al.: A comparison of aprotinin and lysine analogues in high-risk cardiac surgery. N Engl J Med 2008; 358:2319–2331

39. Bayer. (2007). Bayer temporarily suspends global Trasylol® marketing. Available at: http://www.bayerhealthcare.com/scripts/pages/en/press/information_on_trasylol/suspends_global/index.php. Accessed March 12, 2009

40. Sloand EM, Alyono D, Klein HG, et al.: 1-deamino-8-d-arginine vasopressin (ddavp) increases platelet membrane expression of glycoprotein ib in patients with disorders of platelet function and after cardiopulmonary bypass. Am J Hematol 1994; 46:199–207

41. Andersson TL, Solem JO, Tengborn L, et al.: Effects of desmopressin acetate on platelet aggregation, von Willebrand factor, and blood loss after cardiac surgery with extracorporeal circulation. Circulation 1990; 81:872–878

42. Vincentelli A, Susen S, Le Tourneau T, et al.: Acquired von Willebrand syndrome in aortic stenosis. N Engl J Med 2003; 349:343–349

43. Laupacis A, Fergusson D: Drugs to minimize perioperative blood loss in cardiac surgery: meta-analyses using perioperative blood transfusion as the outcome. The International Study of Peri-Operative Transfusion (ISPOT) Investigators. Anesth Analg 1997; 85:1258–1267

44. Levi M, Cromheecke ME, de Jonge E, et al.: Pharmacological strategies to decrease excessive blood loss in cardiac surgery: a meta-analysis of clinically relevant endpoints. Lancet 1999; 354:1940–1947

45. ASA: Practice guidelines for perioperative blood transfusion and adjuvant therapies: an updated report by the American Society of Anesthesiologists' Task Force on Perioperative Blood Transfusion and Adjuvant Therapies. Anesthesiology 2006; 105:198–208

46. Karkouti K, Yau TM, Riazi S, et al.: Determinants of complications with recombinant factor viia for refractory blood loss in cardiac surgery. Can J Anaesth 2006; 53:802–809

47. Weiskopf RB, Viele MK, Feiner J, et al.: Human cardiovascular and metabolic response to acute, severe isovolemic anemia. JAMA 1998; 279:217–221

48. Weiskopf RB, Kramer JH, Viele M, et al.: Acute severe isovolemic anemia impairs cognitive function and memory in humans. Anesthesiology 2000; 92:1646–1652

49. Spence RK, Costabile JP, Young GS, et al.: Is hemoglobin level alone a reliable predictor of outcome in the severly anemic surgical patient? Am Surg 1992; 58:92–95

Index

Page numbers followed by "*f*" denote figures; those followed by "*t*" denote tables.

Acid base balance
  in ESRD, 145–146
  during pregnancy, 230
Acute hypertensive syndromes, 42*f*
β-2 Adrenergic agonists, treatment
    for hyperkalemia, 143
β- Adrenergic antagonists, use
    during pregnancy, 236–237
Adrenoreceptors, effects on PVR,
    187
Airway physiology
  anterior mediastinal mass,
    286–288, 295*t*, 296–297
  in obesity, 248–250
American Joint Committee on
    Cancer's 2002 Tumor-
    Node-Metastasis (TNM)
    Staging System for RCC,
    305, 306*t*
Amiodarone, use during pregnancy,
    236
Anesthesia
  anterior mediastinal masses,
    294–296, 295*t*
  extremely obese patient, 245–266
  general considerations during
    pregnancy, 233–234
  invasive vena caval tumors,
    309–311, 314–316
  lung isolation with a difficult
    airway, 267–284
  pharmacologic considerations
    during pregnancy, 234–235
  positioning of obese patient, 252
  transfusion refusal plan, 343*t*

Anesthetics
  cardiac surgery during pregnancy,
    234–235
  induction in obesity, 255–256
  perioperative management in
    obesity, 252–258
  use in ESRD, 152–153
*Angela Carder v. George Washington
    University Hospital,* 331–332
Angiotensin-converting enzyme
    (ACE) inhibitors, stroke
    prevention, 79
Angiotensin receptor blockers
    (ARBs), stroke prevention,
    79
Anglo-Scandinavian Cardiac
    Outcomes Trial (ASCOT),
    44
Anterior mediastinal mass, 285–302
  airway and cardiovascular
    complications, 286–288,
    296–297
  anesthetic considerations,
    294–296, 295*t*
  CPB and, 297
  perioperative complications, 298*t*
  postoperative complications,
    297–298
  preoperative assessment, 288–293
  pulmonary function studies,
    290–293
  radiological studies, 288–290, 289*f*
  surgical considerations, 293–294
Antiarrhythmic therapy, during
    pregnancy, 237*t*

Anticoagulants
  CPB in pregnancy, 231–233, 232*t*
  intraoperative strategies in HIT, 171–174, 173*t*
  use in HIT, 169–171
Antifibrinolytic therapy, 339–340
Antihypertensive treatment, 38*f*
Antiplatelet therapy, stroke prevention, 75–77
Aorta, atherosclerosis, 5–7
Aortic Placque and Risk of Ischemic Stroke (APRIS) study, 7
Argatroban, use in HIT, 169–171, 173*t*
Arndt Blocker, 269, 270*t*, 271–274*f*
Asymptomatic Carotid Atherosclerosis Study (ACAS), 79–80
Atheromatous instability, biomarkers, 77–78
Atherosclerosis
  aorta, 5–7
  pulse pressure relations, 50*f*

Barbiturates, use in ESRD, 153
Benzodiazepines
  use during pregnancy, 235
  use in ESRD, 153
Bivalirudin, use in HIT, 169–171, 173*t*
Bleeding
  management during surgery, 340–344
  postoperative management, 340–344
Blood pressure
  brachial and central systolic, 45*f*
  clinical management strategies, 50–58
  duration of liability, 58*f*
  in ESRD, 138–139
  management, 12–13, 29–68
  measurements, 43–46
  perioperative control, 55*f*
  postoperative control, 56*f*
  prevalence of high BP, 30*f*
  science to strategy, 46–48
  systolic and diastolic levels, 32*t*
  understanding the risk, 31–35
Body mass index, morbidity and mortality in cardiac surgery, 246–247, 247*f*

Body temperature
  changes in pregnancy with CPB, 223–224, 223*f*
  management, 15–16
Brain, perioperative injury, 2–4
Brain protection
  CPB, 2–17
  pharmacologic, 17–18
  strategies, 6*t*
Bronchial blocker, lung isolation, 268, 269–270*t*, 270*f*

Cardiac surgery
  anesthesia in the extremely obese patient, 245–266
  arterial stiffness and, 49–50
  blood pressure management during, 48–49
  blood pressure management in, 29–68
  dialysis-dependent renal failure requiring, 129–161
  general considerations during pregnancy, 233–234
  glucose management in the diabetic patient, 109–128
  Jehovah's Witness Church and transfusion necessity, 330–331
  kidney injury after, 49*t*
  lung isolation with a difficult airway, 267–284
  management of severe bleeding, 340–344
  material and fetal risks, 219–220
  patient refusing transfusion, 327–347
  pulmonary hypertension and, 185–214
  recommendations for insulin in ICU patients, 121*t*
  timing during pregnancy, 220–222
Cardiopulmonary bypass (CPB)
  with anterior mediastinal mass, 297
  anticoagulation in pregnancy, 231–233, 232*t*
  aortic atherosclerosis, 5–7
  blood pressure management, 12–13
  brain protection and, 2–17
  flow management, 7–9

glucose management, 16–17
hemoglobin/hematocrit targets,
   15
hypothermic *versus* normothermic
   in the parturient, 228–229
impact on fetoplacental unit,
   222–224
maternal and fetal risk during,
   219–220
mean arterial pressure in, 33
mediastinal CO_2 insufflation,
   13–15
myocardial protection in
   pregnancy, 231
myometrium during, 224–225
neuromonitoring, 17–18
obstetric monitoring during,
   225–226
pericardial suction management,
   11–12
pH management during
   hypothermia, 9–11
pregnant patients, 215–244
priming, in pregnancy, 231
pulsatile *versus* nonpulsatile, in
   pregnancy, 224, 226–227
temperature management, 15–16
venal caval invasive tumors and,
   319–320
Cardiovascular disease
anterior mediastinal mass,
   286–288
ESRD and, 149–150
pathophysiology in obesity,
   250–251
Carotid and Vertebral Artery
   Transluminal Angioplasty
   Study (CAVATAS), 74
Carotid artery stenting (CAS)
versus CEA, 74–75
risk factors from stroke from,
   73–74
risk of MI after, 80–81
Carotid endarterectomy (CEA),
   68–69
CABG combined procedures, 83,
   84–98*t*
versus CAS, 74–75
risk factors from stroke from, 73
risk of MI after, 80
stroke prevention by, 79–80
Carotid stenosis, 69–107

concomitant coronary disease,
   70–72, 81–98
risk of stroke from, 79–80
Cell salvage technique, 337–338
Cerebral blood flow
after CABG, 5*f*
autoregulation, 13–15, 14*f*
management during CPB, 7–9
Chemotherapy, invasive vena caval
   tumors, 310*t*
Chronic kidney disease (CKD), 130
physiology and complications,
   136–149
prelude to ESRD, 131–132
stages, 131*t*
Clevidipine (CLV), hypertension
   management, 52, 55*f*
Clopidogrel, stroke prevention, 76,
   76*t*
Clopidogrel in Unstable Angina to
   Prevent Recurrent Events
   (CURE) trial, 76, 76*t*
Cohen Blocker, 269, 270*t*, 271–274*f*
Computed tomography (CT)
anterior mediastinal mass, 287,
   289–293, 296, 298
before cardiac surgery, 3
difficult lower airway, 279, 283*f*
invasive venal caval tumors, 308
Conduit Artery Function Evaluation
   (CAFE) study, 44
Continuous renal replacement
   therapy (CRRT), 133
Cook airway catheter, 276*f*
Coronary artery bypass graft
   (CABG)
brain protection and, 2–4
carotid endarterectomy and, 69
cerebral perfusion after, 5*f*
combined CEA studies, 83, 84–98*t*
versus PCI, 81
rate of adverse outcomes after, 35*f*
risk factors for stroke, 72–73
risk of MI after, 81
Coronary disease
age-adjusted rates, 33*f*
concomitant carotid stenosis,
   70–72, 81–98
morbid obesity and, 245–246

Danaparoid, use in HIT, 169–171,
   173*t*

Diabetes mellitus (DM),
  cardiothoracic surgery and,
  109–128
Dialysis. *see* Hemodialysis
Digoxin, use during pregnancy, 236
Diuretics, treatment for
  hyperkalemia, 144
Double-lumen endobronchial tube
  (DLT), lung isolation, 268,
  269*t*, 275–281

ECLIPSE Trial, 52–58, 53*f*, 54*t*, 57*t*
Efficacy of Volume Substitution and
  Insulin Therapy in Severe
  Sepsis (VISEP) study, 118
Electrocardiography (ECG), in
  hyperkalemia, 140–145
Electrolytes, in ESRD, 146–147
Endarterectomy *versus* Stenting in
  Patients with Symptomatic
  Severe Carotid Stenosis
  (DVA-S3) trial, 75
Endobronchial tube, 268, 269*t*
Endothelial mechanoreceptors, 42*f*
Endothelial shear stress, 40–42*f*
Endotracheal intubation, surgery
  during pregnancy, 234
End-stage renal disease (ESRD), 129
  cardiovascular system and,
    149–150
  epidemiology of, 130–132
  extracorporeal support, 132–136
  pharmacokinetics, 152–153
  physiology and complications,
    136–149
  vascular complications, 151–152
Enzyme-linked immunosorbent
  assay (ELISA), for HIT, 166
Ephedrine, use during pregnancy,
  235
Erythropoietin, 337

Factor VII deficiency, 341–342
Fetal heart rate, monitoring during
  CPB, 225–226
Fiberoptic bronchoscope (FOB), 280*f*
Fibrinogen deficiency, 341
Fondaparinux, use in HIT, 171, 173*t*
Fuji Uniblocker, 269, 270*t*, 271–274*f*
Functional residual capacity (FRC),
  effects of obesity and
  anesthesia, 248*f*

Glidescope video-laryngoscope,
  276*f*
Global Utilization of Streptokinase
  and Tissue Plasminogen
  Activator for Occluded
  Coronary Arteries IV-Acute
  Coronary Syndrome trial
  (GUSTO IV-ACS), 174–175
Glucose management, 16–17,
  109–128
  in extreme obesity, 256–257
  hypoglycemia and, 117–119
  intraoperative, 114
  perioperative strategies, 113–117
  perioperative strategies as a
    quality measure, 122
  postoperative, 114–117

Harrell v. St. Mary's Hospital, Inc., 332
Harrison v. Smith, 332
Health Care Power of Attorney,
  333–336
  medical decision hierarchy in
    North Carolina, 333*t*
Hematologic complications, in
  ESRD, 147
Hemodialysis, 133–136, 135*f*
  complications of therapy, 150–151
  IHD for hyperkalemia, 145
Hemodilution, CPB during
  pregnancy, 225
Hemofiltration, 133–136, 135*f*
Hemoglobin/hematocrit targets, 15
Heparin
  discontinuation, 168
  thrombocytopenia induced by,
    163–184
Heparin antibodies, independent
  risk predictors of HIT,
  174–176
Heparin-induced thrombocytopenia
  (HIT), 163–184
  clinical suspicion for, 168*t*
  general principles of treatment,
    168–171
  heparin antibodies as risk
    predictors, 174–176
  intraoperative strategies in HIT,
    171–174, 173*t*
  laboratory assessment, 166–168
  pathogenesis, 165–166
  presentation, 163–165

pretest probability of, 167*t*
Hyperglycemia
  complications with, 112–113
  morbidity and mortality after
      cardiac surgery, 110–111
  potential causes, 111–112
Hyperkalemia, 140–145
  treatment for, 143–145
Hypernatremia, 139
Hypertension, 12–13, 29–68
  acute management, 35–37
  cardiovascular surgery and, 48–49
  clarification of subtypes, 31*t*
  pathophysiology of, 37–43, 42*f*
  prevalence of different types, 37*f*
  shear forces associated with, 40*f*
  vessel stretch, 41*f*
Hypoglycemia, 117–119
Hypotension, as complication of
      dialysis, 150–151
Hypothermia, pH management
      during, 9–11
Hypoxemia, surgery during
      pregnancy, 234

IHD (in-center hemodialysis). *see*
      Hemodialysis
Infection
  as complication of dialysis, 151
  improvement measures, 122*t*
Inotropic agents, in pulmonary
      hypertension, 201–203
Inotropic and antiarrhythmic
      agents, use during
      pregnancy, 236, 237*t*
Insulin
  perioperative intensive therapy
      protocols, 119–121,
      120–121*t*
  recommendations for cardiac
      surgery ICU patients, 121*t*
  recommendations for noncardiac
      surgery ICU patients, 120*t*
  treatment for hyperkalemia, 143
Intraaortic balloon pump (IABP),
      combination therapy for
      PH and RV, 203–204
Intravenous leiomyomatosis (IVL),
      invasive tumor of vena
      cava, 307–308

Intubation, in obese patient,
      253–254, 254*t*
Isolated diastolic hypertension
      (IDH), 32–34, 33*f*, 34*f*
Isolated systolic hypertension (ISH),
      32–34, 33*f*, 34*f*
Isoproterenol, use during
      pregnancy, 236

Jehovah Witness Church,
      transfusions and cardiac
      surgery, 330–331
Joint National Committee on
      Prevention, Detection,
      Evaluation, and Treatment
      of High Blood Pressure,
      Seventh Report, 31

Kaplan-Meier analysis, cerebral and
      cardiac survival, 36*f*
Kaplan-Meier Surgical curve, 3*f*
Ketamine, use during pregnancy,
      235
Kidney injury, after cardiac surgery,
      49*t*

Left ventricular dysfunction, in
      pregnancy, 218–219
Lepirudin, use in HIT, 169–171, 173*t*
Lung isolation, 267–284
  with a difficult airway, 273–277,
      274*f*, 276*f*
  with a difficult lower airway,
      279–281. 279*f*
  techniques, 268–273, 269*t*

Magnetic resonance imaging (MRI),
      1
  anterior mediastinal mass, 290
  invasive venal caval tumors, 308
  managing pulmonary
      hypertension, 185
  RV and LV volume and function,
      196
Mask ventilation, in obese patient,
      253–254, 254*t*
Mean arterial pressure (MAP), 33, 37
Mechanical ventilation, in obesity,
      256
Mediastinal CO_2 insufflation, 13–15
Mediastinum, anatomy, 285–286,
      286*f*

Medical decision hierarchy, 333*t*
Multiple Risk Factor Intervention
    Trial, 33*f*
Myocardial infarction
    risk after CABG or PCI, 81
    risk after CAS, 80–81
    risk after CEA, 80
Myometrium, during CPB, 224–225

National Health and Nutrition
    Examination
    Survey/National Center
    for Health Statistics
    (NHANES/NCHS), 29
Neurological complications, after
    cardiac surgery, 1–18
Neuromonitoring, 17–18
Neuromuscular blocking agents, use
    in ESRD, 153
Nicardipine (NIC), hypertension
    management, 52
Nitroglycerin, hypertension
    management, 52, 55*f*
Nitrous oxide, use during
    pregnancy, 234–235
Nonsteroidal antiinflammatory
    drugs (NSAIDs), use in
    ESRD, 153
Normovolemic hemodilution,
    338–339, 338*t*
*North American Symptomatic Carotid
    Endarterectomy Trial*
    (NASCET), 75–76, 80
Northern New England
    Cardiovascular Disease
    Study Group, 246

Obesity
    anesthesia in cardiac surgery,
    245–266
    anesthetic induction in, 255
    cardiovascular pathophysiology
    in, 250–251
    glucose management in, 256–257
    hemodynamic monitoring during
    surgery, 251
    mechanical ventilation in, 256
    morbidity and mortality, 246–248
    perioperative anesthetic
    management, 252–258
    pharmacokinetic alterations with,
    251–252

postoperative management, 258
    pulmonary and airway
    pathophysiology, 248–250
    pulmonary hypertension and,
    257–258
Obesity hypoventilation syndrome
    (OHS), 249–250
Observed arterial pulse wave, 38*f*
Obstetric monitoring, during CPB,
    225–226
Obstructive sleep apnea (OSA)
    body mass index and, 249
    morbid obesity and, 246
One-lung ventilation, 273–277, 274*f*,
    276*f*
Oscillatory shear stress, 40*f*
Oxygenation
    effects on PVR, 187
    preoxygenation in obese patients,
    253
Oxygen consumption, during
    pregnancy, 216–217

Patient autonomy, refusal of
    transfusion, 329–330
Patient-related risk factors, stroke,
    72
PDE III inhibitors, in pulmonary
    hypertension, 200–201
Pediatric fiberoptic bronchoscope,
    277, 278*f*
Percutaneous coronary
    interventions (PCI)
    versus CABG, 81
    risk factors for stroke from, 73
    risk of MI after, 81
Perfusion flow and pressure, CPB
    during pregnancy, 222–223,
    229–230
Pericardial suction aspirate, 11–12
Peritoneal dialysis (PD), 133–136
pH, management during
    hypothermia, 9–11
Pharmacokinetics
    alterations associated with
    obesity, 251–252
    ESRD, 152–153
Phenylephrine, use during
    pregnancy, 235–236
Platelet dysfunction, 340
Platelet inhibitors, intraoperative
    strategies in HIT, 173*t*

Potassium, in ESRD, 140–145
Preeclampsia, surgery during
  pregnancy, 234
Pregnancy
  β- adrenergic antagonists, 236–237
  anesthetic considerations during,
    234–235
  antiarrhythmic therapy during,
    237*t*
  anticoagulation in CPB, 231–233,
    232*t*
  blood rheology, 217, 218*t*
  cardiac function and
    hemodynamics in, 216
  cardiac risk assessment during,
    218–222
  cardiopulmonary bypass and,
    215–244
  hypothermic *versus* normothermic
    CPB, 228–229
  inotropic and antiarrhythmic
    agents, 236, 237*t*
  myocardial protection for CPB,
    231
  oxygen consumption, 216–217
  physiologic changes during,
    216–218, 217–218*t*
  pulmonary function, 217–218
  specific CPB considerations,
    226–227
  sympathomimetic agents, 235–236
  timing of cardiac surgery during,
    220–222
  vasodilating agents during,
    237–238
Pulmonary artery pressure (PAP),
  RV function and, 193–196
Pulmonary function studies, in
  anterior mediastinal
  masses, 290–293
Pulmonary hypertension
  anesthetic management with, 197
  cardiac surgery and, 185–214
  evaluation by TEE, 190–191, 191*f*
  in extreme obesity, 257–258
  fluid management, 198
  gas exchange strategies with, 198
  inhaled pulmonary vasodilator
    therapy, 204–206, 206*t*
  inotropic agents in, 201–203
  PDE III inhibitors, 200–201

RV and, combination therapy,
  203–204
  therapeutic options for, 196–197,
    197*t*
  vasodilators in, 198–201, 200*f*
Pulmonary physiology, 185–187
  in obesity, 248–250
Pulmonary vascular resistance
  (PVR), 185
  factors affecting, 187–188
Pulsatile component, blood
  pressure, 37
Pulse pressure
  atherosclerosis relationship, 50*f*
  Kaplan-Meier analysis, 36*f*
  outcomes after cardiac surgery, 4*f*
  stroke after cardiac surgery, 35*f*
  stroke-free survival and, 3*f*
Pulse wave velocity, 44–45*f*

Quality control, perioperative
  glucose control, 122

RCC, invasive tumor of vena cava,
  304–305
Renal failure
  dialysis-dependent, 129–161
  physiology and complications,
    136–149
Right ventricular (RV) failure
  evaluation by TEE, 190–191, 191*f*
  global assessment, 191–193,
    192–194*f*
  PH and, 188–190
  combination therapy, 203–204
  pulmonary artery pressure and,
    193–196
  therapeutic options for, 196–197, 197*t*
Rocuronium, use in ESRD, 153

*Schloendorff v. Society of New York
  Hospitals*, 327–328
Shed mediastinal blood, 11–12, 11*f*
Single-lumen endobronchial tube,
  lung isolation, 268, 269*t*
Sodium and tonicity, in ESRD,
  139–140
Sodium bicarbonate, treatment for
  hyperkalemia, 143–144
Sodium nitroprusside (SNP),
  hypertension management,
  52

Stamford Hospital v. Vega, 332
Statin therapy, stroke prevention, 77
Stenting and Angioplasty with
	Protection in Patients at
	High Risk for
	Endarterectomy
	(SAPPHIRE) trial, 74
Stent-protected Percutaneous
	Angioplasty of the Carotid
	versus Endarterectomy
	(SPACE) study, 75
Stroke
	after cardiac surgery, 35*f*
	preoperative pharmacological
		prevention, 75–79
	risk factors for, 72–75, 72*t*
Surgical approaches
	anterior mediastinal masses,
		293–294
	combined carotid and coronary
		disease, 81–98
	vena caval invasive tumor,
		316–320
Surgical Care Improvement Project
	(SCIP), infection
	improvement measures,
	122*t*
Sympathomimetic agents, use
	during pregnancy, 235–236

Temperature. *see* Body temperature
Testicular carcinoma
	chemotherapeutic agents, 310*t*
	invasive tumor of vena cava,
		305–307
Thrombocytopenia, heparin-
	induced, 163–184
Tocolytics, CPB during pregnancy,
	225
Transesophageal echocardiography
	(TEE)
	atheromatous disease, aortic, 95
	evaluation of PH and RV failure,
		190–191, 191–192–194*f*
	invasive venal caval tumors, 308,
		312–314, 312*f*, 313*t*
	managing pulmonary
		hypertension, 185
	pulmonary hypertension, 185
	vena caval invasive tumor, 308,
		311–316
Transfusion, 327–347

anesthetic plan with refusal, 343*t*
blood conservation modalities,
	337–340
clinical decision making, 336
clinical scenario, 328–330
Jehovah's Witness Church,
	330–331
medico-legal implications of
	refusal, 331–336
pediatric patients, 335–336
Transthoracic echocardiography,
	managing pulmonary
	hypertension, 185

Unidentified factor deficiency, 342
Univent bronchial blocker, 268, 269*t*
Uremic syndrome, 132
Ureteroplacental insufficiency, CPB
	and, 224
Uterine contractions, monitoring
	during CPB, 225–226
Uterine displacement, during CPB,
	233, 233*f*

Vascular remodeling, 38–39, 39*f*
Vascular stenosis, in pregnancy,
	218–219
Vasodilators
	inhaled pulmonary, 204–206, 206t
	intravenous, in PH, 198–201, 200*f*
	use during pregnancy, 237–238
Vecuronium, use in ESRD, 153
Vena caval tumors, 303–326
	cell types, 304–308
	diagnostic evaluation, 308–309
	extent of involvement, 311, 311*t*
	induction and maintenance of
		anesthesia, 314–316
	intraoperative monitoring,
		311–314
	preoperative anesthetic
		evaluation, 309–311
	surgical techniques, 316–320
Venovenous bypass, 318–319
Video MACINTOSH System,
	277–278F
Volume status, in ESRD, 137–138
von Willebrand disease, 341